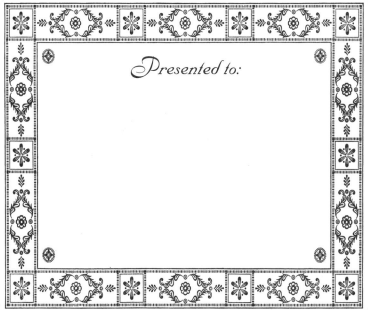

Presented to:

THOMAS F. NEALON, JR., M.D.

Director, Department of Surgery
St. Vincent's Hospital and
Medical Center of New York

Professor of Clinical Surgery
New York University School of Medicine

Illustrated by Ellen Cole Miller

FUNDAMENTAL
SKILLS
IN
SURGERY

Second Edition

Joseph A. Carvelli

W. B. SAUNDERS COMPANY – Philadelphia · London · Toronto

W. B. Saunders Company: West Washington Square
Philadelphia, Pa. 19105

12 Dyott Street
London, WC1A 1DB

833 Oxford Street
Toronto 18, Ontario

Fundamental Skills in Surgery

ISBN 0-7216-6701-5

Print No.:   9   8   7   6   5   4   3   2

To Cay

PREFACE
TO THE
SECOND EDITION

The wide and warm acceptance of the first edition of *Fundamental Skills in Surgery* was a very satisfying experience. I want to thank the reviewers and the many interested physicians who took the time to write to me: many of the changes incorporated in the present edition were initiated by their suggestions. In this edition I have resisted the temptation to expand the scope of the book and have for the most part confined new material to new techniques which advancing medical technology has made available to the house staff.

Major changes have occurred recently in the management of burns. To insure a current appraisal I have asked Dr. Ronald Ollstein of our Burn Service at St. Vincent's Hospital to write this chapter. Because the ready availability of bacterial identification and antibiotic sensitivity techniques has placed specific antibiotic therapy into the hands of the house staff, it seemed appropriate that additional information be made available to assist the house officer in choosing an appropriate antimicrobial agent for use until specific identification of the organism has been made. The table of likely pathogens and potential appropriate antibiotics is included to bridge the two- to three-day gap while the antibiotic sensitivities are being studied.

The new section on ventilatory support is included because the widespread use of this technique demands that the house officer have a good understanding of the underlying physiology as well as the technical details involved. Since parenteral hyperalimentation has been firmly established as a valuable means of nutrition, and everyone caring for seriously ill patients should be familiar with the technique, a substantial discussion is included. Additional, less extensive changes have been made in other chapters, particularly those concerning fluid and electrolyte balance and resuscitation.

v

I am indebted to Eduardo Gonzalez, Nathanial Ching and my entire house staff, particularly Stephen Camer and Randolph Maloney, for their suggestions. Robert Rowan of the W. B. Saunders Company has continued to offer encouragement and invaluable counsel. I appreciate the support and assistance of Eugene Hoguet and Mrs. Carol Cramer, also of Saunders.

I would like to thank my secretaries, the Misses Helen Collamore and Helen Tinti, Mrs. Ruth Lizer and Miss Helen O'Connell for their careful and punctual handling of the manuscripts.

PREFACE
TO THE
FIRST EDITION

Scattered about in the literature there are descriptions of most of the simple technical procedures which the embryonic physician or surgeon is expected to perform early in the years of his clinical training. But no other single source or text provides full details about all, or nearly all, of these techniques. In addition, there are many useful little tricks which are commonly passed on by word of mouth and have not been deemed worthy of formal presentation. Ever since I was a junior resident I have felt the need of compiling such material in one book. The need was further emphasized by repeated requests from students for such a reference book. The present volume was undertaken to fill this need.

As a rule of thumb, the material in this book was initially limited to those procedures which a young physician might be expected to perform on his own whether or not he had had the benefit of watching them done by a more experienced surgeon. The areas where this limited purpose has been exceeded are best blamed on an author's inevitable bias toward problems in which he is particularly interested.

There are other areas where the ultimate result of an acute problem or the very life of the patient depends upon proper management by the first physician who sees him. It seemed very important that all physicians be made aware of these areas and have detailed instructions available for management of these problems. This was the reason for inclusion of much of the material on trauma to the chest and hand, on respiratory and cardiac arrest, and on burns.

No effort has been made to include all methods of performing a procedure; I have selected one which has been satisfactory in my hands. Many of the procedures described are routine and their manner of operation has become firmly established. On the other hand, such matters as use of antibiotics and treatment of severe infections are constantly changing and an effort has been made to present entirely current information of these topics.

The author assumes all responsibility for any errors in the text. Credit for anything worthwhile should probably go to my teachers—John H. Gibbon, Jr., who saw fit to train me as a surgeon, Frank F. Allbritten, Jr., George Willauer, Adolph Walkling and John Y. Templeton, III. I am indebted for suggestions as to content and review of some of the material to Francis Sweeney, Charles Fineberg, Robert Johnson, Rudolph C. Camishion, Walter Ballinger, Jerome Sandler, and Kalman Faber. This book would never have become a reality were it not for Robert Rowan of the Saunders Company. In addition to inducing me to stop talking about the project and do something about it, he went over every bit of material personally and made many valuable contributions. Eugene Hoguet and all others of the Saunders staff with whom I had contact were wonderfully cordial. The editorial assistance of Dr. Esther Montgomery was invaluable and is much appreciated. I am indebted to Miss Ellen Cole for her excellent artwork and the gracious and pleasant manner in which she accomplished all this. She produced all the artwork except for some of the material on knot tying and the drawings on pediatrics. I did not think the drawings on tying one hand and two hand knots could be improved over those in the Ethicon Manual and the plates for these were loaned to us through the generosity of Mr. Gus Bee, president of Ethicon. All other illustrations in the book are original, but in many cases inspiration and stimulation came from figures which had already appeared in the literature. To the many authors and artists who thus assisted us I now express my debt and my gratitude.

The arduous task of typing and retyping the manuscripts never fell behind, thanks to the tireless and uncomplaining efforts of my secretaries, Misses Anne Wittmer and Florence Berlin.

Thomas F. Nealon, Jr.

Philadelphia, Pa.

CONTENTS

Chapter One

Care of the Surgical Patient

The physician's relationship with the patient may have an important effect upon the results of treatment. If good rapport is established early, treatment will be more satisfactory. The physician who makes an effort to put the patient at ease, and is courteous, polite, straightforward and yet decisive, will gain his confidence at first meeting. It is very disconcerting to the patient to sense that the doctor is unsure or uncertain of the proper course, and this is particularly true in a surgical situation. If the patient is ill at ease it is sometimes worthwhile to discuss generalities until he seems to relax and is ready to talk about his medical problems.

PREOPERATIVE EVALUATION

Many of the recent advances in surgical accomplishment are due to our appreciation of the importance of preoperative study and planning. An un-derstanding of the particular surgical problem and a thorough knowledge of the physiological state of the whole patient are vitally important. The latter is best accomplished through a good history, a complete physical examination, and pertinent laboratory and roentgenologic studies.

HISTORY

The history should be taken completely, carefully, and in a leisurely fashion. If done well, and if it includes a thorough review of all systems, pertinent information may be uncovered which might not be available in any other way.

PHYSICAL EXAMINATION

It is a good policy to do a complete physical examination at the outset.

1

However, it is best to defer the entire examination if you do not have sufficient time to complete it when you first see the patient. If portions of the examination are postponed, too often they are never carried out. The only exception is when it may seem advisable to delay a pelvic examination in an apprehensive female. All areas should be systematically examined, even though no specific symptoms are referable to that area. The survey should include a neurological examination, a rectal examination, a pelvic examination in adult females, and an examination of the peripheral pulses, as well as the usual examination of the head, chest and abdomen. All data, including normal findings, should be noted on the chart to provide a base line which can be compared with subsequent changes during the period of hospitalization.

LABORATORY STUDIES

The only laboratory studies which should be done routinely before all surgical procedures are a red blood cell count and urinalysis. The condition and age of the patient and the nature of the anticipated operation will suggest other studies. The indications for these studies should be developed in the course of the work-up of the patient; one should not routinely order a batch of unnecessary studies on each patient who comes into the hospital. Some concept of the high cost of laboratory studies would help discourage their use except when indicated. However, no study should be avoided because of its high cost, nor should one be included because of its low cost.

Any correctable abnormalities discovered during the work-up should be treated prior to operation. Any electrolyte or fluid imbalance or an anemia is corrected if possible. If the patient has lost a substantial amount of weight the possibility of a diminished blood volume must be considered. A routine blood count in such a patient is deceiving and may lead to the conclusion that he is not anemic when in reality there may be a serious hemoglobin deficit as result of a diminished circulating blood volume.

PREOPERATIVE PREPARATION

OPERATIVE SITE

The patient should arrive in the operating room with the skin of the operative site as sterile as is practical. Patients who are prone to skin inflammations or who are having operations performed on areas which are difficult to keep clean should be encouraged to scrub the operative area with an antiseptic soap periodically for several days prior to operation in order to increase skin cleanliness.

Through the years most hospitals have made it policy to shave and thoroughly cleanse the operative site and a generous area about it the night before operation. The area is then covered with a sterile towel which is left in place until the patient arrives in the operating room. Ideally the shaving should be done in the operating room area immediately prior to operation in order to avoid possible infection from nicks in the skin. The surgeon's preoperative orders must indicate the exact area which is to be prepared.

PATIENT

Most patients are concerned about their approaching operation and are best put at ease by sedation the night before operation. The dosage must be adjusted to the age and general condition of the patient. Elderly, senile, or debilitated patients require less medication than do younger, healthy patients. A healthy patient is usually given 100 to 200 mg. of a barbiturate by mouth at bedtime. This helps him to relax and sleep comfortably the night before operation. This may be repeated in the morning in a healthy adult. An hour before the anticipated time of induction of anesthesia the patient should be given further sedation. This may be morphine or Demerol, with the dosage adjusted to the individual patient. If general anesthesia is planned, atropine or scopolamine is given to reduce the secretions in the respiratory tract.

Catheterization

Before the patient leaves for the operating room he should be encouraged to void; otherwise, he will arrive at the operating room with a full and often distended bladder. If the operation is to involve the pelvic organs or the colon, it is advisable to insert an indwelling catheter prior to operation. If the patient is highly nervous or apprehensive with a low pain threshold, the catheter may be inserted in the operating room after he has been anesthetized.

Preparation of Gastrointestinal Tract

If the patient is to have general anesthesia he should take nothing by mouth after midnight. If the operation is to concern the upper gastrointestinal tract or one of its accessory organs—the gall bladder, liver or pancreas—a nasogastric tube should be passed and attached to suction early on the morning of operation.

The contents of the upper gastrointestinal tract are relatively sterile because of the action of the gastric acid (except in patients with gastric anacidity). The lower intestinal tract contains many bacteria so that spillage of gastrointestinal contents during surgery of the lower bowel is far more serious than spillage from the upper bowel. This danger can be minimized in operations on the lower bowel by preoperative preparation and sterilization of the bowel contents in the following manner: The patient is put on a low residue diet when he enters the hospital. This is changed to a liquid diet the day before operation. He is given 4 Gm. of Sulfasuxidine every six hours the first day. Daily enemas are given until the return is clear. It takes a minimum of four days to prepare the patient for operation by this routine.

A more rapid method is to combine the use of Neomycin and a saline cathartic. This makes it possible to prepare the bowel in 24 hours. Put the patient on a liquid diet. Start by giving a saline enema. Give 1 Gm. of Neomycin hourly for a total of four doses; after this give 1 Gm. of Neomycin every four hours. Give castor oil the afternoon before operation and another saline enema the night before operation.

Cathartics before operation are unnecessary for most patients. The habit of giving all preoperative patients an enema is overdone; an enema should be given prior to operation only when there is a positive reason for evacuating the lower gastrointestinal tract, e.g., the necessity for removing traces of barium from the gastrointestinal tract following contrast x-ray studies, and the proper preparation of the colon for operations in that area.

POSTOPERATIVE CARE

The postoperative care of the patient begins as soon as the dressing is applied. A draw sheet, which lies transversely across the middle of the operating table beneath the patient, is used to move him to the carriage. Two persons, each lifting one end of the draw sheet, with an additional person to support the patient's head, can readily lift him. The patient should be transferred slowly and gently. If there is an intravenous needle and/or drainage tube, care must be taken to avoid dislodging them.

In the recovery room, to which he is accompanied by an intern or resident, the patient should be properly positioned in bed. Tubes should be checked to see that they are functioning properly. If intravenous solution is running, the apparatus should be checked to see that it continues to function properly at the desired rate of flow. The postoperative orders should be reviewed in detail with the nurse who will care for the patient. It is, unfortunately, common practice to write postoperative orders before the operation is performed. In many routine, uncomplicated procedures no harm may result but, on the other hand, an unanticipated situation may arise. The surest way of avoiding a tragic error is to delay writing the postoperative orders until after completion of the operation.

Pulse, blood pressure, and respirations should be measured periodically until the patient has completely recovered from the anesthesia. Although the frequency varies with the condition of the patient and the magnitude of the operation, these signs are usually checked every fifteen minutes for at least an hour or two, every thirty minutes for a similar period, and then hourly until stable. The patient must be watched carefully until (1) he is able to swallow, (2) there is no longer danger of his tongue falling back into his pharynx, and occluding his airway, and (3) he is sufficiently alert that he will not aspirate any vomitus. If a nasogastric tube is in place or if the patient is receiving parenteral fluids, the intake and output must be carefully measured and charted. If the patient does not void within twelve hours after operation he should be catheterized. He should be encouraged to breathe deeply and, if necessary, to sit up and cough occasionally in order to keep his chest clear. To relieve pain a narcotic should be ordered. The dosage will depend upon the condition of the patient, but it should be allowed every three or four hours for approximately 24 hours; the order must then be rewritten. The patient will rest better if he takes a barbiturate at bed time; usually 100 mg. is adequate. Usually the patient is allowed nothing by mouth

and the barbiturate must be given intramuscularly. If the patient is unable to sleep, it is permissible to repeat the dosage once.

The patient should be seen periodically by a physician to ascertain that his condition is satisfactory. This may vary from once a day to as often as every hour depending upon the patient's condition. His chart, which includes a record of his temperature, pulse, blood pressure, and respiration, should be examined. Any figures which do not seem compatible with the patient's condition should be verified. The dressing should be examined, but should not be disturbed unless (1) there is evidence of bleeding, (2) the dressing is wet or soiled, or (3) there is reason to examine the wound, such as an unexplained temperature elevation. The patient who has had an abdominal operation should be examined at each visit for evidence of abdominal distention and, by auscultation, for the reappearance of peristalsis. The chest should be routinely examined to be sure that ventilation is satisfactory. The calves should be palpated for evidence of phlebitis and the peripheral pulses checked in the groin, popliteal areas and feet. The patient should be quizzed as to any particular complaints. The dietary intake should be noted as well as the urinary output if it has been measured. One must continually be on the lookout for the development of any complications. Any untoward findings and all treatment must be noted on the patient's chart.

POSTOPERATIVE COMPLICATIONS

HEMORRHAGE

A. External

Hemorrhage is the earliest complication which may occur after operation. It may be readily evident or concealed.

One of the commonest sites of external hemorrhage is the drain site. The drain is usually brought out through a separate stab incision and there may be continuous oozing from a vessel either in the skin or immediately beneath it. This incision is made immediately before the completion of the operation and the bleeding may not be noticed at that time. It is usually detected the first time the dressings are inspected. When dressings are saturated with blood the wound should be examined. If there is oozing from the skin edges, injection of the area with one per cent procaine solution will distend the tissues and compress the bleeding vessels (p. 259). This is usually sufficient treatment, but if the bleeding recurs it may be necessary to clamp and ligate the vessels.

The dressings may be saturated with blood coming through the drain from the wound itself. If this bleeding persists and the patient's general condition cannot be stabilized with one bottle of blood, immediate reoperation to control the bleeding is indicated. It may take some time to determine the extent of the bleeding; the decision is best made by frequent review of the condition of the patient. Nurses should be instructed to save all bloody dressings for the surgeon's inspection. If these indicate the presence of sanguineous oozing, which will cease in a short time, the physician is justified in first giving the patient a blood transfusion and waiting to see whether the bleeding stops. If a second transfusion is needed, reoperation is indicated.

There are two sites of external bleeding that require special consideration: the thyroid and hemorrhoidal areas.

POST-THYROIDECTOMY BLEEDING. Bleeding into the wound after a thyroidectomy predisposes to formation of a hematoma which, if not evacuated immediately, can asphyxiate the patient. The safest course is to open the wound immediately and decompress the hematoma. This procedure is done in the patient's room if his condition is serious enough. He is then returned to the operating room where clots are removed from the wound and bleeding is controlled. Often, after all clots have been removed from the wound no bleeding site is evident, and if the wound remains dry it can be closed without fear of recurrence. If the patient's condition seems good enough to allow his return to the operating room before the wound is opened, a physician should accompany him, prepared to open the wound if his condition should change suddenly.

HEMORRHOIDAL BLEEDING. Severe bleeding may develop after a hemorrhoidectomy. The best treatment is to return the patient to the operating room and, with the patient anesthetized, grasp the bleeding vessel and ligate it. Occasionally, the bleeding may be due to hemorrhagic defect. When this is the case the patient must be given blood transfusions, preferably fresh blood, and the specific defect treated as indicated.

B. Internal Hemorrhage

It is more difficult to recognize internal hemorrhage because the clinical manifestations may develop slowly. The classical signs of hemorrhage are pallor, falling blood pressure, rapid pulse of poor quality, sweating and thirst. They rarely appear early in the course of the bleeding. The commonest error is to mistake hemorrhage for delayed surgical shock. There is really no such thing as delayed surgical shock; shock as a result of operation appears during operation. If the patient returns to his room after operation with a normal blood pressure and pulse and later shows a drop in blood pressure and an elevation of pulse, this is not delayed surgical shock but concealed hemorrhage. The only exception is the occasional cardiovascular or pulmonary accident.

Hemorrhage may occur at the time of operation or during the postoperative period. The hemorrhage may be due to a bleeding ulcer; a patient who never had ulcer symptoms may develop a bleeding ulcer postoperatively. The psychological trauma of the operation can aggravate an ulcer sufficiently to produce bleeding. Whatever the cause, treatment consists of stopping the bleeding and replacing the blood loss if it exceeds 500 ml. The cardiovascular system should be kept filled with any suitable, available fluids—glucose in water, saline, plasma, or a plasma expander. All of these expedients are temporary; blood, in an amount sufficient to replace the loss, must be given as soon as possible. If the patient's condition has not been stabilized by a liter of blood, operation for direct control of the bleeding is indicated.

Shock

The patient may be in shock as a result of (1) trauma of the operation, (2) hemorrhage, (3) intracranial injury or (4) interference with ventilation. These various possible causes must be considered and either ruled out or remedied.

While the patient's blood pressure is low, he should be kept in a Trendelenburg position unless this position interferes with proper ventilation. The shock should be treated with intravenous plasma, a plasma substitute, or blood. If the hematocrit is below 55, whole blood should be used; if above 55, plasma. The patient should be kept covered, but heat should not be used. If narcotics are required to relieve pain, they should be given intravenously in considerably smaller doses (8 mg.) than for the normotensive patient.

Pulmonary Complications

Pulmonary complications are the next possibility in the order of postoperative complications. Usually, the initial complications are retained secretions and atelectasis. While these can develop after any operation, they are most common after thoracic and upper abdominal procedures. Because of the discomfort of the operative incision the patient splints his chest and does not breathe deeply, thereby allowing secretions to accumulate. The problem is further complicated if the patient is dehydrated. An early tachycardia, a marked elevation in temperature, and tachypnea may then develop. These dysfunctions lead to a further loss of fluids, the patient has difficulty expelling the thickened secretions, and the situation worsens.

The complication is best prevented by encouraging the patient to breathe deeply, by giving him sufficient narcotics to relieve his pain and by keeping him properly hydrated. When atelectasis develops the patient should be treated by adequate hydration, by encouraging him to cough, by the use of intermittent positive pressure breathing and by relieving his pain. If these measures are not successful, nasotracheal intubation (p. 241) should be used and, if this fails, bronchoscopy. If the patient requires bronchoscopy more than twice, tracheostomy (p. 202) is indicated. If the atelectasis is not properly cleared, pneumonia and a pulmonary abscess may develop. Postoperative atelectasis is marked by an elevation in temperature, pulse and respiration within the first forty-eight hours after an operation, the fever also being caused by retained secretions. Antibiotics are of little or no value in controlling the temperature elevation, but if the vigorous treatment described above is begun immediately, this condition can be cleared without sequelae.

Distended Bladder

Most patients have some difficulty voiding after a lower abdominal or pelvic operation, or when they have injuries or diseases of the central nervous system. The patient's bladder becomes distended and he becomes restless and noticeably uncomfortable. The distended bladder can be palpated and percussed through the abdominal wall. If the patient does not void within twelve hours after operation he should be catheterized (p. 285). If the patient is a male with an enlarged prostate it is probably wise to insert an indwelling catheter at the time of the initial catheterization. In all instances when the patient requires a second catheterization, an indwelling catheter should be used.

When a patient has difficulty voiding for several days postoperatively and then voids a small amount, this may erroneously be considered evidence that he is able to void satisfactorily. However, this may be merely overflow from a distended bladder. Such an individual requires prolonged catheter drainage and possibly some specific urological treatment. After a patient who has required prolonged catheterization voids spontaneously for the first time, it is wise routinely to catheterize him again in order to rule out retention. This provides an opportunity to measure the residual urine in his bladder. The symptoms of an overdistended bladder are frequency, inability to void more than 50 to 100 ml. at a time, and pain. The pain is not the discomfort normally associated with the desire to void, but rather a generalized abdominal discomfort. Examination will reveal a lower abdominal mass which may be somewhat fluctuant. Disappearance of the mass after catheterization is proof of diagnosis.

ABDOMINAL DISTENTION

Abdominal distention in a postoperative patient may be due to one of several causes. The more serious causes, peritonitis and gastrointestinal obstruction, will be discussed later in this chapter.

The more common reason for abdominal distention in the early postoperative period is acute gastric distention, often an iatrogenic disorder. The surgeon, to prevent pulmonary complications, encourages the patient to drink large amounts of liquids. The overzealous patient who drinks copious volumes will distend his stomach. A similar type of distention may occur if a patient is fed before there is satisfactory gastrointestinal motility to move secretions along, or before a gastrointestinal anastomosis has opened up and become functional. Another common cause of abdominal distention which is not generally appreciated is the use of straws for drinking. A patient may draw in considerably more air than fluid when using a drinking straw. A straw should be used only when a nasogastric tube is in place and the excess air can be drawn off, or when this is the only simple way in which a patient whose jaws are wired can get sustenance.

If the stomach is distended a nasogastric tube should be passed (p. 174), all secretions removed, and the nasogastric tube withdrawn. The fluid and nutritional requirements of the patient for that day should be given intravenously. The gastrointestinal tract should be slowly reactivated by administering per os small and gradually increasing amounts of liquids.

FECAL IMPACTION

Fecal impaction is most likely to occur in patients who have had x-ray studies of their gastrointestinal tract using barium, or in those using aluminum hydroxide for the treatment of ulcer, or in debilitated patients. The kneading action of the abdominal muscles, which occurs only with considerable activity, is important to intestinal motility. Consequently, the normally active patient who lies quietly in the hospital bed must tend to become constipated. Fecal impaction may develop in any patient whose bowels have not moved properly for a few days.

The commonest symptom of fecal impaction is diarrhea. The patient experiences a desire to defecate but is able to pass only a small watery stool which does not relieve his discomfort. He may complain of lower abdominal pain which is not well localized to the rectum, or he may merely complain of constipation. If his daily bowel function is not normal for him or if he complains of diarrhea, and if enemas do not seem to solve the problem, rectal examination is indicated and will immediately establish the diagnosis.

The hard mass of the impaction must be removed from the rectum. Enemas should be repeated until the return is clear. At the completion of the treatment the results should be checked by a digital examination. In an occasional, stubborn case, one may have to digitally remove the impacted mass.

INFECTION

Infection is a common postoperative complication. This is frequently first manifest by an elevation of temperature. If an elevation of temperature occurs, one must examine the chest, the wound, the legs and the urine to rule out the usual causes. As indicated earlier (p. 6), the commonest cause of a temperature elevation in the first 24 hours is retained pulmonary secretions. Later in the convalescent period pulmonary infection can occur.

Pulmonary Infection

Physical examination and/or a chest x-ray may identify the area of infection. Sputums should be studied for identification of bacteria and their antibiotic sensitivity. If the smear of the sputum demonstrates bacteria, antibiotics should be started empirically based on the type of bacteria seen. These are changed when sensitivities are reported.

Wound Infection

Wound infection first manifests itself by elevation in the patient's temperature. The temperature may rise suddenly and remain high, but this is uncommon. More commonly the temperature curve will be spiking, falling in the morning and rising in the afternoon.

Whenever the temperature rises the wound should immediately be examined. With infection, tenderness may or may not be present but there is always induration. The commonest site of the infection is the fatty tissue superficial to the fascia, but sepsis may occur at any tissue level.

The diagnosis is made by the presence of pus. The wound should not be opened unless a definitely suspicious area can be demonstrated. If there is doubt, a large bore needle, inserted after proper preparation of the skin with antiseptics, can be used in an attempt to aspirate pus from a suspected pocket. If pus is found, it is cultured in the laboratory for identification of the organism and assessment of antibody sensitivity. While awaiting the laboratory report the wound should be opened along the full length of the infection and warm moist saline compresses applied four times a day. If need be, a rubber drain can be inserted to keep the wound open. As soon as the antibiotic sensitivity of the organism is known, specific therapy should be instituted. Attempts to solve the problem without adequate drainage will only prolong the infection.

Urinary Tract Infection

When there is no evident cause of a temperature elevation, the urinary tract must be suspected. A urinalysis will give some information but a culture of a sterile urinary specimen is more helpful. This will identify the causative organism and the antibiotics to which it is sensitive. Usually specific antibiotic therapy is all that is necessary. When the infection does not clear readily, one must consider the possibility of some obstruction to the urinary tract.

Peritonitis

Peritonitis is inflammation, usually bacterial, within the peritoneal cavity. The most common cause is the rupture of a hollow viscus, but it can result from breakdown of an anastomosis of the gastrointestinal tract. A patient who seems to be doing moderately well postoperatively may suddenly complain of abdominal pain. There is an abrupt rise in temperature and pulse and possibly a drop in blood pressure. On examination there is abdominal tenderness, usually generalized, and guarding and rigidity of the abdominal muscles. The gastrointestinal tract is usually distended, as evidenced by a distended abdomen and also by x-ray demonstration of gas in multiple loops of the bowel. The abdomen is silent, no peristalsis is audible. On rectal examination there is tenderness in all directions. Treatment consists of administration of specific antibiotics, continuous gastrointestinal suction, oxygen, correction of any fluid and electrolyte imbalance and keeping the patient in semirecumbent position to avoid the accumulation of pus under the diaphragm. The areas where pus is most likely to accumulate are under the diaphragm, in the pelvis or at the site of the wound infection. If there is evidence of localization of the pus in any of these areas, drainage of the collection is indicated.

Subphrenic Abscess

One of the most distressing developments from generalized peritonitis is a subphrenic abscess, which is caused by a localization of pus under the leaf of the diaphragm. An effort is made to avoid this by placing the patient with generalized peritonitis in a semirecumbent position so that gravity drainage will be away from the subdiaphragmatic area. As a subphrenic abscess develops a patient who seems to have been doing fairly well begins to show temperature and pulse elevation without evident cause. There is first a sterile effusion in the pleural cavity above the abscess which becomes infected and then a frank empyema which, if not treated, proceeds to form a lung abscess and ultimately a bronchopleural fistula. One of the first studies in making a diagnosis of subphrenic abscess is a chest x-ray. If an abscess is present, there will be some evidence of pneumonitis and of pleural effusion on the affected side. If there are no changes in the lung it is unlikely that there is a subphrenic abscess. Fluoroscopy will show whether the diaphragm moves well on that side. The abscess itself is treated by external drainage.

Phlebothrombosis

The blood of the postoperative patient is frequently hypercoagulable. This factor, combined with bed rest, increases the possibilities of phlebothrombosis. Phlebothrombosis is evidenced by tenderness of the calf. You can detect this by daily examination of the calves; otherwise, the patient may bring it to your attention by complaining of pain in his calf when he first stands. This is particularly dangerous because it can result in pulmonary embolism.

Pulmonary Embolism

The patient who develops a pulmonary embolism suddenly experiences a pain in the chest followed by hemoptysis and shortness of breath. Occasionally, the insult may be so severe as to cause immediate death. Generally, however, the initial embolus is not lethal, in which case it is important to find its source and to prevent its recurrence. The source is usually a phlebothrombosis in the leg; this should be treated by either anticoagulation or vein ligation, usually at the superficial femoral level or, rarely, at the level of the inferior vena cava. Some life-threatening emboli have been removed from the pulmonary artery with the aid of a heart-lung machine.

WOUND DISRUPTION

Wound disruption is most common after upper abdominal operations and appears to be more often associated with a vertical incision. The incidence is higher among patients who are in poor condition. Disruption can be caused by coughing, vomiting, hiccupping, or wound infection. A common cause not generally appreciated is the development of partial intestinal obstruction with a consequent rise in intra-abdominal pressure. Whenever there is any question of intestinal obstruction the wound should be examined for evidence of disruption.

Most wound disruptions are not evident until the seventh to tenth postoperative day, although many probably develop earlier. The first indication of disruption is the appearance of a copious amount of pink serum; the dressings, which were dry until that time, are suddenly saturated. There may be complete breakdown of the wound or there may be only a very small opening from which the serum is flowing. Regardless of the size of the defect, the leakage is pathognomonic of disruption and should be treated as such. If the patient's condition is so poor that operative intervention is out of the question, one must compromise and merely support the wound. However, the safest course is to cover the wound with a sterile towel supported by a dressing, and make arrangements to take the patient to the operating room immediately. In the operating room, satisfactory general anesthesia is ob-

tained, the entire area is prepared, the wound is opened, the possibility of intestinal obstruction investigated and the obstruction corrected if found, and the wound reclosed. The wound is best closed in a single layer with through-and-through wire sutures which are left in place for two weeks. The sutures should be placed approximately one-half inch apart. Remarkably, almost all such wounds heal without a second disruption.

UREMIA

Uremia is the result of inadequate renal excretion of the nitrogen breakdown products. This most commonly occurs after operations on elderly patients with poor renal function, in patients with peritonitis or intestinal obstruction, and in individuals with longstanding kidney disease or longstanding obstructive jaundice. Dehydration is associated with this condition. A patient may excrete the urea, but only if he has an excessive urinary output; if urinary output after an operation is inadequate the urea content of the blood will rise. Early symptoms are drowsiness and confusion; later the patient may begin to hiccup, lapse into coma and develop a typical uremic odor. The diagnosis is established by a blood urea determination. Treatment is aimed at lowering the production of urea and encouraging its excretion. The production can be lowered by correcting any chloride deficiency. If chloride is deficient, protein metabolism rises, causing the production of more urea. The urinary output can be stimulated by correcting existing dehydration and by the administration of extra fluid. If the patient is already edematous, concentrated glucose solution given intravenously will absorb the fluid and at the same time stimulate diuresis. If the patient is edematous and has an associated hypoproteinemia, the intravenous administration of concentrated plasma or albumin is helpful.

Intestinal Obstruction

The first sign of intestinal obstruction is abdominal distention. The patient also complains of cramplike abdominal pain and commences to vomit. On auscultation of the distended abdomen one can hear peristaltic rushes and high pitched tinkles.

The common type of postoperative obstruction is due to a combination of factors, prominent among which is edema. The edema can usually be corrected without operating on the patient. The preferred treatment is gastrointestinal suction with a long limb drainage tube such as a Cantor tube or a Miller Abbott tube, the idea being to get this to pass through the area of obstruction. So long as there is no evidence of any strangulation of the bowel (temperature elevation, increase in pulse or increase in leukocyte count), prolonged gastrointestinal intubation may be carried out. In most instances the edema subsides, clearing the obstruction. In the meantime, of course, the patient must have his fluids and electrolytes properly regulated. If signs of strangulation appear, or if prolonged suction does not correct the situation, operative intervention is indicated. Prolonged nonoperative treatment of gastrointestinal obstruction is used only in early postoperative obstructions. Since edema has a lesser role in the causation of late obstructions nonoperative success is less likely.

Chapter Two

Instruments

The multiplicity of surgical instruments which have been designed for the same purposes is evidence of the dissatisfaction among individual surgeons with the instruments already available. However, until one becomes very experienced, any variant of a standard type of instrument is adequate for a given task. Early in his career the surgeon should learn the specific use and proper manipulation of each instrument.

SCALPEL

A scalpel is the best instrument for division of tissue. The sharp blade allows one to divide structures with minimal trauma to surrounding tissue. The blades are of different shapes, each designed for a specific purpose.

The scalpel must be held in a way that permits full control of the instrument and, at the same time, freedom of movement. The handle of the scalpel is grasped between the thumb and the third and fourth fingers and the index finger placed over the back of the blade to provide firm control. For cutting, a smooth sweep is made with the rounded portion of the blade, rather than the point. Since the blade is sharp very little pressure is required; a light stroke over the tissues with the middle of the blade is adequate.

The drawing on the right illustrates some of the most useful blades for a scalpel with a detachable handle. There are also many scalpels which are made of one solid piece of steel; these require periodic sharpening. The commonest type of blade has a straight ribbed back and an oval cutting side. This is available in many sizes (#10, #20, #21, #22).

The size of the blade does not change the technique of its use. A small blade (#15) is used in plastic surgery, allowing more precise turns when making the incision. Blades designed for specific purposes have quite different configurations. A bistoury blade (#12) looks like a hook and is used for draining infection of the middle ear; the tip sweeps through the drum in an arc. A bayonet

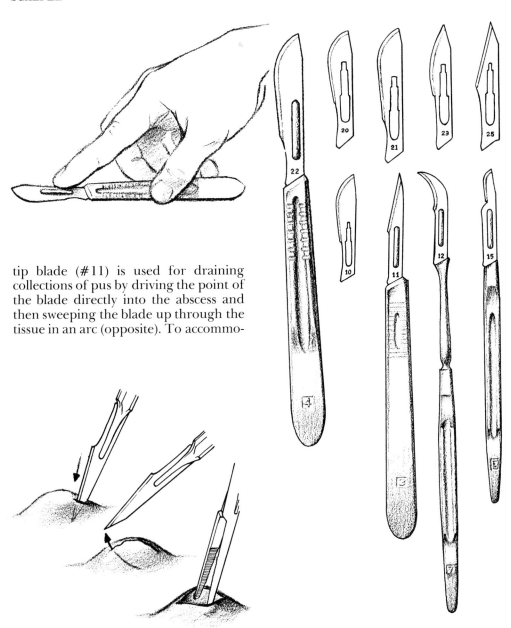

tip blade (#11) is used for draining collections of pus by driving the point of the blade directly into the abscess and then sweeping the blade up through the tissue in an arc (opposite). To accommo-

date detachable blades of various sizes, two different size handles are available. The #4 handle takes the larger blades (#20) and the #3 handle the smaller blades. The ends of the #7 and #9 handles are similar to that of a #3, and fit the same size blades. The #7 handle is commonly used in eye, ear, nose and throat work and the #3 handle in plastic surgery.

The detachable blades of the scalpels pictured can be discarded when they become dull. To remove the blade hold the scalpel in your left hand with the sharp side of the blade away from you. Grasp the proximal end of the blade with a hemostat, lift the posterior edge of the blade to clear the hub of the handle and free it by pushing it up over the end of the handle.

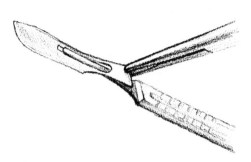

To replace a blade reverse the maneuver. Hold the scalpel in the same way, and slide the blade back onto the handle. The purpose of handling the blade thus is to keep one's hand in such a position that a slip will not cut the hand.

SCISSORS

Next to a scalpel scissors are the instruments most commonly used to divide tissues. Scissors are also used to cut sutures and dressings. Tissue scissors are usually lighter, made of better steel, and have a much finer cutting edge and smoother points than the suture scissors. A good surgeon zealously cares for his tissue scissors because the blades must be kept sharp for effective dissection. On the other hand suture scissors may cut sutures even when the blades are in only fair condition. Tissue scissors should never be used as suture scissors. Straight scissors are used for work on the surface; curved scissors are used deeper in the wound.

To hold the scissors the thumb and fourth finger are inserted through the rings, the middle finger is rested in front of the ring finger, and the index finger is set against the blades. The index finger placed well forward on the

scissors provides more control of the instrument.

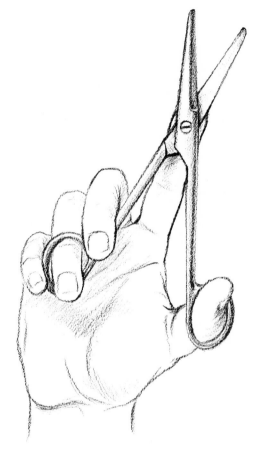

Usually only the distal portion of the blade is used for cutting. When a tough structure must be cut, the heel or the back portion of the blade is used so as not to spoil the blade near the tip. To avoid damage to vital structures, the scissors should never be closed unless the tips of the blades can be seen clearly. In areas where this danger exists, sharp tipped scissors should not be used. Sutures should be cut only when they can be seen clearly. The person who is cutting should have full control of the scissors before attempting to use them. The scissors should not have a handle longer than the available hemostats; this removes the danger of transecting a vessel beyond the reach of a hemostat.

DISSECTING SCISSORS

Among the many different kinds and sizes of dissecting scissors, probably the most popular are the Mayo type, with straight or curved blades. These rather heavy scissors with rounded tips are the first three scissors shown below.

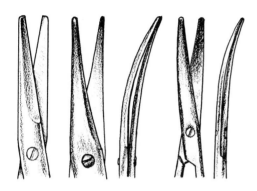

My favorite is the lighter Metzenbaum scissors (the two on the right above). This is a longer finer instrument with a gentle curve near the end. Usually the tissues to be divided are held with a forceps while being cut with scissors. The tip of the scissors is sometimes used as a blunt dissector to spread tissues before dividing.

SUTURE SCISSORS

The commonest type of suture scissors is an ordinary, general purpose scissors with blunt ends.

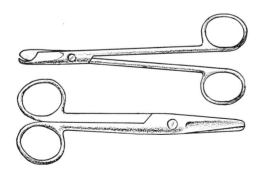

With such a scissors there need be no worry that the tips will puncture a viscus. One variation has a notch in one blade into which the suture to be cut is held taut while the suture scissors, with tips open, are slipped down along the suture to the point where it is to be cut.

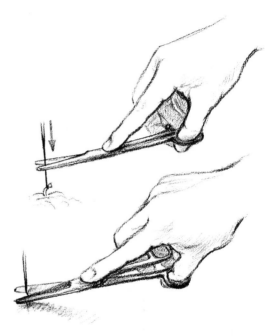

If the suture material is nonabsorbable, slip the scissors down to the knot, turn the blade slightly, and cut. If the suture material is catgut leave the end about one-quarter inch long because the catgut will loosen up a bit after it becomes moist. Never attempt to cut a suture unless (1) you are in good position; (2) you have full control of the scissors; (3) you can see the suture to be divided and (4) you can see that you are not likely to cut any other structure.

BANDAGE SCISSORS

The commonest type of bandage scissors has one blade with a flat blunt prow which can be inserted beneath a dressing and slid forward without fear of penetrating the skin.

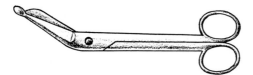

When the blades are in the proper position they are closed. As its name implies, this instrument is used mainly to cut bandages. It is rarely used at the operating table but is an essential item of equipment for every surgical interne or resident. (If carried in the pocket the scissors is naturally not sterile and should never be allowed in direct contact with a wound.) The bandage should be divided at some point other than over the wound. If the bandages are soiled or wet, the scissors should be sterilized before use near another patient. When dealing with an open wound a fresh sterile set of instruments must be used.

General Purpose Scissors

There are several types of general purpose scissors. In one type both blade tips are sharp, in another both are blunt, in still another one is sharp and one is blunt.

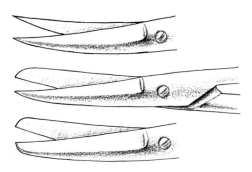

The scissors with both blade tips blunt are commonly used as suture scissors. The scissors with one or both blade tips sharp are used where it is necessary to push a sharp end of a scissors beneath

tissues in order to divide them. For instance, if one is removing a portion of a finger nail, a scissors with at least one sharp point is required.

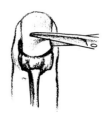

A pair of scissors with either edge pointed should not be used in a cavity where it can perforate an organ or a vessel.

THUMB FORCEPS

A thumb forceps consists of two strips of metal joined at one end and is used to pick up tissue or to hold tissue between the apposed surfaces. If there are teeth in the apposing surfaces the forceps can hold the tissue without slipping and without exerting undue pressure. For this reason the tissue or dissecting forceps has teeth. On the other hand, a forceps to be used about vital structures, which should not be perforated should not have teeth. To provide additional grasping strength this forceps has a wider head.

The forceps is held between the thumb and the middle and index fingers of either hand.

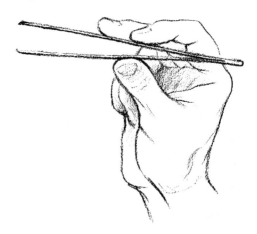

During an operation it is more commonly used in the left hand to hold tissues which are to be dissected or divided by a scalpel or scissors held in the right hand.

TISSUE FORCEPS

The tissue forceps has teeth which prevents it from slipping. Since the teeth bite into the tissue, only a small amount of pressure is required to grasp the tissue firmly. The teeth vary in number from one to a dozen and in size from very fine to fairly large.

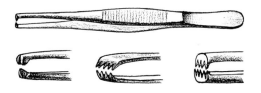

The specific design of the head of each instrument depends upon the particular purpose for which it is intended. This type of thumb forceps can be used to handle most tissues, but never when one is dealing with a hollow viscus or a blood vessel. It should always be used when handling skin.

RING TIPPED FORCEPS

The ring tipped forceps is desirable when handling large structures which might be punctured by a sharp point.

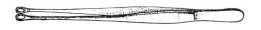

This instrument has a considerable grasping surface which decreases the amount of pressure required. It is commonly used when manipulating the major vessels of the lung.

DRESSING FORCEPS

A dressing forceps has a blunt end with coarse cross striations to give it additional grasping power.

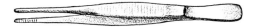

This is used routinely in applying and removing dressings and it is also used to handle a hollow viscus which might be punctured by a sharply pointed forceps. It is improper to use this instrument to grasp the skin when putting in skin sutures; since there are no teeth on the grasping edges the force required to hold the skin firmly may be enough to cause necrosis.

SPLINTER FORCEPS

A splinter forceps has a plain sharp point.

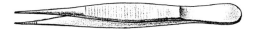

The apposing surfaces meet principally at the tip, enabling one to get a good hold on the splinter and to extract it from the tissue. This is an example of a tip designed for a specific purpose.

GRASPING FORCEPS

These instruments are designed primarily to take hold of tissues and allow one to exert traction. The apposing surfaces of the individual heads vary a great deal depending on the specific purpose. All have a set of finger rings and a locking mechanism.

BABCOCK FORCEPS

This instrument has a smooth grasping surface with a bar on each blade.

The bars appose gently without damaging the grasped tissues.

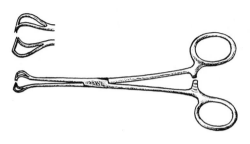

A forceps like this can grasp delicate tissue, such as the wall of the gastrointestinal tract, without perforating it. The instrument is also handy for holding tubular structures which are not really grasped; when the instrument is closed it creates a loop to hold a tubular structure without exerting any pressure on it.

ALLIS FORCEPS

The tip of this forceps consists of apposing serrated edges with fairly short teeth.

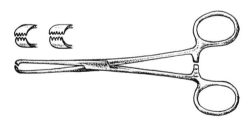

This type of traction forceps is used for grasping fascia, and for traction on the skin. The instrument is not applied to the skin itself because this would cause necrosis; the tissue immediately beneath the skin is picked up and used for traction purposes. The Allis forceps has considerably more grasping power than the Babcock forceps. It is also used to hold wound drapes in place.

KOCHER FORCEPS

The blades have transverse serrations running along the full length and at the tips there are long sharp points.

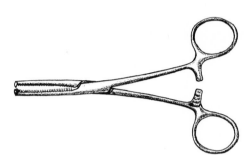

This forceps has considerable grasping power and allows one to exert a considerable amount of tension on tissues. It is commonly used on heavy fascia. When fascia is grasped with a forceps of this nature it is unlikely to pull free.

THYROID TENACULUM

The thyroid tenaculum is also called a Lahey thyroid forceps. The blades have long prongs which bite deep into the thyroid tissue so that traction can be exerted on the gland.

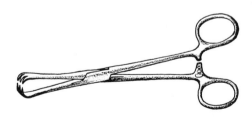

HEMORRHOIDAL OR LUNG CLAMPS

This forceps has triangular tips with serrated approximating surfaces.

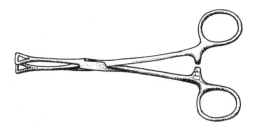

As the names imply, this type of clamp is used to grasp hemorrhoidal varicosities or lung tissue prior to excision. Since they traumatize tissue, these clamps should be applied only to tissues which are to be excised.

Towel Clip or Towel-Holding Forceps

This consists of a grasping forceps with two sharp points which hold the edges of a towel in place.

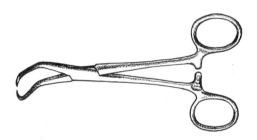

This is the most common means of approximating the towels on the wound when first draping it.

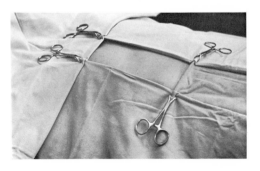

This instrument is used to grasp ribs when external traction is applied to the chest wall.

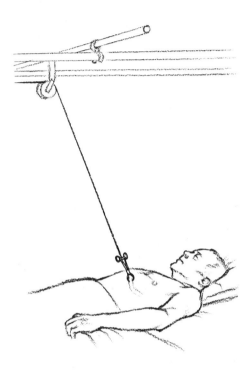

Sponge-Holding Forceps

This large grasping forceps has large rings with serrated apposing surfaces.

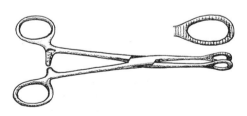

These are commonly used to hold sponges to: (1) use as a retractor, (2) sponge fluids from deep within a body cavity and (3) prepare the operative site. The flat four-by-four gauze sponge is doubled on itself twice so as to make it only one-fourth its normal size. This is then grasped by the forceps. When used for preparing the wound, the sponge is dipped into the antiseptic solution, the excess fluid allowed to drip off, and then the wet sponge is applied to the skin. A fresh gauze is used if the application is repeated. Sometimes cotton balls are used instead of the gauze sponge.

HEMOSTATIC FORCEPS

These instruments are the main means of establishing hemostasis during an operation. There are numerous variations.

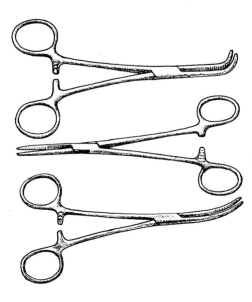

In some of them the serrations are parallel with the direction of the blades, while in others they are perpendicular. The depth and breadth of the serrations also vary. Most hemostats close with considerable force, so that they can grasp securely small amounts of tissue. As a result, any tissue within the blades is crushed. For specialized situations, such as in cardiovascular surgery, it has been necessary to develop noncrushing clamps. Such clamps exert sufficient ten-

sion to hold vessel walls in apposition, but not enough to damage the clamped tissue. Traction is increased when a knitted cotton sleeve is placed over the ends of some noncrushing clamps. Such instruments may be straight, curved or sharply angled.

The noncrushing and crushing clamps are used quite differently. The *noncrushing clamps* are applied across tissue where damage is to be avoided because later function is expected, for example, the ends of blood vessels which are to be sutured together.

The *crushing clamp* is used to establish hemostasis at the divided ends of blood vessels of all sizes. Since the clamped tissue will be destroyed, the tip of the clamp should grasp the end of the blood vessel, the tip of the vessel only and not the adjacent tissue. Continued hemostasis is assured if the end of the vessel is tied. A tie is passed around the vessel at the tip of the hemostat and the first half hitch is set.

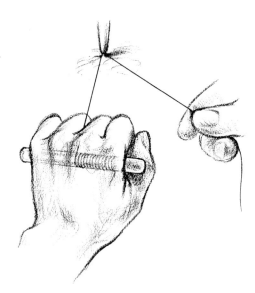

While this is being done, the assistant should hold the clamp in such a way that the tip of the instrument is exposed to the operator. To elevate the tip of the clamp the handle is depressed. After the

first half hitch is set, the assistant removes the hemostat; the first half hitch
is tightened further before the second is
begun.

RETRACTORS

Retractors are used to hold tissues
aside in order to improve the exposure
in the operative field. There are two
major types of retractors: One type is
held by an assistant and the other (mechanical or self-retaining retractor) is
held in position by counterpressure
against opposite sides of the wounds.

PLAIN RETRACTORS

There are numerous varieties of plain
retractors. Many plain retractors consist
simply of metal strips fashioned into different shapes. The simplest of these is a
malleable retractor which is really a strip
of chromium plated copper.

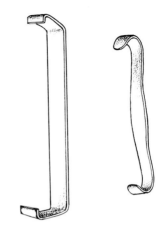

A Deaver retractor, which is shaped in a
long gentle sweep, is popular for retraction deeper in wounds.

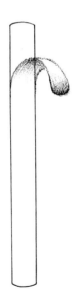

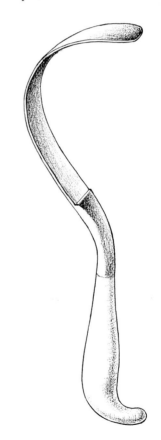

This can be shaped into any configura-
tion which best accomplishes the desired
retraction. Others have a gentle curve
or a right angle and are used to hold
back superficial tissues.

The many variations of this have to do
mainly with the width of the blade, its
overall length and types of handles.

Another common type has a broad head with rounded edges at right angles to the handle of the retractor. Richardson, Eastman, and Sims retractors are examples. Deep in the wound it is best to interpose a gauze sponge between the retractor and the tissues. When the sponge is in contact with the bowel it should be moistened.

RAKE RETRACTORS

When one wants the retractor to grasp the tissue and to pull it back, it is common to use a rake retractor because it will dig into tissue rather than slide over it. The points of the retractor may be blunt or quite sharp.

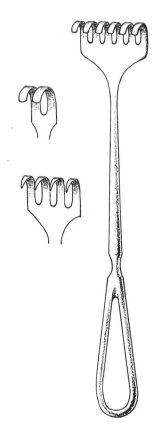

There may be two, four or six points. The sharper points can exert greater traction because they are better able to

penetrate tissue, but they can only be used in areas where there is no concern that the point of the retractor might penetrate a blood vessel or a hollow viscus.

SELF-RETAINING RETRACTORS

Self-retaining retractors are placed against both sides of the wound and spread apart so that one side is an anchor against which counterpressure is exerted from the opposite side of the wound.

A gauze sponge should be placed between the retractor and the tissues at the edge of the wound. The Balfour retractor, which consists of such a self retaining retractor plus an additional side retractor that can be used to retract the bladder is one of the commonest types used in abdominal operations.

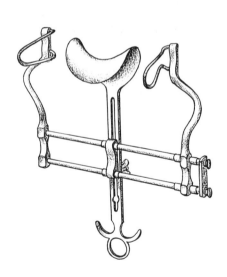

The Finochietto retractor, which is rolled up by a ratchet arrangement on one blade, is typical of the most commonly used retractor for holding open wounds in the chest wall. This type of retractor has a considerable mechanical advantage when the ratchet is turned and thus a small amount of pressure on the ratchet can cause enough pressure by the blades to fracture the ribs. This is less likely to take place if one turns up the retractor slowly and intermittently rather than all at one time.

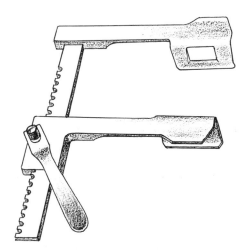

There are other, smaller kinds of self-retaining retractors, many of which are of the rake type, and allow satisfactory retraction of the superficial tissues of the neck or the mastoid area.

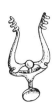

NEEDLE HOLDERS

The simplest method of sewing is to use a straight needle, which can be held and pushed through the tissue with the fingers. When a straight needle is used sewing is done in a direction away from the operator. A straight needle can only sew in a straight line, hence it can only be used in tissues where it is possible to distort the tissues sufficiently to allow the straight needle to project from the

desired point of egress. However, since much of the suturing during operation must be done within a wound, in tissue which cannot be distorted, a curved needle must be used. Such curved needles must be manipulated with a needle holder.

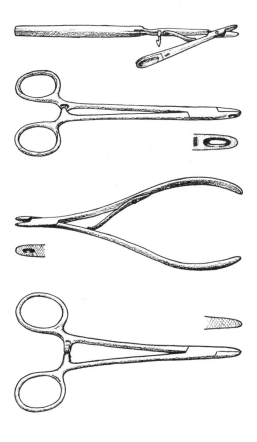

All needle holders have wide heads and there are many different types of serrations of the head. The needle holder is applied at approximately one quarter of the distance from the blunt end of the needle. In most situations the needle should protrude from the left side of the needle holder for a right handed surgeon. Suturing with a curved needle is done toward the surgeon. Holding the needle holder as he would hold a scissors, the surgeon inserts the needle into the tissue with a sweeping arc-like motion, attempting to follow the general arc of the needle. When the needle protrudes from the tissue, he grasps the point with a forceps and holds it while removing the needle holder from the blunt end and reapplying it to the portion of the needle protruding from the tissue. The needle is lifted free of the tissue in a continuing sweeping motion. One should learn to tie knots while holding the needle holder. This reduces the number of motions necessary and thus saves time.

SUCTION APPARATUS

A means of suction is useful during operation to aspirate blood from the wound, to empty a hollow viscus, or to collect fluid from the peritoneal or the pleural space. At the operating table the suction consists of some modification of a hollow tube. A tonsil suction is a hollow tube with a molded handle and a blunt tip with multiple holes.

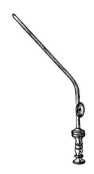

These instruments are used to aspirate blood from open areas. Such apparatus does not function well in the abdomen because the bowel is sucked against the openings, occluding them and interrupting the suction. There are special types of suction apparatus which use the sump principle in which an inner suction tip is contained within an outer jacket that has multiple perforations. This prevents the bowel from being sucked against the openings in the inner suction tube.

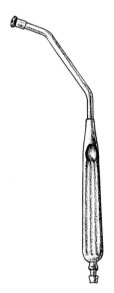

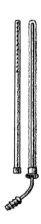

A brain sucker is a small narrow tube which has a side vent near the base; when a finger is placed over the vent, the suction increases.

A regular tip can be used in the peritoneal cavity if a gauze sponge is put over the suction tip. The gauze sponge will prevent the tissue from being sucked against the opening, but the fluid can be sucked through the sponge.

Chapter Three

Operating Room Conduct

PREPARATION OF PERSONNEL FOR OPERATION

ATTIRE

An essential principle of surgery is that wound infection be prevented insofar as is humanly possible; introduction of microbes into the operating room must therefore be reduced to a minimum. This is why personnel must be properly outfitted before entering the operating room area. No one should enter the area wearing street clothes or clothes worn elsewhere about the hospital. Furthermore, anyone who participates in an operation on a patient who has an infection should shower and don clean operating room clothes before helping in another operation. Before leaving the operating room after an infected case, personnel should put gloves, cap, mask and gown in the containers provided specifically for this purpose.

Conventional operating room attire is the short-sleeved cotton suit. The shirt is tucked inside the trousers, not allowed to hang loosely. Underwear should be made of cotton. Other material such as silk, wool, nylon, dacron, orlon, and rayon can carry a high electric charge and retain it for a long period of time. A spark from these can be very dangerous in the presence of the highly inflammable anesthetic gases.

If the floor is conductive, conductive shoes must be worn. If you do not have these, temporary overshoes are available in every such operating room. The conductivity of the footwear can be checked at the conductometer located at the operating room door.

Before entering the operating room cap and mask should be donned. The cap should completely cover the hair. The mask must be up over the nose.

25

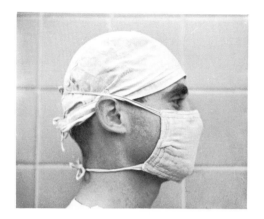

the type of detergent used and the condition of the hands. Take a sterile brush in one hand and fill the palm of the opposite hand with soap solution if you are using a liquid. If you are scrubbing with bar soap you can hold the soap behind the handle of the brush when not actually using it.

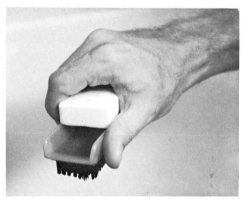

Begin by scrubbing the lateral aspect of the thumb, then scrub over the tip, then the medial aspect.

A person who wears glasses may have difficulty with their fogging when wearing a mask. Masks that have a lead reinforcement along the top edge may be shaped snugly about the nose so that exhaled gases cannot drift up and fog the lenses. Another method is to tape the upper end of the mask to the nose. Rubbing ordinary soap on glasses and then polishing them is the most satisfactory method of preventing fogging. More than one shrewd medical student has earned money by selling ordinary soap, cut in small squares and wrapped in tinfoil, as a special antifog preparation.

SCRUBBING

Scrubbing for an operation is a considerably more elaborate procedure than ordinary washing. The scrubbing is done at special deep sinks having special faucets that make it possible to adjust the flow of water without touching the faucets with one's hands. Turn the tap and adjust the water to a proper temperature. Wet your hands and apply a few drops of detergent or soap, then mix with water; make a good lather and scrub the hands and forearms to 3 inches above the elbows for 35 to 60 seconds, depending upon

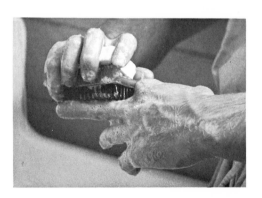

Continue this routine over each finger until you have cleaned all five. Next scrub the nails by rubbing the tips of the fingers and the nails against the bristles.

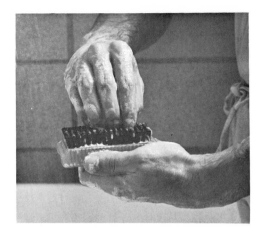

more vigorously and more rapidly can accomplish the same effect in a shorter period of time. Conversely scrubbing more slowly and less vigorously requires a longer period.

Rinse the suds from the hands and forearms, holding the hands higher than the elbows so that the water will run off the elbows and the fingers will not be contaminated. If the faucets have arm levers, turn them with the brush or an elbow.

Finally scrub the flat surface of the dorsum and the palm of the hand.

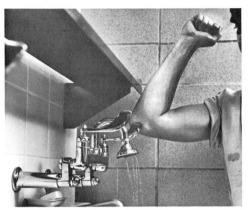

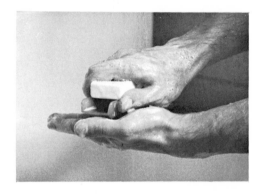

If ordinary soap was used, soak the hands and forearms for one minute in a basin containing an antiseptic. This is unnecessary, and for that matter is contraindicated, if you have scrubbed with Septisol or Phisoderm. Keep the hands higher than the flexed elbows to allow the water to drip off the elbows and to prevent water from running from the upper forearm down on the hands.

Now shift the brush to the other hand and repeat the procedure. After all the fingers have been brushed well, take a nail file or a sharpened wooden stick and scrape the subungual spaces. The nails should not be more than 1 mm. in length. Discard the stick in the sink. Continue to scrub the hands and arms in this manner for the total time prescribed for the type of soap being used. If you use conventional soap scrub for 10 minutes. If you are using one of the special scrub preparations containing hexachlorophene scrub for 10 minutes if there has been a lapse of more than 2 days between scrubs, 5 minutes if this is the first scrub of the day, 2 minutes between cases and 1 minute when the gloves have just been removed. Time is not the only consideration; the number of strokes makes a difference. Scrubbing

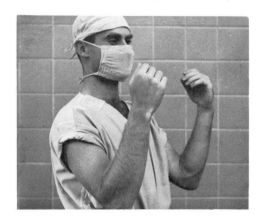

DRYING THE HANDS

Dry your hands with a sterile towel before you put on a sterile gown. To dry the hands and forearms grasp the folded towel with the fingers of both hands, step back away from the table and other persons so that you are not likely to touch anything and open the towel. Place one end of the towel over one hand and blot dry the free hand and wrist making sure that the towel does not touch any unsterile object.

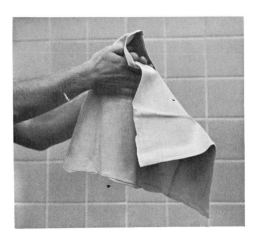

The used (unsterile portion of the towel) is never brought back onto the dry area. Grasp the remaining sterile portion of the towel with the free hand and proceed to dry the opposite wrist and hand. Discard the towel in the receptacle designated for this purpose, being careful not to touch anything in doing so. It is not necessary to dry the elbows.

GOWNING

You may have help in gowning, or it may be necessary to gown yourself. The gown is so folded that the inner surface is exposed to you when you pick it up.

Never touch the outer surface. If you are gowning yourself pick up the gown, hold it out away from your body and sufficiently high so that it will not touch the floor.

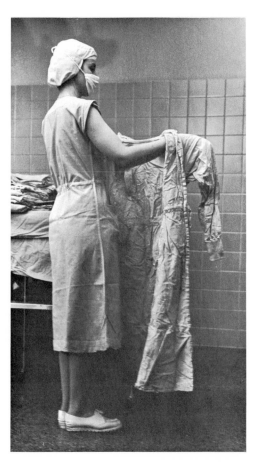

Then allow the gown to drop open. Insert your arms into the armholes, keeping your arms extended as you do so. Then flex your elbows and abduct your arms and wait for the circulating nurse to assist you. In the operating room the scrub nurse is usually the only one who gowns herself. She will then help you gown by handing the gown with the inner side toward you. Insert your arms and wait for assistance.

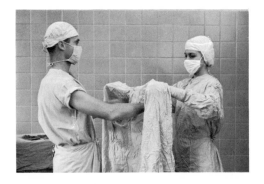

By rubbing the hands together spread the powder over the entire surface of the hands.

Take one glove from the glove container by placing the fingers of the op-

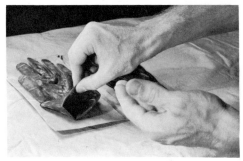

The circulating nurse grasps the inner side of the gown at each shoulder and pulls the gown over the wearer's shoulders and the sleeves up over the wrists.

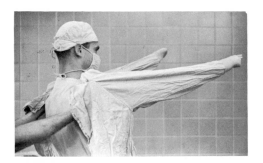

posite hand on the turned down cuff of the glove.

You thus touch the portion of the glove which is on the inner surface when the glove is properly applied. Grasping the glove in this manner at the point in line with the palm of the hand, pull the glove onto the opposite hand.

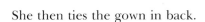

She then ties the gown in back.

GLOVING

Talcum powder or Biasorb powder is used to diminish friction between the skin and the glove. The gloves have been lightly coated with the powder. Powder for the hands is now available in individual tubes of grease glove lubricants, which eliminate dust in the operating room. The gloves are packed individually in a container consisting of two pockets, one for each glove. Open the container of lubricant and squeeze the material into the palm of your hand.

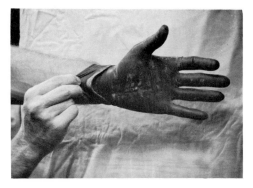

Make no effort at this point to turn up the cuff. Now take the second glove from the envelope by placing the gloved fingers under the inverted cuff.

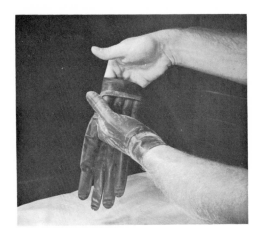

tion, grasp the cuff from the outside and turn it down over the palm.

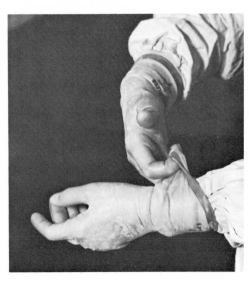

Pull on the glove and then turn up the cuffs on both hands. If necessary you can now adjust the glove fingers. If a sterile nurse is available she can glove you. She does this by holding the glove open with the palm facing you while you slip your hand into the glove.

Do not attempt to remove the glove yourself because you will contaminate the gloved hand. Hold out your hand to the circulating nurse who should grasp the edge of the cuff and pull off the glove.

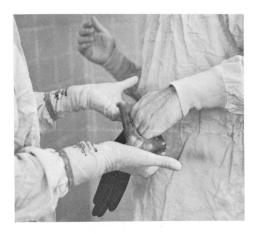

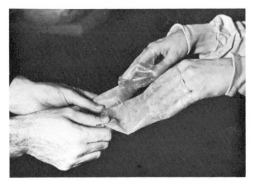

She can hold the glove open with her fingers beneath the cuff so that her glove does not come in contact with your hand. She will glove you only if you are already gowned.

Removing Gloves

If it becomes necessary to remove a glove during the course of the opera-

The glove should be removed if you inadvertently contaminate it or if you tear the glove. Occasionally you may make a small hole in the glove which is not easily found. This is evident, however, if a thin layer of blood spreads about the finger within the glove. The glove should be changed even though the hole cannot be located. Good operating room manners dictate that you wash the blood from your gloves before removing them at the completion of the operation. This is not necessary if disposable gloves are used. When regowning and regloving during an operation remove the gown before the gloves. This is also the proper procedure between cases.

PREPARING THE OPERATIVE SITE

To prevent wound contamination, a wide area of skin around the operative incision must be meticulously prepared and properly covered with sterile drapes. The area is scrubbed and shaved. Fine thin hair must be removed where an incision is to be made; obviously the heavily-haired skin on the abdomen or back, pubic and axillary regions must be shaved if the operation involves these areas. If the guard is removed from the safety razor, one can shave long hair without clogging the razor. Formerly the preoperative preparation was done most commonly the night before operation. More commonly this is now being done immediately prior to operation to avoid nicks in the skin which could get infected in the interim period.

In the operating room, the particular method of skin preparation depends upon the preference of the individual surgeon. At St. Vincent's Hospital, skin preparation is carried out from a separate table called a "prep" table. The member of the operating team who is chosen to do the "prep" dons a pair of sterile gloves. He then goes to the "prep" table which carries a bowl containing 70 per cent alcohol and another containing tincture of Zephiran and four sponge-holding forceps. The sponge holder is dipped into the alcohol. The alcohol is applied directly to the area where the incision is to be made

and then, with gradually widening sweeps, over the entire area. Areas most likely to be infected or heavily infested with bacteria, such as the armpits, groin, or perineum, are done last before each swab is discarded. The alcohol is not simply painted on, but is vigorously rubbed on so as to produce mechanical as well as chemical cleansing. The skin is kept wet with alcohol for a period of five minutes. The same area is then painted twice using tincture of Zephiran. The area prepared should be quite wide; for all abdominal surgery the entire width of the abdomen should be prepared. In inguinal operations the preparation should extend from midthigh to the rib cage. In other abdominal procedures the preparation should extend from below the inguinal ligament to the nipple line.

Draping the Patient

The patient is draped after the surgeon has donned gown and gloves. A doubled towel is laid horizontally across the lower margin of the operative field. A second towel is laid doubled on the medial aspect of the sterile field. A towel clip is then applied to attach the two towels where they cross. The third towel is then applied to the lateral aspect of the operative field, and the fourth towel is doubled and placed at the upper border of the operative field. The towels are clipped together where they intersect.

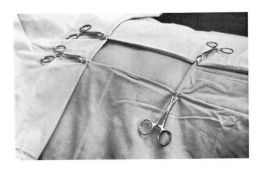

The use of an adherent transparent plastic drape has become common. This avoids the necessity of applying wound towels, providing the plastic drape remains attached to the skin edges. The incision is made directly through the plastic. This probably has its greatest advantage when used to exclude the discharge of a colostomy or a draining fistula from the operative site.

A special full sheet is positioned so that a hole incorporated in it lies over the operative site. This covers the full length of the patient. The upper end extends up over a guard which shields the patient's head and the anesthesiologist from the operative field.

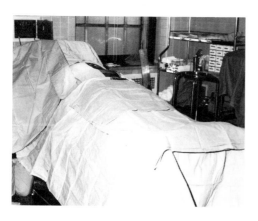

(There are many variations of this procedure, depending upon individual hospital customs.) When the draping has been completed the operative instruments are moved into place, a Mayo-type table is usually brought over the lower portion of the patient, and the large table where the additional instruments are stored is moved within reach of the suture nurse.

THE OPERATION

POSITION AT OPERATING TABLE

The position of the operating team at the table will vary depending upon indi-

vidual circumstances. In general, however, the surgeon usually stands on one side of the operating table with the suture nurse beside him. The first assistant is usually opposite the surgeon and if there is a second assistant he stands beside the first assistant opposite the suture nurse. As the occasion arises for retraction in various directions the second assistant may be moved above the first assistant or around to either side of the surgeon.

PROPER HEIGHT OF OPERATING TABLE

The height of the operating table should be adjusted to produce the least physical strain on the operating surgeon. If the table is too low (and I think it is a common tendency to have the table too low), the operator has to bend over throughout the procedure and may develop a very tired back. The ideal height places the operative field approximately at the level of the surgeon's elbow when his arm is at his side. An assistant who finds the table too high may request one of the stools which are available at various heights for just such a purpose. The tall assistant who works with a short surgeon is at a disadvantage unless the surgeon himself chooses to stand on a stool. It is the responsibility of the first assistant to position the operating table and the light so that the field will be properly illuminated.

PROPER CONDUCT AT OPERATING TABLE

Conduct at the operating table is important. There should be no talking unless initiated by the operating surgeon. He carries a great responsibility and he should not be distracted by non-essential conversation. Furthermore, it has been shown that bacterial contamination of the atmosphere of the operating room increases proportion-ately with the amount of talking. This rule of conversation should be observed even more rigorously if the operation is being done under local or spinal anesthesia. An overheard remark can be very disturbing to the patient. When the patient is conscious it is a good idea to rely heavily upon hand signals in requesting instruments from the scrub nurse.

Make an effort to keep the operating table neat, passing instruments back to the suture nurse immediately after they are used and removing soiled sponges from the field. (Sponges should be dropped into containers at the side of the table.) Do not reach for instruments on the trays, but rather depend upon the suture nurse to pass them to you. Do not lean on the patient. This could be particularly harmful if you lean on the patient's chest restricting his respiration.

Duties of the Individual Assistants

The duty of the assistants is to help the operating surgeon. The primary function of the *first assistant* is to anticipate the needs and moves of the surgeon, and to help him proceed quickly, surely, and without interruption or irritation. The first assistant is allowed considerable opportunity to act as he thinks necessary, unless advised otherwise by the surgeon. The good first assistant anticipates the moves of the surgeon and tries to facilitate them. He attempts to create maximum exposure of the operative site with proper retraction and keeps the field clear of obstruction, removing blood and clots. He keeps the operative field from being cluttered with instruments. He prevents drying of exposed tissues by covering them with moist packs or periodically wetting them. He makes suggestions with discretion when indicated.

The *second assistant* carries out the wishes of the surgeon or the first assistant. He should restrict his activities to holding instruments and retractors as instructed by either the first assistant or

the surgeon; he should make suggestions only when sure of his ground and of the temperament of the operating surgeon.

Passing Instruments

Instruments should be passed in a positive and decisive manner. When an instrument is properly passed the surgeon will know he has it and will not have to move his eyes from the operative field. The suture nurse and the assistants should know what he wants by his signals. When he extends his hand the instrument should be slapped firmly into his palm, in proper position for use when he closes his hand on it.

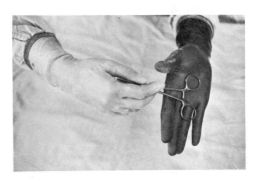

Hand Signals

There are some widely accepted hand signals used at the operating table. These speed up the passage of instruments and eliminate much talking. The signals are as follows:

Hemostat. Extend the hand supinated. This is the position in which most

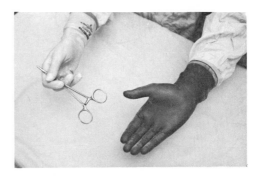

instruments are received. Even when signals are not being used routinely this maneuver should be answered with a hemostat unless the surgeon specifically asks for another instrument.

SCISSORS. Extend the index and middle fingers and adduct and abduct the two fingers in a shearing motion.

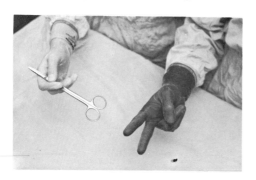

SCALPEL. Hold the hand pronated with the thumb apposed against the distal phalanx of the fingers and flex the wrist.

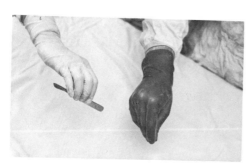

This simulates holding the scalpel and a cutting maneuver.

FORCEPS. Hold the hand pronated and appose the thumb and index finger.

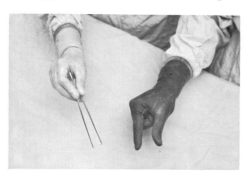

This simulates the position of the hand when holding a forceps.

SUTURE. Extend the hand in a position of bringing the hand from pronation to supination.

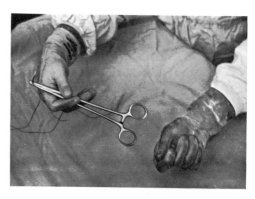

This simulates holding a needle holder and the motion used in inserting the suture.

TIE. Hold the hand elevated with the palm toward the suture nurse.

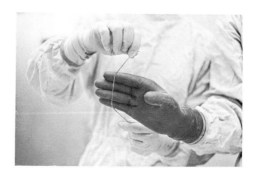

The nurse grasps the tie at each end and sets the mid portion in the surgeon's palm.

COMPLETION OF THE OPERATION

The operation does not end with the placing of the last suture but only when the patient has left the operating room. When the operation is over do not leave until the surgeon leaves, or advises that you may do so. Usually, proper dressing of the wound requires coverage of more skin space than is exposed with the drapes in place. Thus the wound is covered with the initial dressing but completion of bandaging may not be possible until the drapes have been removed. In such a circumstance you may be asked to hold the dressing in place. If you should contaminate your gloves in the removal of the drapes before the wound has been properly protected, notify the surgeon. If you are asked to obtain adhesive plaster to hold the dressing in place remove your gloves before you handle the adhesive side of the plaster.

Remain available to help move the patient to the stretcher. Moving should be done slowly and gently; it is facilitated by placing a sheet beneath the patient. Before moving the patient ascertain that individual members of the team have been designated to support his head and to safeguard any intravenous or drainage tubes.

Remove your gown and place it in the receptacle provided for that purpose. If you plan to participate in another operation do not remove your gloves. While this is not general practice, I think it advisable to change all attire—cap, mask, and suit—between cases.

Chapter Four

Sutures

MATERIALS

Sutures are made of many different materials which can be divided into two groups, absorbable and nonabsorbable.

ABSORBABLE SUTURE MATERIAL

Catgut is the only absorbable suture material in general use. It is made from strands of submucosa of the proximal portion of the small bowel of sheep.

Catgut is available "plain" or in a form treated by chromicizing to slow its rate of absorption. Each type of "chromic" catgut is treated individually to allow absorption over different pre-determined periods. The gut will usually hold at least as long as specified, but some body fluids (such as bile) retard absorption and the gut may last considerably longer than planned. Plain catgut is absorbed rapidly and, therefore, causes a greater amount of tissue reaction. All catgut swells because it absorbs some water from the surrounding tissues. This

swelling has a tendency to loosen knots and longer ends must be left in knots in catgut sutures.

Catgut is supplied in various lengths, the 54-inch length being the most common, and is available either in a plastic tube and envelope, or in glass tubes. The sutures are sterile when packed and the packages are kept in sterilizing solution. Catgut has the following advantages:

1. It will ultimately be absorbed.
2. It can be used as a continuous suture, thereby shortening the time required for its placement.
3. When used as an interrupted suture, it is the material of choice for working in an infected field.

NONABSORBABLE SUTURE MATERIAL

While catgut is still the most commonly used suture material there has been a gradual swing of preference to nonabsorbable suture materials. The most commonly used nonabsorbable materials, in order of popularity, are silk, cotton, stainless steel, and dermal, followed by the synthetics such as nylon. Silk was the first nonabsorbable suture material used extensively and it is still widely used. It was once almost universally used in blood vessel suturing. Some of the plastic sutures have become popular for blood vessel and cardiac sutures because of their strength and in spite of their small size. While very strong, the knots have a tendency to loosen. Many additional throws should be put in knots made of these materials. Cotton produces even less tissue reaction than silk, but the difference is not significant. It can be used wherever silk is appropriate except for blood vessels. Stainless steel gives the least reaction of all suture material. Occasionally a surgeon will employ steel even in gastrointestinal work but its major use is in bringing together strong fascial layers. Some surgeons refuse to bury it, using it only in the skin. It is an ideal skin suture material, if one plans to leave the sutures in for a long time, because it evokes a minimal reaction. Braided wire suture is even stronger than a single strand and is easier to work with. Dermal, particularly the finer sizes, is also popular as a skin suture.

Cotton and silk are available in tubes of multiple strands of 18 or 30 inches. They may also be obtained on rolls in 54-inch lengths for use in multiple ties. Stainless steel comes in individual lengths of 18 or 30 inches as well as on spools. Nonabsorbable suture material offers the following advantages:

1. It has a known strength which will not change in a few days.

2. It produces less tissue reaction.

3. Knots of this material will not slip. Sutures can be cut right on the knot and less suture material is left in place.

Preparing Suture Material

Suture material is usually prepared by the suture nurse. The individual unit (tube or envelope) is transferred with sterile forceps from the sterilizing solution to the sterile field. If the suture is in a glass tube, a sterile four-by-four gauze dressing is wrapped around the tube for protection and the tube broken with the fingers.

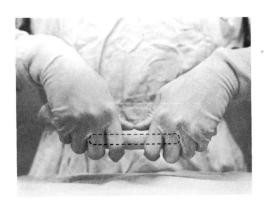

If the suture is in a plastic envelope, the end of the envelope is cut off with a scissors after the suture has been moved back from the edge of the envelope so that the suture is not cut.

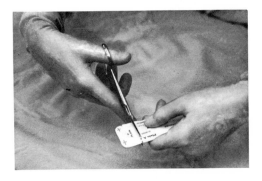

When catgut is removed from its container, it is unraveled and stretched to remove the kinks. It is cut to the desired length and stored under a towel, with only the tip of each piece protruding. Thus each length will be easily accessible but not in a position to become entangled with the instruments. The full length catgut suture is cut into quarter-lengths for free ties. A quarter-length, pulled about four inches through the eye of the needle, is used for an interrupted suture. A continuous suture is usually a half-length pulled about four inches through the needle. For tying clamped vessels the surgeon keeps a full length suture wrapped around a container tube. Since this can be held in the hand while placing ligatures about hemostats, the number of motions necessary is reduced. Full lengths of sutures are now processed in rolls or spools.

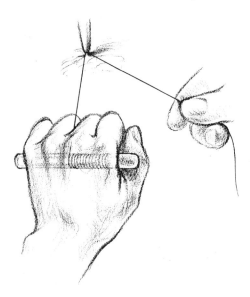

Nonabsorbable suture material already has been cut in the desired lengths before packing. These are merely placed beneath the towel. The long suture for continuous ties has already been rolled before packing.

Size of Sutures

The suture material should never be stronger than the tissue it is expected to hold together. Representative sizes are as follows:

Catgut: Gastrointestinal anastomosis —#000 and #00000 chromic
    Fascia—#0 chromic
    Skin—#0 chromic

    Tying small vessels—#000 plain
Silk: Blood vessel anastomosis—#000 and #00000
    Gastrointestinal anastomosis—#000
    Fascia—#000 and #00
    Skin—#0000
    Retention sutures—#2
Cotton: Fascia—#30
    Subcutaneous tissues—#50
    Skin—#80
Wire: Skin—#34 or #36
    Fascia—#30 or #32
    Retention—#28

NEEDLES

Needles can be classified according to shape and to the nature of their point.

Shape

Needles may be straight or curved.

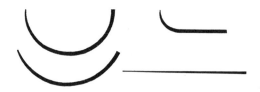

The curved needle allows the surgeon to dip in and out of tissues and to work in deep holes. A needle holder is necessary in most instances when a curved needle is used. The straight needle can only be used where there is adequate exposure and where the tissue can be distorted to allow the straight needle to be pushed and pulled through the tissue. Since a straight needle does not require a needle holder, suturing can be done with considerably less motion and consequently more rapidly.

Point

The point of the needle may be tapered or it may have a cutting edge.

The cutting edge needle is used for suturing skin, periosteum, or perichondrium. The sharp cutting edge facilitates pushing the needle through firm tissue. When suturing deeper structures and organs, a needle with a tapered tip is used. Use of a cutting edge in these deeper tissues would make undesirably large holes and might lacerate vessels, causing troublesome bleeding.

Head

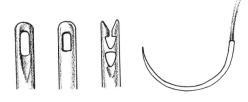

Minimal trauma needles are available; in these, suture material is swaged into the needle. The French-eye needle has a unique eye arrangement which allows threading of heavy suture material on relatively small needles. The suture material, held taut, is slipped through the notch into the eye of the needle.

Placing Suture in Needle

About four inches of suture material is threaded through the eye of the needle. The straight needle needs no holder. To attach the needle holder to a curved needle the needle is grasped in the left hand with the concave or inner surface up and the point on the left. With the right hand the needle holder is applied approximately one quarter of the distance from the eye end of the needle. The needle is threaded from within its curvature so that the short end falls away from the outside curvature to prevent an easy pull-out.

With the left hand, the two ends of the suture are grasped and laid in the jaw of the needle holder distal to the needle. This will prevent the suture from pulling out.

TYING KNOTS

Every surgeon must learn to tie knots easily, quickly and well. To do this one first learns the technique and then develops facility by practice. To hold properly, all knots should be set down as square knots otherwise they are likely to loosen. In a square knot the half-hitches are made so that both ends of the suture fall under the same loop. This is accomplished by making the second half-hitch in the direction opposite to that of the first half-hitch. Proper technique in setting the knot down determines how well it will hold and the importance of this cannot be overemphasized.

The well trained surgeon will know how to tie knots by several different methods.

Two Hand Knot

This is the surest way of tying a knot properly. It is particularly useful when continuous pressure is required while the knot is being tied. Either half-hitch can be made first. The tying can be done about the fingers of either hand, but is more commonly done about the fingers of the left hand.

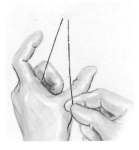

Grasp the long end of the suture with the flexed middle, fourth, and little fingers of the left hand. With the other hand bring the short end back between the extended thumb and index finger of the left hand.

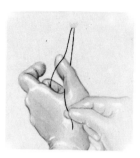

Cross the thumb of the left hand over the short end and under the long end. Continue to hold the ends of the suture as before.

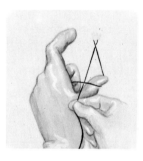

Hook the thumb of the left hand about the long end and pull it across the short end by extending the thumb. In this way a loop is created.

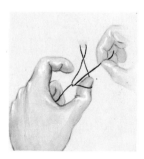

Bring the short end being held by the right hand forward over the long end and place it on the palmar surface of the distal phalanx of the thumb.

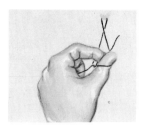

Grasp the short end of the suture between the thumb and index finger of the left hand.

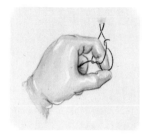

Bring the short end of the suture through the loop by advancing the index finger and allowing the thumb to slip out of the long end. You now have the first half-hitch, with the index finger through the loop made by the hitch.

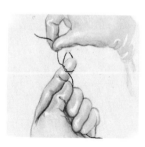

Since the ends of the suture are crossed at this point it is necessary to cross your hands to uncross the suture after the short end is grasped by the right hand.

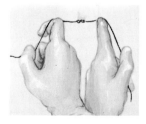

The first half-hitch is set down. Note that the long end which was on the left side as the knot was begun is now on the right side. However, the left hand is still grasping the long end.

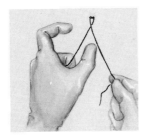

Begin the second half-hitch by uncrossing the hands, but continuing to hold the long end with the middle, fourth, and little finger of the left hand and the short end with the thumb and index finger of the right hand.

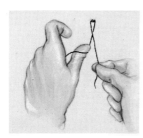

Hook the thumb of the left hand under the long end which is being held by that same hand.

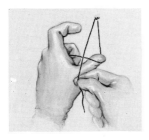

Bring the short end in the right hand across the left thumb to midway between the thumb and index finger thus producing a loop.

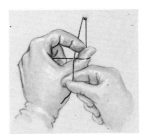

Appose the index finger of the left hand against the thumb.

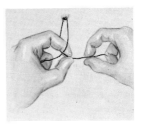

Pass the apposed thumb and index finger through the loop. Bring down the short end held by the right hand and place this end between the thumb and index finger of the left hand.

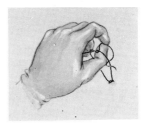

Release the short end from the right hand and bring the index finger and thumb of the left hand back through the loop carrying the short end along.

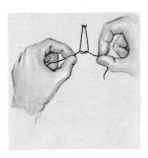

Grasp the short end again with the right hand.

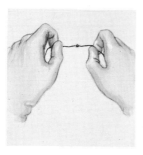

Set the second half-hitch in place.

When you first begin to tie knots you will have difficulty holding the first half-hitch in position while you begin the second half-hitch. This problem is solved by holding one end taut but not pulling on it, or by making two turns about the suture on the first half-hitch. The latter is called a surgeon's knot and is acceptable when you first begin to tie, but after you develop proficiency it should not be necessary.

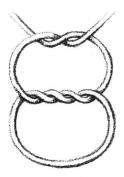

The experienced surgeon usually resorts to such a knot only when he is tying down on some elastic structure like a drainage tube.

A young surgeon should learn first to tie the two hand knot. However, he will find that there are certain advantages in the one hand knot. He does not have to put down all his instruments to tie this knot, consequently fewer motions and less time are required. It also is convenient when tying in a deep hole.

ONE HAND KNOT

The knot may be tied with either hand. However, it can be done more expeditiously with the left hand. If you tie with the left hand you can keep the needle holder in your right hand, thereby reducing the number of motions necessary. The technique will be described as if the short or free end of the suture lies on the right side. If the short end happens to lie on the left side, the second half-hitch should be made first. Whichever half-hitch is made first, the other should follow.

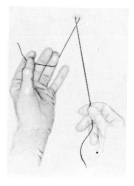

Grasp the short or free end which is on the right with the left hand and bring it across to the left under the long end which is held by the right hand. Hold the short end between the thumb and index finger of the left hand with the proximal portion lying on the volar surface of the middle and ring fingers.

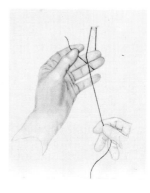

Bring the left hand under the long end until the long end crosses the short end between the index and middle fingers of the left hand.

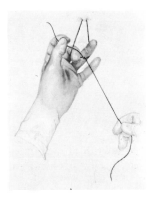

Flex the middle finger and get it beneath the short end.

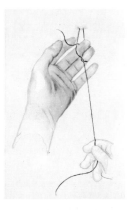

Catch the short end between the middle and ring fingers of the left hand. When you have hold of the suture with these fingers you can release the end which was held by the thumb and index finger of the same hand.

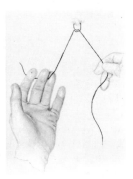

Withdraw the middle and ring finger through the loop bringing the short end along with them.

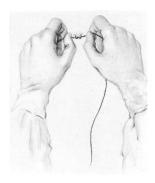

Set this half-hitch in place by pulling on both ends.

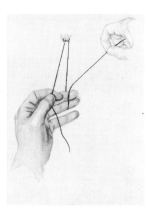

Continue to hold the short end between the thumb and index finger of the left hand. With the right hand, bring the long end beneath the ring finger of the left hand and up over the volar surface of the middle and ring fingers of the same hand.

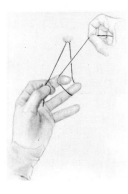

Flex the middle and ring fingers of the left hand and move them over beneath the short end.

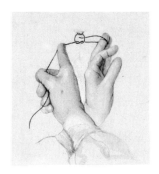

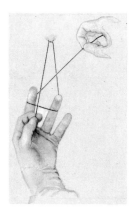

To set the knot down properly you must cross your hands after pulling the short end through the loop.

Extend the middle and ring finger so that there is one finger on either side of the short end of the suture.

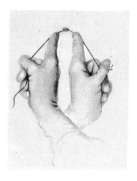

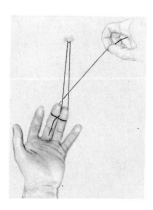

The knot is then set in place with proper traction in the plane of the loop. To develop proficiency in tying in a hole, take a cylindrical container, such as a cereal box, remove both ends, secure a piece of cloth over one end, and then practice tying sutures into the cloth, working through the box.

INSTRUMENT TIE

The third type of knot is the instrument tie which requires the use of a hemostat. This is of value when one end of the suture is short (as, for example, when it has been accidentally broken), when tying a knot in a deep cavity or when using a "no touch" technique when working in a joint cavity.

Bring the middle and ring fingers of the left hand together, grasping the short end of the suture. Release the hold by the index finger and thumb on the same suture. Pull the middle and ring fingers from the loop with the contained short end of the suture.

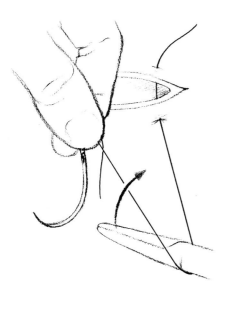

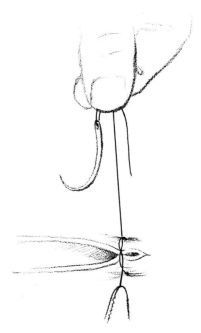

The short end can be pulled quite short. Make a loop of the long end of the suture about the instrument beginning with the instrument in front of the suture.

Pull the suture through the loop and set the knot down properly using only the instrument for traction. The traction must be exerted in the plane of the knot. Pull the short end toward you and the long end away.

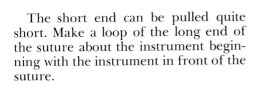

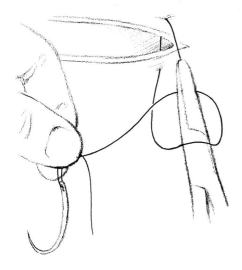

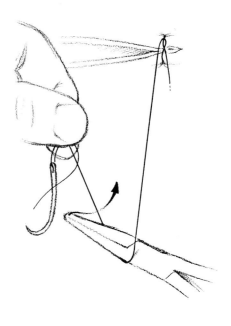

Grasp the short end of the suture by the hemostat which is through the loop.

Start the second half-hitch by again wrapping the long end about the instrument, but in this instance do it in the opposite direction. Begin with the instrument behind the long end of the suture.

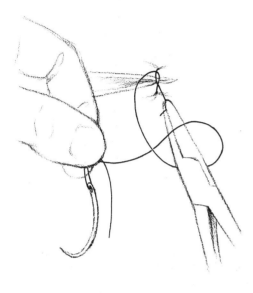

After making the loop about the instrument grasp the short end of the suture with the instrument and pull it though the loop.

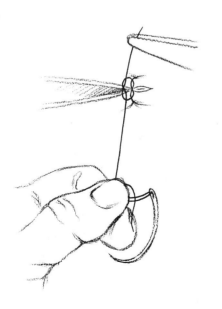

After pulling the short end through the loop, set the short end in place, pulling the short end away from you and the long end toward you.

Beginning surgeons have a tendency to rely on an instrument tie because it seems easier to tie a square knot this way. It is best to learn to tie knots in the order in which they have been presented here.

SUTURES

INSERTING SUTURES

The suture material need be only as strong as the material it is holding together. A straight needle is preferable for suturing the skin or a very superficial area, because less motion is required. On the other hand, if one is working in a deep field or if the nature of the work requires dipping the needle in and out of the tissue, a curved needle is preferable. A needle holder should be used with a curved needle. Grasp with a forceps the tissue to be sutured. If working on a hollow viscus or vessel, use plain forceps to hold the tissues. When working on fascia or skin use forceps with teeth; holding skin with plain forceps requires so much force that the skin will be damaged. While holding the tissue with a forceps insert the needle. If you are using a curved needle you will find that the needle will slip through the tissue more easily if you exert pressure in the line of the needle. In other words, to insert the curved needle exert a turning force on the needle holder. Practice tying the suture while holding the instruments. This will reduce the number of motions necessary and materially cut down on over-all operating time.

Set the knots down so that they lie properly or you will not have a square knot. Both ends of the suture must be either above or below the loop at each end (opposite). Do not tie the knots with excess tension. The tissues need only be approximated.

After an incision has been sutured edema of the skin and subcutaneous tissues always ensues, so that sutures that appear to firmly approximate the tissues when they are placed will be causing too much tension the following day.

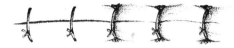

In this figure the first two sutures were placed with proper tension. The latter three were too tight but probably appeared satisfactory when tied. Proper approximation of the tissues depends upon the point of placement of the suture on each side. For example, in skin sutures the needle should include the same amount of tissue on each side of the wound. If the needle is inserted at different depths on apposing sides of the wound the skin edges will overlap when the suture is tied.

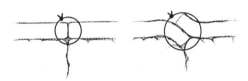

It is also important to approximate all tissues as a wound is closed. Leaving "dead" space will encourage the accumulation of fluid which predisposes to wound infection.

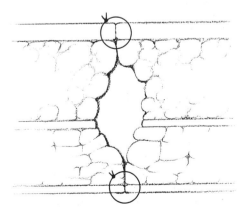

The distance of the needle insertion from the edge of the wound is dependent on the tissue being sutured; about ¼ inch is a good average. The distance from one suture to the next should be approximately the same as the distance from the edge of the wound to the suture.

Cutting Sutures

When cutting sutures, close the scissors most of the way; slip the small portion still open over the suture and run it lightly down to the knot; twist the tip to allow the desired length of tail and cut the suture.

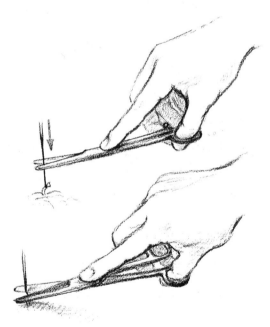

Keep the tip of the scissors in sight and do not close them unless you can see that the tips are clear of tissue. If you are not certain that you can properly and safely cut the suture *do not attempt* to do it. Tell the surgeon you are not in position to do it properly.

Remove the ends of the suture from the field as they are cut. Buried catgut sutures should be left with a ¼ inch tail. Buried sutures of nonabsorbable suture material can be cut right beside the knot. The tail of an interrupted skin suture should be cut short enough that it will not become entangled in the next suture.

Removing Sutures

The length of time sutures are left in place is variable. The preference of the individual surgeon enters into the decision and the sutures should never be removed without his approval. A general rule regarding time is as follows:

Skin sutures about face and neck	2 to 5 days
Other skin sutures	5 to 8 days
Retention sutures	10 to 14 days

The difference in time is related to the rate of healing in individual areas and the purpose for which the sutures were initially inserted. Naturally the skin of the head and neck, with its excellent blood supply, heals most rapidly. Regardless of the suggested time of removal, sutures should be left in place if the wound is not properly healed. The only exception to this rule applies when there is evidence of infection about a suture.

Technique of Suture Removal

1. Cleanse the area carefully with alcohol. Use hydrogen peroxide to remove any dried serum crusted about the sutures.
2. Pick up one end of the suture with a thumb forceps and divide the suture where it dips beneath the skin.

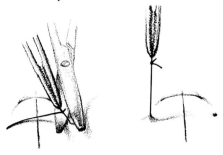

3. While holding the suture with the forceps, gently pull it out through the other skin orifice. If a continuous suture is to be removed, cut the suture at each skin orifice on one side and remove the suture through the other. The objective in each instance is to remove the suture without pulling through the skin any portion of the suture which had been outside the skin.

TYPES OF SUTURES

Interrupted	Continuous
Skin	
Over-and-over	Over-and-over
Vertical Mattress	Vertical Mattress
Horizontal Mattress	Horizontal Mattress
Subcuticular	Subcuticular
Michel Clips	Lock
Inverting	
Lembert	Lembert
Halsted	—
—	Cushing
—	Connell
—	
Purse-string	
Everting	
Horizontal Mattress	Horizontal Mattress
Retention	
Over-and-over	
Far-near-near-far	
Special Purpose	
Hemostatic	
Figure-of-eight	
Suture ligature	

In this listing the sutures are categorized according to the common site of usage, except the over-and-over suture which is used both superficially and deep. The sutures are further divided as to whether they are continuous or interrupted; some sutures, of course, may be used in either continuous or interrupted form. The continuous suture has the advantage that it can be placed more rapidly. However, if one knot slips the entire suture line loosens, whereas, if a knot slips in an interrupted suture, only that one suture loosens; time is thus sacrificed to added safety.

In infected areas *only interrupted sutures of catgut* should be used.

Sutures

Over-and-Over Suture

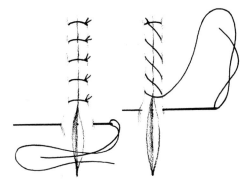

This is probably the most commonly used suture. It may be interrupted or continuous. It can be used, as illustrated, in the skin or in approximating deep tissues. Equal bites of tissue should be taken on each side. In deep tissues, the interrupted suture is usually used. However, the continuous suture may be used to close peritoneum or layers of the abdominal or chest wall, particularly when speed is indicated. In superficial layers, the suture may be interrupted or continuous.

Vertical Mattress Suture

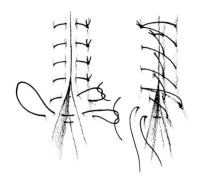

Since this suture takes both deep and superficial bites, it is useful in closing deeper wounds. The superficial bite makes for a more exact apposition of the skin edges and probably gives the best approximation of skin edges short of a plastic closure. It may be either interrupted or continuous. If one inserts two over-and-over continuous sutures, one close to the wound edge and the other further back, a continuous vertical mattress suture will result.

Horizontal Mattress Suture

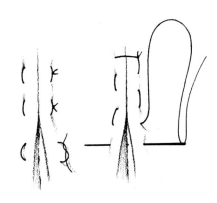

These sutures are placed horizontally. Since the suture lies parallel with the wound edges, any single suture takes the place of two. These may be interrupted or continuous. The suture only crosses over the wound edge at each end.

Subcuticular Suture

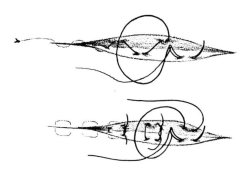

This gives a satisfactory skin closure by approximating the subcuticular tissues. The suture must be anchored at one end of the wound, either by a conventional tie or by perforated buck shot. The suture is then inserted in the subcuticular tissue in a line parallel with the wound. The suture is not pulled tight until the full suture has been placed. After it has been pulled taut the distal end is anchored in the same manner as the proximal end. When the suture is pulled taut it is evident only at each end. It can be used as an interrupted suture, but usually is continuous.

Lock Stitch

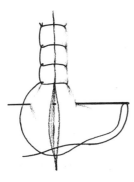

A continuous hemostatic suture, it is most commonly an over-and-over suture through all layers of the bowel in which the loop is made to fall over the point of emergence of the needle so that the needle comes up through the loop forming a self-locking stitch when pulled taut. This controls most of the bleeding. Some surgeons lock an over-and-over suture in the skin.

Michel Clips

Skin edges can be well approximated by means of Michel clips. The skin edges are held together with a pair of toothed forceps and the clips are inserted with a special clip applicator.

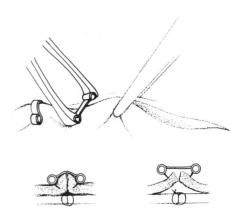

Clips are used only on the skin, they are never buried. When they are to be removed, one end of the clip is grasped with forceps; the clip remover is inserted beneath the clip and closed. The clip will open free from the skin.

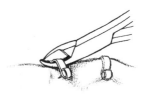

The clip remover should not be lifted until the barbs are free of the skin. This will pull on the skin and cause pain. The angle of the tips is such that closure will cause the points to come out of the skin in the proper direction without discomfort.

INVERTING SUTURES

All sutures described thus far are used to appose tissues. Certain circumstances require a suture which will invert the edges of the tissues; an example is anastomosis of the bowel. If mucosa is apposed to mucosa the surfaces will not seal, but serosa will readily seal to serosa. Furthermore, if a suture penetrates all layers of the bowel wall, infection may follow the needle hole outside the bowel. For this reason, the bowel closure must involve a layer which apposes serosa to serosa and should not penetrate all layers of the bowel. A single layer could achieve this but most bowel anastamoses are made up of two layers, an inner layer through all layers of the bowel and an outer layer through only the outer layers (serosa and muscularis), apposing serosa to serosa. Either interrupted or continuous sutures may be used. If a continuous suture is used it should be of catgut, preferably swaged to a needle. If interrupted sutures are used, catgut, silk or cotton is acceptable. Since the inner layer penetrates the mucosa it is commonly catgut.

Lembert Suture

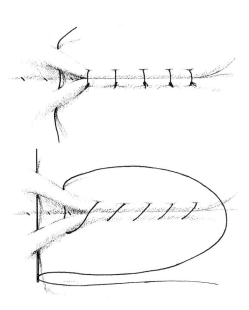

This is one of the most commonly used sutures in gastrointestinal surgery. It may be used as an interrupted or as a continuous suture. Insert the needle from the outside 2.5 mm. lateral to the incision and direct it down through the wall to penetrate the serosa and muscularis, but not the submucosa. Change direction and bring out the needle near the edge of the incision. Reinsert the needle close to the edge of the incision

in the apposing piece of bowel, carry it through the serosa and muscularis, and then back out of the bowel wall without having entered the lumen of the viscus. Then tie the suture just snugly enough to appose the serosa but not so tight as to strangulate the bowel wall. Place the sutures 3 to 5 mm. apart.

The continuous suture is placed exactly as the interrupted, but sometimes is placed obliquely. It requires less time to place and is more watertight than the interrupted suture, but it is also more strangulating. A Lembert suture is most commonly used in the outer layer of a gastrointestinal anastomosis.

Halsted Suture

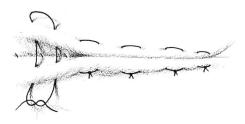

This is an interrupted suture which is a modification of the Lembert suture. It consists of a horizontal mattress suture, so applied that the loop end is on one side of the wound and the two free ends are on the other. Each limb of the mattress suture is placed in the same manner as a Lembert suture—an inverting seromuscular suture placed perpendicular to the line of the wound edge. This suture is valuable when approximating friable tissue.

Cushing Suture

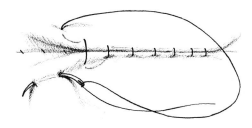

This is a continuous inverting suture used for closing the outer layers of gastrointestinal anastomosis. The needle is inserted approximately 2.5 mm. back from the edge of the bowel. The needle is faced parallel to the incision. The suture is carried through the serosa and muscularis and then brought out again. A similar stitch is then made on the other side of the bowel and is begun exactly opposite to where the suture came out on the first side so that the suture crosses the wound at right angles.

Connell Suture

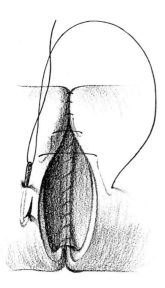

This is a U-shaped continuous suture which penetrates all layers of the bowel. It is placed approximately 4 mm. from the edge of the wound and parallel with the wound. It is placed in a manner similar to the Cushing suture except that it penetrates all layers of the bowel.

After the first suture is placed, it is tied with the knot on either the inside or the outside of the bowel, depending on the placement of the suture. If the knot is within the bowel the suture is brought to the outside through the wall of the bowel. Sutures are then placed on each side of the bowel, running parallel with

the wound 4 mm. from the edge. The suture is inserted through all layers of the bowel, carried within the lumen about 3 mm. and then brought back and on the same side. This is repeated on the other side of the wound. The suture is tied at the end. The suture crosses the incision only from the outside of one wall to penetrate the outside of the opposite wall.

This suture is used to close the first layer in a gastrointestinal anastomosis. Since it penetrates all layers of the bowel wall it is hemostatic. It is always made of catgut and is reinforced by an outer layer of inverting sutures.

Purse-String Suture

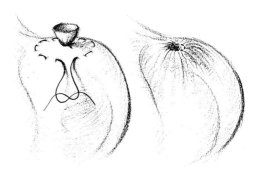

This is an inverting suture placed in a circle about a circular opening which is to be inverted and is commonly used to bury the stump of the appendix. The sutures are really interrupted Lembert sutures placed about the opening. After the suture is placed, the first hitch of a square knot is placed in the free ends and upward traction exerted while the appendix is inverted into it. It is helpful to have an assistant grasp that part of the purse-string suture exactly opposite the knot, and to exert upward traction on this portion of the suture. When the stump is satisfactorily inverted, the suture is pulled snug and tied. This suture should not extend through all layers of the gut, but if it does it must be reinforced with inverting sutures.

Everting Sutures

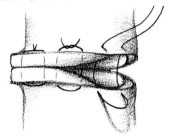

In the early days of blood vessel anastomosis it was thought that apposition of the inner surface was required. Eversion with either interrupted or continuous sutures is most satisfactory, but many surgeons now merely use a continuous over-and-over suture with equally good results.

Retention Sutures

An over-and-over retention suture is inserted and tied in the same manner as any other over-and-over suture. However, it includes considerably more tissue, extending completely through the abdominal wall. Clearly the suture must be of a strong material. Some surgeons use braided silk, but others claim that this acts as a wick or medium of entry for infection. Stainless steel wire, #28, is a far better material for retention sutures. Steel causes minimal tissue reaction and can be left in place for a prolonged period without concern. Braided wire is even stronger and easier to handle because it is more pliant. Unfortunately, it is common practice to place a small rubber covering over the retention suture supposedly to prevent pressure; frequently the rubber cover only causes more necrosis. The best means of preventing necrosis is to avoid excess tension on the suture. A gauze wick under the suture may also be helpful. An inadequate number of retention sutures will give the patient no support and the surgeon a false sense of security. A few scattered retention sutures are worthless; they should be placed no more than one-half inch apart. The most common use of reten-

tion sutures is to reinforce an abdominal wound in which individual layers have also been apposed by sutures. However, a sufficient number of retention sutures, properly placed, can accomplish satisfactory closure without the support of sutures in underlying layers. As a matter of fact, this is the only method of closing a wound dehiscence when one cannot identify individual layers. As many retention sutures are necessary when they are used for reinforcing a closure as when they are the only method of closure. The commonest cause of failure of retention sutures is an inadequate number. I have seen more wound disruptions in wounds closed with both a layer closure and retention sutures than with either closure. This occurs because retentions are put in to reinforce an inadequate layer closure. Because of the layer closure an inadequate number of retention sutures are inserted. A combination of two inadequate closures is not as good as one proper closure.

Far-Near-Near-Far

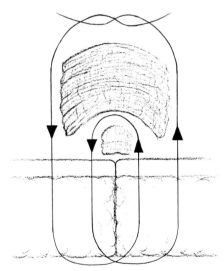

This is another type of retention suture. All points mentioned above about retention sutures pertain here also. This suture has the advantage of producing better apposition of the wound edges. A gauze wick placed under both sutures prevents cutting of the skin and no other dressing is necessary.

Special Purpose Sutures

Hemostatic Sutures

On occasion one will encounter raw areas which continue to ooze, although there are no spurting blood vessels. A hemostatic suture, consisting of two loops of an over-and-over suture placed at right angles to each other, will help to stop the oozing.

Suture Ligature

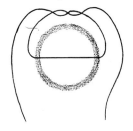 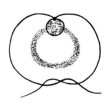

This is a second tie placed on an important vessel to avoid slipping. Since it cuts through the vessel a conventional tie must be proximal to it, otherwise it may cause bleeding or even tear the vessel. It must be placed back on the vessel sufficiently far to preclude the possibility of one side of the suture slipping over the end of the vessel. A suture is passed through the middle of the vessel. It is tied first around one half of the vessel and then around the entire vessel.

Metal Staples

Various mechanical gadgets have been designed for inserting metal staples to approximate tissues. These have been available for some time for gastrointestinal anastomoses and have recently become available for blood vessel anastomoses.

Chapter Five

Dressing of Wounds

TYPES OF DRESSING

All wounds should be protected from contamination and many require support. The dressing serves both purposes. The type of dressing varies with the nature and position of the wound. A dry wound must be covered and kept dry. Raw areas must be protected by dressings which will not adhere. Some wounds require pressure, either to appose large undermined areas or to compress a small area. Draining wounds may require irrigation and indurated wounds compresses, affecting the type of dressing. Wounds which require drainage present other problems.

DRY DRESSINGS

Wounds in which the skin is intact or in which the skin edges are approximated present a dry surface to which a dressing will not adhere. Wide mesh gauze is most commonly used in this situation; it protects the wound and allows

free circulation of air through the dressing. Moisture from the skin can thus evaporate and the dressing remains dry.

NONADHERENT DRESSINGS

If the wound has a raw surface, a nonadherent dressing should be used. In the past the most commonly used nonadherent dressing was petrolatum gauze, which was prepared by autoclaving strips of two-inch roller bandage in a container with a large amount of petrolatum. This was done in the individual hospital and there was often far more petrolatum than necessary on the gauze. The excessive lubricant irritated and caused maceration of the skin. Where this type of dressing is still used, one can remove the excess petrolatum by drawing the strip of prepared gauze between two pieces of dry sterile gauze before applying it. A single layer of petrolatum gauze is sufficient; it should be no larger than necessary to cover the raw area.

Nonadherent gauze dressings which have been impregnated with wax are now commercially available. Another satisfactory product has, on the surface which will touch the wound, a thin layer of cellophane-like material perforated with many fine holes. Before lubricated gauze was used silk, which was so tightly woven that dried serum could not impregnate it, and silver foil were used. Any of these makes a satisfactory nonadherent dressing; the preference of the individual surgeon will determine which is selected. Any nonadherent dressing is backed with gauze squares, fluffed gauze or mechanic's waste, as indicated by the nature of the particular wound.

CARE OF DRESSINGS

The length of time a particular dressing is left in place depends upon the individual circumstances. A wound which has been closed need not be covered for long. Some surgeons remove the dressing 24 hours after the operation because they believe this affords the patient more freedom of movement and more comfort. On the other hand, some leave the wound covered until the sutures are to be removed. Experience has shown that the rate of infection in wounds is about the same. With either course there are several precautions to take. First, the daily removal of the dressing and replacing it with a clean one is of no advantage and may be a disadvantage. This change involves handling the wound and the possibility of infection is really greater than if the dressing had simply been removed altogether. The surgeon, in going from wound to wound, is likely to introduce bacteria other than those already present on the patient's skin.

The dressing should be inspected daily. It should be removed and the wound examined if the dressing is saturated with blood or if the patient's course suggests that the wound might be infected. Profuse pink drainage from an abdominal wound is pathognomonic of an impending dehiscence. If the wound becomes wet, either from drainage or from the patient's sweat, the dressing should be changed in order to avoid maceration of the skin. Never completely cover a dressing with adhesive plaster; some ventilation through the dressing is necessary to evaporate perspiration. When removing adhesive plaster always pull toward the wound. When cutting off a dressing do not cut the bandage directly over the wound. If the dressing adheres to the wound, it can be freed with hydrogen peroxide.

When there is profuse drainage, dress the wound with bulky absorbent dressings. These should not be allowed to become saturated. Instruct the nurses to change the dressings sufficiently often to prevent this. If you do not want the wound exposed have the nurses replace only the superficial layers of the dressing.

METHOD OF HOLDING DRESSING IN PLACE

The wound dressings may be held in place by adhesive plaster, by collodion spray, or by bandaging.

ADHESIVE PLASTER

Adhesive plaster will stay in position and will keep the patient from dislodging his dressings. It has the disadvantages that it sometimes causes skin irritations and is uncomfortable to remove; when repeated applications are required the skin becomes raw and tender. To minimize these unsatisfactory features the area to which the plaster is to be applied should be shaved. The plaster should not be applied over an area covered with antiseptic solution, particularly iodine. Painting the skin with tincture of benzoin and allowing it to dry before applying the adhesive plaster will give some protection. When repeated dressings are required use adhesive straps, known as Montgomery tapes.

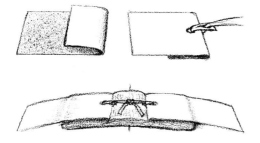

These consist of adhesive plaster with cotton tape attached. To make such a strap fold a two-inch strip of adhesive plaster partially back on itself, make a hole near the end of the doubled portion and insert a cotton tape. Tie this over the wound in such a way that the dressing is covered by the doubled portion of the adhesive. To change the dressing, just untie the tapes. The adhesive strips may be left in place for a week or two without replacement. Readymade tapes of this type are available in most hospitals.

Another method of protecting the skin is to remove only the plaster immediately over the dressing, leaving intact the plaster adhering to the skin and applying plaster for the new dressing directly over it. This maneuver can be repeated five or six times before removing the layer adherent to the skin.

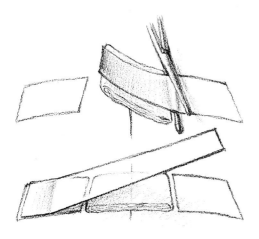

If the patient is sensitive to adhesive, Scotch Tape makes a very good substitute. Several new surgical adhesive plasters and papers have been produced commercially. These can be applied more easily and, while waterproof and firmly adherent, they are readily removed without irritation to the skin.

Method of Application

The purpose of the adhesive is either to support the wound or to hold a gauze dressing in place. The skin where the plaster is to be applied should be intact, dry, and free of grease. Ideally it should be shaved, painted with tincture of benzoin and allowed to dry. Apply one end of adhesive to the shaved, dry skin, well away from the wound. Hold the free end up in the air and run the flat of your hand from the adherent end toward the free end, setting the tape in place by pressure of the moving hand.

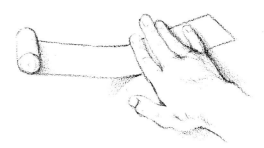

It should lie smooth and without wrinkles. The tape can be made to adhere to the skin more firmly if the ends are bifurcated. The wound is covered with wide mesh gauze to provide protection and at the same time allow circulation of air through the wound. If the gauze is completely covered by airtight adhesive the wound cannot dry; the dressing then becomes essentially a wet compress because of the patient's perspiration. Maceration of the skin will always ensue if a wet dressing is kept against the skin for a prolonged period of time. To avoid this leave some space between the strips of adhesive plaster.

Method of Removal

The adhesive plaster can be removed with less discomfort to the patient if the skin was cleared of hair and protected with tincture of benzoin before the dressing was applied. The strips should have been applied perpendicular to the line of incision. Pick up one end of the strip of adhesive plaster and pull it towards the incision, using the fingers of your free hand to gently push the skin away from the adhesive.

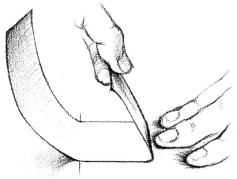

Remove one side as far as the incision, then go to the other side and repeat the procedure. This avoids pulling on the wound which can cause pain. When the dressing must be changed frequently the adhesive in contact with the skin can be left in place or adhesive straps can be used (see p. 57).

COLLODION SPRAY

Collodion spray is another method of holding dressings in place. Several layers of gauze are placed directly over the wound, the dressing is saturated with collodion and, after it dries, the excess gauze is cut away. This is an excellent type of dressing for small lacerations, particularly of the scalp. Several commercial preparations have recently been offered which combine a plastic with an antibacterial agent made up in an aerosol base. These are sprayed directly on the wound where they dry rapidly, and provide satisfactory protection.

BANDAGES

Types of Material

GAUZE. This material, in a 32×28 mesh, is the type of bandage generally used to hold dressings in place. It can be obtained in rolls one, two, and three inches wide. There is also a variety of "special" bandaging materials. In the main these are made in such a manner that they "give" in different directions, so as to allow firm application of the bandage even if the proper principles of bandaging have not been observed. These special materials are more expensive than ordinary gauze and in the hands of an expert they do not produce a better dressing. However, they do make up for the shortcomings of an inexperienced bandager.

MUSLIN. This is used as straps (as the T-binders of the perineum) and to hold traction tape in place on extremities. Muslin may be obtained in three-, four-, and six-inch widths.

OUTING FLANNEL. This material has been used for some years in the treatment of traumatic injury to the extremities and, particularly, to the joints. The material is usually three or four inches wide. Cotton elastic bandage has now largely replaced outing flannel.

COTTON ELASTIC BANDAGE. A cotton bandage, so woven that it has considerable elastic properties, has become very popular. It is available in two-, three-, four-, and six-inch widths. It has generally supplanted the flannel bandage. Cotton elastic may be applied satisfactorily with little knowledge of bandaging; the elastic properties of the dressing allow it to conform to the contour of any portion of the body being dressed. It is used to give support and to apply even pressure. These bandages are expensive, but they can be washed, dried, and reused. Persons requiring reapplication of these bandages should have two sets available.

ELASTIC ADHESIVE BANDAGE. This type has considerable value for fixation of dressings in areas where it is difficult to hold a bandage in place and where expansion and contraction are necessary, e.g., the chest. This type of bandage has a tendency to unroll at the end, a deficiency the bandager can overcome by placing a piece of plain adhesive plaster over each end or by rounding the ends of the elastic adhesive bandage.

General Considerations of Bandaging

Bandaging should be done neatly and carefully. The appearance of the bandage is an indication of the proficiency of the person who applied it and has an effect also on patient morale. A properly applied bandage, which carries out the purpose for which it was applied and remains in position for the period desired, makes a good impression upon the patient. The bandage should be snug, but not so tight as to leave marks in the skin after it has been removed. On the other hand, it should remain firmly in place until it is time for the wound to be redressed. The amount of pressure should be merely sufficient to hold it in place.

The bandage should be applied evenly without wrinkles. Turn the roll 180 degrees when necessary to make one side or the other more firm. (This is not necessary with elastic bandage.) Always maintain proper control of the roll of bandage. Dropping the roll has a bad psychological effect, to say nothing of the fact that you must discard the roll and start over again.

Since the mesh of gauze bandage is wide to allow air to circulate, completely covering such a dressing with adhesive is senseless. Adhesive, when used, should merely secure the end of the bandage to help hold it in place. When applied over a gauze bandage on an extremity the adhesive is best wrapped in a spiral to avoid constriction of the circulation. There is a common tendency to use bandage that is too narrow. Use the widest bandage with which you can properly do the job; for example, one-inch bandage should only be used

in wrapping the fingers; two-inch bandage should be used on the hand and in head dressings. For all other areas, three-inch bandages should be used with the exception, of course, of the feet where one- and two-inch widths are indicated on the toes and foot.

An elastic bandage should not be stretched to its limit before it is applied, or it becomes, in essence, a nonelastic bandage. When used to wrap an extremity, the elastic bandage should be tightest at the distal end and looser as it is applied proximally. It should never be so tight as to leave marks when it is removed. An elastic bandage on the lower extremity must include the toes; otherwise the unbandaged limb distal to the elastic dressing will swell. If pressure over a wound is required, additional dressings should be applied and the bandage wrapped tighter. However, under such circumstances the area must be examined at frequent intervals to ensure that the pressure is not injuring the tissues.

Methods of Bandaging

Bandages can be applied in many different ways. Circumstances peculiar to the various areas of the body require different types of applications.

CIRCULAR BANDAGE.

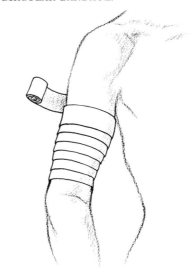

This is used over a tubular area such as the arm. The bandage is fixed by several turns about the part and it is then advanced by circular turns in the direction desired. Each successive turn overlaps the preceding one by ½ to 1 inch. If it begins to be loose at one edge, the bandage may be tightened by applying a reverse spiral (the bandage is rotated clockwise 180 degrees).

FIGURE-OF-EIGHT BANDAGE.

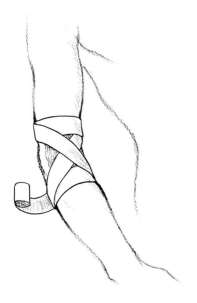

Used over joints, it is anchored at one end by making several turns about the limb below the joint. The bandage is then carried obliquely across the joint and is again anchored above the joint by a complete turn. The dressing is then taken obliquely across the joint to the lower part of the extremity and again anchored with a complete turn. This process is repeated until coverage is adequate. A joint should never be covered by a circular turn unless an elastic bandage is used.

RECURRENT BANDAGE. This bandage is used on distal stumps. It can be used as a bulky dressing over the hand, over any distal area, such as the finger, on an amputation stump, or as a head dressing. The bandage is anchored by several circular turns and then, while one holds the bandage at the point

where it is anchored, the direction is changed 90 degrees and the bandage is applied over the end and down to the other side of the anchoring bandage.

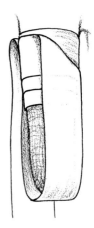

It is again anchored here and the direction reversed back to the initial anchoring point. When bandaging a finger you can anchor the ends with the thumb and another finger of your free hand; when bandaging larger structures, you need additional help to anchor the ends. The dressing is continued back and forth until adequate coverage is accomplished. The bandage is locked by a circular turn.

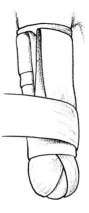

Circular turns over the length of the stump complete the bandage.

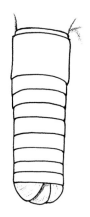

REVERSED SPIRAL BANDAGE.

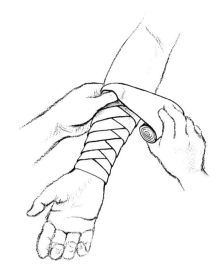

This bandage is used for tubular structures of changing diameter such as the leg or forearm. The bandage is fixed by two or three circular turns and then, on each turn, is rotated counterclockwise 180 degrees, creating a reverse spiral as it is advanced along the extremity. This bandage is likely to slip and is unsuitable for use over joints.

SPICA BANDAGE. This is used to cover the junction of two parts of unequal size such as at the groin, the shoulder, or the thumb. This is a very effective method of applying firm pressure to any of these areas. It will be described in detail in discussions of the areas mentioned.

"T" BANDAGE. A firm material, such as muslin, is used to hold perineal and scrotal dressings in place. This is described on page 68.

DRESSINGS OF SPECIFIC AREAS

HEAD

Scalp

For minor lacerations of the head, a conventional type of dressing is undesirable because it necessitates the removal of a considerable amount of hair. There are two simple types of scalp dressings which can frequently be hidden by rearranging the hair. The first is the collodion scalp dressing. This consists of several layers of gauze which are saturated with collodion and applied directly to the wound. After the collodion dries the wound is satisfactorily protected. An alternate type of dressing can be used readily on women because of their long hair; put a few small squares of gauze over the wound and then fasten with twisted ropes of hair which are drawn across the dressing and held in place with a postage stamp of adhesive.

Head

For more extensive wounds of the scalp, gauze squares are applied to the wound and held in place with a skull cap or a stocking night cap. In another method the wound is covered with gauze four-by-fours and a piece of gauze approximately 20 inches square is draped over the head.

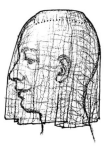

This is anchored at the level of the forehead by two turns of two-inch roller bandage.

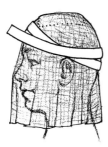

The gauze is turned up over the bandage toward the top of the head.

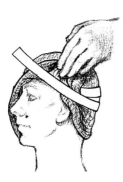

Several more turns of gauze secure this

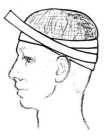

and the dressing is completed by application of adhesive strips.

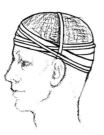

A recurrent bandage is commonly used for extensive lacerations of the head. After you apply gauze dressings to the wound, anchor a two-inch gauze roller bandage by two turns about the head at the level of the forehead. Next, commence in the midline to run the bandage from anterior to posterior using the occiput and the point above the nose as the anchoring points. In this procedure an assistant must hold the bandage tips at one end while it is being applied.

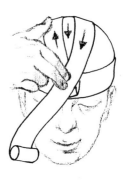

On successive sweeps move the bandage across the head until the entire surface has been covered, then lock the bandage in position by making several more turns about the head at the forehead level where the initial anchoring had been done.

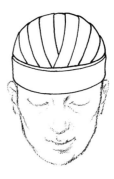

Finally, fasten the bandage in place with a one-inch strip of adhesive plaster brought completely around the anchoring bandage and then with two strips across the head, one from anterior to posterior and the other from side to side in the temporal area.

Head and Neck

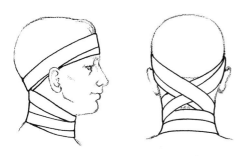

Dressings about the back of the head or about the eyebrow can be held in place by two-inch roller gauze brought around the head, anchored at the forehead level anteriorly and the occiput posteriorly. After several sweeps about the head, begin a figure of eight over the posterior surface of the neck; make one and one-half turns about the neck before bringing it back up again to the forehead line. Repeat the maneuver as often as necessary.

Jaw

To hold dressings in place beneath the jaw, a Barton type of bandage is used.

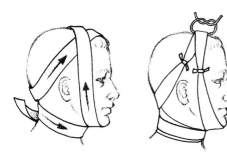

Start a two-inch bandage at the occiput and run it up over the top of the head and down on the opposite side of the face anterior to the ear to a point beneath the jaw. Cross under the jaw and come up on the proximal side of the face anterior to the ear, crossing over the head posteriorly and going down over the occiput. Anchor it by encircling the neck. The entire process can be repeated as often as necessary. At the point where the bandage crosses the top of the head the two strips should be tied together with an additional piece of gauze.

Thyroid

Gauze squares are opened to a four-by-eight size and held in place with two-inch adhesive plaster. The plaster is cut approximately two feet in length. The middle third of the strip is cut in a half inch on each side and turned on itself so that the middle portion is not adherent.

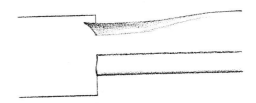

Place the nonadherent portion at the back of the neck where it is in contact with the skin; bring each end around over the gauze dressing placed in position on the neck, crossing the adhesive in the midline and continuing each end over the edge of the gauze and on to the skin of the anterior chest wall.

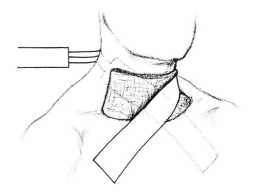

Upper Extremity

Shoulder

The most satisfactory and firm dressing about the shoulder is a spica.

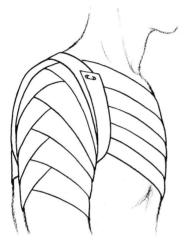

After covering the wound with dressings, apply several reverse spiral turns about the upper arm until the bandage is as high as possible in the axilla. Bring the bandage through the axilla, over the shoulder, around the chest (passing under the opposite armpit) and then back to the starting point. Repeat this second maneuver until an adequate dressing has been applied.

Axilla

Because of the contour of the area the more commonly used dressings do not function well. With the patient's arm abducted away from the chest wall, apply elongated layers of gauze (such as 4 × 4s opened to 4 × 16) to cover the axilla, the apposing surfaces of the chest wall, and the inner aspect of the arm. Hold this in place with strips of adhesive plaster applied perpendicular to the long axis of the dressing at the upper end of the axilla and at appropriate points on the chest wall and the arm. Make the adhesive plaster on the arm short of complete encirclement to avoid constriction of the arm and the underlying vessels.

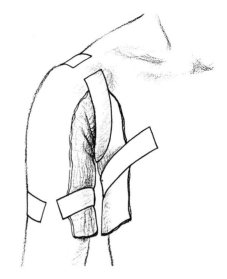

Upper Arm

The upper arm is essentially a tubular structure. Use either a circular bandage (p. 59) or a reverse spiral bandage (p. 61) of three inch gauze bandage to hold the dressing in place. This should be sufficiently snug to hold the dressing as desired but not so tight as to interfere with circulation. Examine the forearm and hand after the dressing has been completed. If there is any question of interference with the circulation the dressing must be changed.

Elbow

The most satisfactory dressing of the elbow is a figure-of-eight bandage.

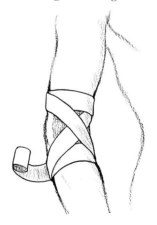

Apply a gauze dressing directly to the wound. Anchor a three-inch roller gauze bandage with two turns about the arm below the elbow. Cross the elbow joint and anchor the bandage with a complete turn on the arm before crossing the joint back to the forearm. Repeat as many times as necessary.

Forearm

A wound here should be covered with a dressing held in place by either a reverse spiral (p. 61) or a circular bandage (p. 59) of three-inch roller gauze.

Hand

A hand dressing is really a combination of several methods of bandaging.

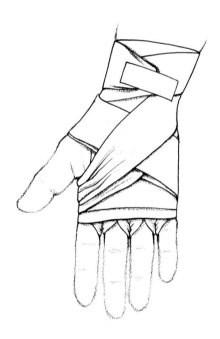

Cover the wound with gauze squares. Anchor the gauze with several turns about the hand with a two-inch gauze bandage. Cover the webs between the fingers with a recurrent bandage held in the palm and on the dorsum of the hand. Anchor the recurrent bandage with several turns about the hand and complete the dressing with a figure-of-eight bandage over the hand and the wrist, passing diagonally over the wrist joint on the palmar surface. This may be repeated as often as necessary to get the desired coverage. You can secure the dressing by going back to the wrist in the figure of eight where the bandage is tied, or you can anchor the end with adhesive plaster Crisscrossing the dressing with narrow strips of adhesive plaster will also hold it in place.

Finger

A finger wound requires a recurrent type of dressing and essentially the same type can be used for an amputation stump, the only difference being that for an amputation stump of the leg or arm three-inch gauze should be used, instead of the one-inch gauze used for a finger dressing. Cover the area with gauze of appropriate size. You can get neater coverage if you bifurcate the dressing and then overlap the bifurcated ends to get better molding about the finger. Anchor the gauze and the roller bandage at the base of the finger with several turns of the bandage. Hold the bandage and reverse the direction to make multiple turns upward anteriorly over the tip of the finger and back dorsally to the circular bandage.

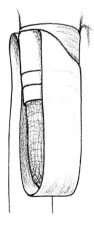

Repeat this recurrent movement until the finger is covered. Anchor the bandage and cover the entire length of the finger with circular turns.

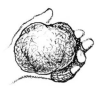

Put the hand in a position of function and cover the entire hand and the wrist with several layers of loose gauze dressing, which is circular over the wrist and recurrent over the hand.

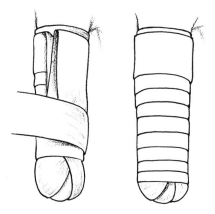

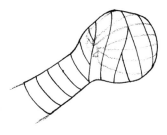

Cover the entire dressing with a two- or three-inch cotton elastic bandage.

This dressing may be secured in one of two ways: (1) It may be held with adhesive. A narrow strip of adhesive plaster should be carried from the volar aspect of an uncovered portion of the finger, over the bandaged portion and down posteriorly to an uncovered portion of the finger on the dorsal surface. A similar piece of strapping should be applied from the lateral to the medial aspect of the finger. It is completed with two circular strips of adhesive. (2) Should the bandaged finger require treatment with wet compresses, secure the dressing with a gauntlet type of dressing instead of holding it with adhesive, which will come off when wet. Bring one of the circular turns of bandage down posteriorly over the hand and about the wrist, anchor it at the wrist with two turns and bring it back over the hand to the finger in a figure-of-eight. This should be done at least twice. Fasten by tying the bandage.

To apply a pressure dressing to the hand, first cover the wound, then put gauze between the fingers and place a large amount of mechanic's waste over the palm of the hand and about the fingers.

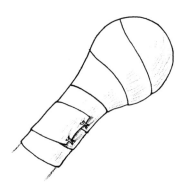

The dressing should be put on in a manner that will allow you to get at the tips of the fingers to ascertain that the circulation is not compromised.

TRUNK

Chest

For satisfactory dressing of the chest choose elastic adhesive bandage in order to permit easy breathing. A typical example is the dressing of a posterolateral incision. Cover the wound with gauze. Paint the surrounding skin with tincture of benzoin and allow it to dry. Hold the dressings in place with strips of three-inch elastic adhesive bandage applied parallel to the ribs and extending about four inches beyond the midline, both anteriorly and posteriorly. The elastic adhesive should be snug but not tight. Cover the end with plain adhesive to prevent the elastic adhesive from unraveling.

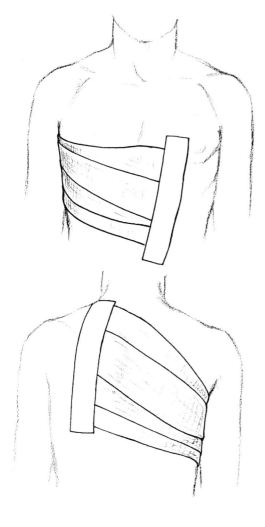

Simple incisions of the chest primarily closed can be covered with gauze dressings held in place by a single strip of elastic adhesive bandage.

Breast

Simple incisions in the breast can be covered with gauze dressings held in place by a few strips of adhesive plaster placed perpendicular to the incision. Additional support is best provided by a brassiere. If the dressing is bulky a larger size than the patient usually wears will be more comfortable.

Radical mastectomy requires a pressure dressing. First cover the wound with gauze dressings. If skin has been grafted it is covered first with nonadherent gauze and a pressure dressing tied over the grafted area. Then cover the entire area with generous amounts of mechanic's waste or fluff gauze. This material must be spread evenly over the area where compression is desired; otherwise the pressure will be uneven. Lay the forearm encased in a layer of absorbent cotton across the abdomen. Add gauze as necessary to protect any protruding points on the arm. Cover the entire area with two six-inch elastic bandages, applied firmly but not tightly. Allow the hand to protrude between the folds of dressings. A few vertical strips of adhesive plaster will keep the bandage in place.

Suction Drainage of Breast

Since the major purpose of the dressing on a radical mastectomy is to avoid accumulation of fluid under the flaps so that they will heal properly, many surgeons now use continuous suction. Two catheters are inserted under the flap, and continuous suction is supplied by a plastic drum-shaped container with springs inside that press on the ends, developing a negative pressure. This can be attached to the patient's clothing. Since this portable apparatus, which does not immobilize the patient, has become available, suction is used much more often.

Abdomen

Uncomplicated, primarily closed abdominal wounds need merely be covered with gauze squares held in place by a few strips of adhesive. There is a tendency to overdo the amount of dressing on abdominal wounds.

Groin

Wounds of the groin may be dressed with a spica which is applied in essentially the same manner as a spica of the shoulder.

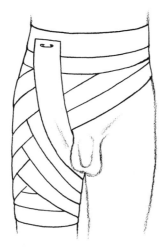

Cover the wound with a gauze dressing. Using three-inch gauze bandage make several reverse turns from within outward, around the top of the thigh. Carry the bandage over the groin to just below the iliac crest. Continue around and bring it obliquely across the symphysis, crossing over the starting point; this is repeated for as many layers as are necessary. The spica dressing has been less often used since elastic adhesive bandage became available. The elastic adhesive bandage, placed to run parallel to the inguinal ligament, may be easily applied over a gauze dressing covering the wound.

Perineum

Dressings are held in place with a T-binder.

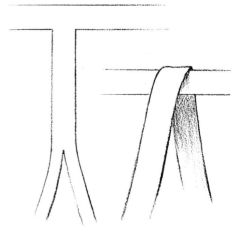

This is usually of muslin, but may be made up of strips of three-inch gauze roller bandage. Secure the horizontal limb of the T about the abdomen at the waist with the vertical limb in the midline posteriorly. Cover the wound with gauze squares. Hold these in place with the vertical limb of the T which is brought anteriorly between the legs and tied to the horizontal limb at the waist. For male patients the vertical limb is bifurcated and one portion is brought up on either side of the scrotum.

Lower Extremity

Dressings are essentially the same as those to the upper extremity, i.e., circular or a reverse spiral to the calf or thigh, a figure-of-eight about the knee, figure-of-eight about the ankle, and recurrent dressings and a figure-of-eight for the foot.

SPECIAL PURPOSE DRESSINGS

Pressure Dressings

There are two types of pressure dressings: (1) those which provide a considerable amount of pressure over a limited area, and (2) those which provide limited pressure over an extended area. To apply pressure over a limited area cover the wound itself with gauze, then build up bulk over the wound (preferably with sterile sponge rubber; if this is not available, with several four-by-four gauze pads rolled up). Hold this in place with elastic adhesive dressing, with some tension on both sides of the wound; bifurcate the ends of the elastic adhesive dressing so that it will adhere more tightly.

Limited pressure is required over a wider area in wounds where skin has been grafted or when there is a wide area of potential dead space where it is necessary to maintain the superficial tissues firmly apposed against deeper structures. The dressing after a radical mastectomy is an example of this. Cover the wound with dry or nonadherent gauze as indicated. Cover this with fluffed gauze or mechanic's waste, evenly distributed, and apply mild compression with cotton elastic bandage.

Wet Applications

Wet Dressings

When an infection of an extremity is drained it is common practice to immobilize the extremity and utilize a wet type of dressing. The site of drainage is left wide open, several loose gauze dressings are placed about the wound, and then gauze fluffs or mechanic's waste, loosely placed. This is then loosely covered with roller gauze bandage in a recurrent type of dressing. Before the extra dressings are applied, two #8 urethral catheters are inserted down deep into the dressings. One may even be placed in the open wound. A thin layer of wax paper is wrapped over the gauze and the entire area is then wrapped snugly but not tightly with bandage. Irrigations can be carried out through the catheters which are led out through the dressings. If you plan to irrigate directly into the wound, you can keep the interior of the catheter sterile by inserting a sterile medicine dropper into the end protruding from the dressing. The nurse then irrigates by inserting the irrigating solution through the rubber bulb of the medicine dropper with a needle and syringe. If heat is also required, the entire area can be wrapped in a plastic or rubber sheet, over which an electric heating pad can be applied. The wet compress dressing should be removed daily and the extremity allowed to dry completely before re-application in order to avoid serious maceration of the skin.

Wet Compresses

Superficial application of wet compresses is indicated in many circumstances, even when the skin is intact as in cellulitis. First place a rubber sheet beneath the part. Place a liberal quantity of loose gauze directly over the area. Wet this with sterile warm solution using an asepto syringe to transfer the solution from its container. Cover this with large cotton pads and then with a layer of wax paper. Place a hot water bottle over this and enclose the whole, first with the rubber sheet and then a large towel.

Do not use wet compresses continuously more than 24 hours because serious cutaneous maceration may occur. The most desirable management is to use such compresses for 20 to 30 minutes four times a day. Remove the compresses and allow the area to dry in the intervals. A thin coating of vaseline protects the skin during the compress.

Drainage

Wounds are drained to remove excessive air and fluid. Tubes are placed to encourage drainage either around or through the tubes. Drainage from the chest and from hollow viscera, such as the gall bladder, common bile duct, or bladder, passes through the drainage tube. Drainage from the peritoneal cavity, or drainage of collections of pus or blood passes primarily around the tube. Another problem requiring drainage is the wound that has a wide area of potential oozing; in this instance one wants to avoid the accumulation of fluid which will keep apposed tissues apart. Catheters are inserted and suction is applied, as demonstrated after a radical mastectomy.

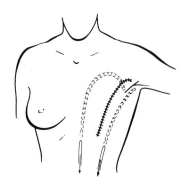

Draining a Collection of Fluid

The commonest type of drainage tube is a thin-walled rubber tube which may or may not contain a gauze wick. The tube is inserted into an area of infection or an area where excessive secretions or oozing is expected. The purpose of the tube is to create an artificial passage about the tube along which the drainage can work its way out. With the exception of the thoracic cavity, the pressure within all areas of the body is higher than atmospheric; consequently secretions flow outwards. A gauze wick is inserted in a tube which is deeply imbedded in order to give more strength and make it possible to pull out the tube without danger of tearing it and leaving part of it in place. This is called a cigarette drain or Penrose drain. Contrary to common belief, the wick does not materially increase the drainage.

When a tube is inserted at the time of operation a suture should be placed through the skin to anchor it in place, and this suture should remain until the tube is to be shortened. Long tubes should not be removed all at once, but rather shortened a quarter to a half their length at a time. Obviously, how much the tube should be shortened depends upon individual circumstances. When the tube is shortened a sterile safety pin should be placed through the stump of the tube just at the level of the skin. The pin is taped to the skin to keep the tube from slipping in or out.

Draining wounds of the chest or of the abdomen should be covered in such a way that they can be uncovered without completely removing the adhesive holding the dressing. To accomplish this use Montgomery straps.

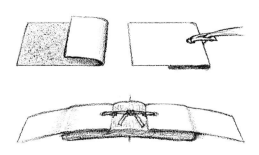

These consist of adhesive with tapes incorporated into the ends so that the tapes merely need be untied in order to remove the dressing. The dressing itself should consist of multiple layers of soft, fluffy gauze directly in contact with the draining area, the amount depending upon the amount of drainage anticipated. This should then be covered with large cotton pads. If drainage is excessive it is sometimes helpful to put a layer of paraffin paper beneath the outermost dressing in order to keep the patient's clothes dry. Such dressings must be changed frequently if drainage is profuse.

Draining a Hollow Viscus

Hollow, hard rubber tubes are used when it is expected that drainage will come through the tube. Tubes for this purpose are anchored in place with a suture. A conventional skin suture is placed, then a second square knot is placed about a centimeter distal to the knot of the skin suture and this is tied about the rubber tube. To make this snug, one must usually resort to a double throw or to a surgeon's knot.

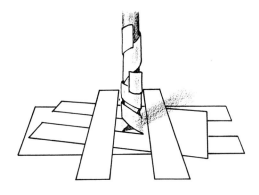

Sump Drain

Occasionally there may be excessive and/or irritating drainage from the peritoneal cavity either from a large abscess or from a fistula of the biliary tract or pancreas. This problem is best managed by a sump drain of which there are two types. One type consists of two perforated tubes, one within another; the other is a single tube with multiple perforations.

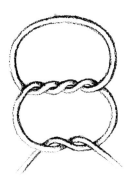

The tube should then be taped to the skin. Trifurcate a piece of two-inch adhesive plaster to half its length. Set this so that the middle strip can be wrapped about the tube. Attach the remainder to the skin.

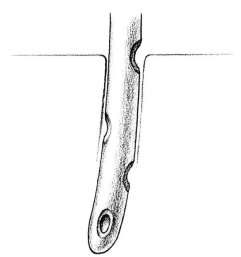

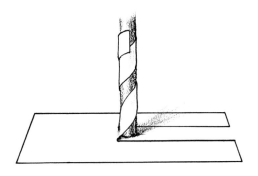

Repeat on the other side. Anchor each with a strip of adhesive plaster.

When using the latter tube it is important that the most proximal opening be positioned at the skin edge so that there is no danger of the tube becoming plugged by pulling the wall of the tract against the hole. Furthermore, the material which escapes to the surface can then be aspirated. Either type of sump drain is attached to constant suction.

Homemade double lumen sumps were not very satisfactory. There are now many good plastic commercial tubes available.

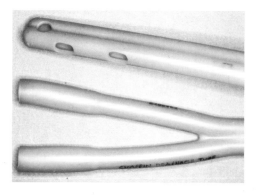

If you are unable to get one and need deep suction, cut the tip off a Foley catheter. The tube to the bag allows air to get to the wound, allowing continuous suction.

DRESSINGS FOR SUPPORT

In addition to providing protection, some dressings have also the function of supporting an injured area. Examples are wounds associated with fractures of bones or injuries where tendons have been divided and repaired. Support may be effected by (1) wooden splints, (2) metals splints, (3) plaster of paris, and (4) plastic splints.

Wooden Splints

The wooden splint is usually a straight piece of wood; its application is limited but it has the advantage of being readily available. All types of wooden splints are prepared in the same fashion. The size ranges from tongue depressors for fingers to long pieces of wood for support of a lower extremity. The wood should be of appropriate size,

no thicker or heavier than necessary as the patient must carry the extra weight. Ideally, sharp corners should be removed from the splint, but in an emergency this can be overlooked. The wood should be covered with cotton padding held in place with roller bandage, circular over the central portion of the splint and recurrent over the ends. A single piece of tape at the end of the gauze will suffice to secure the bandage. The size of bandage used to wrap the splint depends upon the size of the splint. Three-inch bandage should be used on wide splints and one-inch bandage without padding is all that is required on a tongue depressor. The splint is held in place on the patient's body with a circular roller bandage. Where the hand and wrist must be splinted, they should be held in a position of function. Obviously, a straight splint would be unsatisfactory. Tape a roll of three-inch bandage near the end of the splint. Set the arm on the splint so as to have the palm of the hand over the roller bandage. Secure with roller bandage.

In the main, wooden splints should be used only as an emergency measure until better devices are available. This is particularly true when fingers are splinted. For long-term splinting the fingers should always be in flexion. If they are splinted in extension the lateral ligaments of the interphalangeal joints will shorten and the fingers will be in permanent extension. For this reason, fingers should be splinted on tongue depressors for no more than a few days.

Metal Splints

It is now possible to obtain metal splints in almost any shape or form. They are usually made of aluminum because of its light weight and ease of forming. They are most commonly used for the arm and hand and are particularly handy in circumstances where the splint must be periodically removed and reapplied. The splint is applied to the desired area with a minimum amount of padding and held in place by a few strips of adhesive and covered with a roller bandage.

Plaster of Paris

Plaster of Paris is the most versatile material for splinting because it can be molded into any shape desired. It is used as a splint to support soft tissue injuries and simple fractures. It is used as a tubular cast to immobilize complicated sprains and fractures.

POSTERIOR SPLINT. This consists of a single slab of plaster which is applied to one surface of the extremity. This can usually be applied directly to the skin of the hand and leg, or over no more than a thin layer of cellulose wadding. Casts directly in contact with the skin should not encircle the extremity. Make a slab the desired length by unrolling the Plaster of Paris bandage and making several passes back and forth. Now take each end of the slab and immerse it in a basin of warm water. When the entire slab is wet lift it out of the water and squeeze out the excess water. Apply the plaster to the area to be supported and wrap it in position with roller gauze bandage. Hold the joint in the desired position until the plaster is completely dry. Remove the gauze and hold the splint in place with cotton elastic bandage. You may want to pad the splint with cellulose wadding.

TUBULAR CAST. This is used where more support is required. Proper immobilization of a fracture requires immobilization of the joint proximal and distal to the area of fracture. Plaster of Paris is available in widths of one, two,

and three inches. Since it completely surrounds the extremity, the plaster should not be in contact with the skin. There should be at least one-quarter inch of padding beneath the cast. Furthermore, points of pressure should be padded. The cast should be strengthened by a splint or a slab. Apply the slab as described above. Hold it in place with plaster bandage. Set the roll of plaster bandage in warm water and allow it to stand until bubbles cease to rise. Grasp the bandage at each end and squeeze out the excess water. Roll the bandage on, smoothing each layer with the palm of your hand as you go. Do not reverse the bandage to tighten up one end, but rather pleat the gauze. Do not use a figure-of-eight about a joint; roll the gauze directly over the joint, pleating as necessary. After sufficient gauze has been applied, smooth the cast by rubbing vigorously with the palm of your hand. If necessary you can use some excess plaster to smooth. Hold the part in proper position until the cast is dry. Trim off any excess plaster with a scalpel. Instruct the patient to recognize any evidence of circulatory impairment—pain, swelling, or discoloration. If this occurs have him elevate the extremity. If this condition has not completely cleared in one hour he is to come back; if he cannot reach you he is to remove the cast himself.

Plastic Splints

Many ready-made plastic splints are available. They are attractive, light and comfortable. Plastic material is also available to mold splints. Directions for use are included with the material.

Chapter Six

Anesthesia

GENERAL CONSIDERATIONS

A fundamental principle of surgery is that the surgeon performs the smallest procedure which will allow him to correct the problem. A similar principle pertains in anesthesia: only the smallest effective amounts of the safest available agents should be used.

LOCAL ANESTHESIA

ADVANTAGES

Local anesthesia is suitable for most outpatient surgery. Since general anesthesia carries definite risks of itself the patient should not be put to sleep unless his disease, injury or condition so requires. Furthermore, patients requiring more extensive surgery, but who have eaten shortly before they come into the hospital, might vomit under a general anesthesia and aspirate the vomitus. If a local anesthetic can

provide proper working conditions this is the method preferred.

Operations on elderly debilitated patients, or on any patients who tolerate the complications of general anesthesia poorly, may be safely and painlessly performed with local anesthesia.

On the other hand, there are contraindications to local anesthesia. The patient who is too young to understand and cooperate during the operation should be put to sleep. Furthermore, an attempt to operate on a child under local anesthesia may cause him undue psychological trauma. The patient who gives a history of reaction to a local anesthetic should not be exposed to the risk again. A highly nervous patient or one who has hysterical tendencies is a very unsatisfactory candidate for the use of local anesthesia. If a patient has any affections of the nervous system (neuritis, paresthesias, etc.), it is probably better to use a general anesthetic. Patients suspected of malingering should not have local injections of anesthetic solutions because such individuals commonly complain of an inordinate amount of discomfort at the site of the injections. Any infection in the area where the anesthetic is to be injected represents a contraindication.

Anesthetic Drugs

The most commonly used local anesthetic drug is *procaine hydrochloride* or *novocaine*. Its popularity is due to the fact that it is the least toxic of the anesthetic drugs available. This drug begins to act in 5 to 15 minutes and its duration of action ranges from 45 to 90 minutes. It is available in concentrations of 0.5 to 10 per cent; the drug is dissolved in either physiologic saline solution or distilled water. For spinal anesthesia, crystals of the drug can be dissolved in spinal fluid. The 0.5 and 1.0 per cent concentrations are used for local infiltration and field blocks. An average of 150 ml. of 0.5 per cent or 75 ml. of 1.0 per cent solution should be the maximal amount used at one time. The 2 per cent solution is used for specific nerve and ganglion blocks. The total amount used should be approximately 30 ml.; under no circumstances should this exceed 50 ml. For spinal anesthesia, 5 and 10 per cent solutions are used and the total dosage ranges from 50 to 150 mg.

The other widely used local anesthetic agent is *pontocaine*, also called *tetracaine*. Attitudes toward this drug are divided; those who use it regularly are very enthusiastic about it while those who do not, believe it is too toxic. Volume for volume it is more toxic than procaine. On the other hand, since considerably less of the drug is needed there is little difference in toxicity. Pontocaine is seven times as toxic as procaine, but it is effective in concentrations one tenth the strength of procaine. This drug is particularly popular for use in spinal anesthesia. Its onset of action is slower than that of procaine, but the over-all duration is much longer, extending 3½ to 6 hours. Consequently, the surgeon has

more operating time. It is used in 0.1 per cent solution for infiltration and field block; the maximum dose should not exceed 1.0 mg. per pound of body weight. Dosage for spinal anesthesia ranges from 5 to 20 mg. It is also used in 2 per cent solution as a topical anesthetic.

Cocaine enjoyed an earlier popularity which has since waned because of the incidence of side effects. It remains a very effective topical anesthetic agent in 4 per cent solution.

Metycaine can be used for local infiltration, field blocks, nerve blocks, spinal and epidural anesthesia and topical anesthesia. It is used for nerve blocks and local infiltration in 1 per cent solution, in spinal anesthesia using 75 to 125 mg. and as a topical anesthetic in 3 per cent solution. It has very little advantage other than being a substitute when the patient reacts to procaine. It has a duration of action slightly longer than that of procaine but is also slightly more toxic.

Because it is of low toxicity and has a longer duration of action than procaine, *xylocaine* has been gaining popularity as a local infiltration and nerve block anesthetic. Analgesia begins in 5 to 15 minutes and persists for 1 to 3 hours. A total dosage of 0.5 gm. should never be exceeded. It is available in 0.5, 1.0 and 2.0 per cent solutions; the first two are more commonly recommended. This is my drug of choice for nerve blocks and infiltration.

Vasoconstrictor Drugs

The anesthesia can be prolonged by incorporating a vasoconstrictor drug in the solution, thus decreasing the rate of absorption of drug from the area. This prevents accumulation of drug in the blood stream, thereby decreasing the possibility of a toxic reaction. The most commonly used and most effective drug is Adrenalin or epinephrine. Usually 0.1 to 0.25 ml. of the stock solution, 1 : 1000 (U.S.P.), is added to each 100 ml. of anesthetic solution. The dosage is not varied on the basis of the concentration of the anesthetic solution. The addition of a vasoconstrictor to the local solution is contraindicated (1) in the presence of hypertension or cardiac disease, (2) in a highly nervous patient, (3) in operations on the extremities particularly when the patient has peripheral vascular disease, (4) in obstetrics, and (5) in combination with general anesthesia.

Hyaluronidase

Hyaluronic acid, which is found in the interstitial spaces of the tissues, is thought to interfere with diffusion; hyaluronidase, an enzyme which inactivates the hyaluronic acid, improves diffusion but only in the subcutaneous and areolar tissue and not across fascial planes. Since the hyaluronidase allows for more rapid diffusion, smaller amounts of anesthetic drug can achieve a desired amount of anesthesia, but the reaction will be more short-lived because the drug is more rapidly picked up by the general circulation. The hyaluronidase itself produces little reaction; most of the reactions which occur when hyaluronidase is used are related to the fact that it allows a rapid rise in the circulating blood level of the anesthetic agent, thereby increasing the incidence of drug reactions.

EQUIPMENT

The equipment needed for local anesthesia includes syringes, needles, containers to hold the anesthetic solution, and, as a precaution, auxiliary resuscitation equipment.

SYRINGES. The syringe should be the Luer-Lok type so that the needle can be firmly fixed and is not pushed off when pressure is exerted on the barrel of the syringe. Finger rings allow one to better control the syringe and to exert more pressure on the fluid in the syringe with one hand, thus leaving the other free.

There should be several additional syringes on the tray.

NEEDLES. Needles used for local anesthesia should have a short bevel and preferably have a bead on the shaft of the needle. A needle is most likely to break at its weakest spot, where it joins the hub. If a needle breaks when it is inserted to the hub, the needle will be buried in the tissue. The bead prevents the needle from being inserted so deeply. Needles are designed in varying lengths and diameters for specific purpose. Spinal needles have obturators. This is a solid piece of steel which fills the lumen of the needle preventing material from becoming engaged in the needle. After the needle is properly placed the obturator is removed. Most needles are inflexible, but spinal needles which are to be left in place are malleable, allowing them to be bent without occluding the lumen. Check the needles and syringes before beginning an injection. The barrels should fit the syringes and move easily. The needles must be patent, have sharp points with no burrs, and have no weak points where they are likely to break.

Makeup of a Tray for Nerve and Field Blocks

The makeup of a tray varies depending upon its purpose. However, one which will meet most needs includes:

1. Three containers (preferably stainless steel) to hold the alcohol, skin preparation solution, and local anesthetic solution.

2. A sponge-holding forceps and cotton sponges for preparation of the skin.

3. Four towels for draping the operative field.

4. Four towel-holding forceps.

5. Syringes: one 10 ml. Luer-Lok syringe with finger rings; one 5 ml. syringe; one 2 ml. syringe.

6. Needles: two 2 cm., 25 gauge for raising a skin wheal; two 3.8 cm., 22

gauge; two 5 cm., 22 gauge; two 10.2 cm., 22 gauge.

7. Local anesthetic solution or crystals.

8. One ampule of epinephrine solution (1:1000 USP).

9. Physiologic saline for diluting the drug.

10. An ampule of a short-acting barbiturate.

Additional needles and syringes are included where indicated by the specific nature of the procedure to be performed.

Prophylactic Resuscitation
Equipment

Untoward reactions to local anesthetic agents are rare, but when they do occur immediate specific treatment is required and is ready in time only if it has been made available beforehand. Therefore, the following prophylactic equipment should be included:

1. Oxygen-administering equipment. The simplest is a face mask and bag with a source of oxygen.

2. Suction apparatus. A source of suction and a urethral catheter (about #18 French) are sufficient.

3. A laryngoscope (with batteries that work).

4. An endotracheal tube.

5. One ampule sodium pentothal.

COMPLICATIONS

The untoward reactions from local anesthetics fall into two categories: Sensitivity to the drug employed, and reactions to a high level of the drug injected.

Sensitivity to the Drug

Sensitivity to the drug itself causes typical allergic reactions such as angioneurotic edema, urticaria, itching, hypotension, or asthma.

PROPHYLAXIS. Take a careful history of sensitivity to drugs. If the patient has ever had a reaction to a local anesthetic drug, do not repeat it. If there is a history of possible allergy to a particular agent, you must perform drug sensitivity tests before using that agent.

Cleanse the skin on the volar surface of the forearm with alcohol. Raise a small intradermal wheal with saline solution and a similar wheal with the anesthetic drug to be tested. If, after 5 minutes, there is no difference in appearance of the two wheals the test is negative. If the wheal containing the drug is red and spreading this represents a positive reaction and the drug should not be used. A sensitivity test should also be performed with the agent considered as a substitute.

TREATMENT. The treatment is symptomatic. As soon as there is any evidence of reaction, stop administration of the drug. Give an antihistamine, such as benadryl (50 mg.), intravenously. This may be repeated if necessary. Local antipruritic drugs can be used and sometimes the injection of calcium gluconate is worthwhile. If the patient has difficulty in breathing give him oxygen. Aminophyllin (450 mg.) given intravenously will help. Hypotension can be controlled by intravenous ephedrine sulfate (10 to 15 mg.).

Reactions to High Levels of the Drug

A high level of the drug in the blood stream is responsible for the majority of reactions and can be due to (1) the accidental injection of the drug directly into the blood stream, (2) the injection of an excessive amount of the drug, (3) the erroneous injection of a stronger concentration of the drug than planned, (4) the use of a highly toxic drug with too small a margin of safety or (5) the injection of the drug in combination with a substance to improve absorption, such as hyaluronidase, without an appreciation of the rapidity with which the drug can be absorbed.

In the early stages of reaction the patient becomes excited or apprehensive, and complains of sudden headache. He may experience nausea and vomiting and have twitching of the small muscles, particularly of the face and fingers. The pulse changes in character, generally becoming irregular and slow but sometimes quickening. The blood pressure falls with concomitant pallor, clammy skin, perspiration and syncope. The depth and rate of respirations increase. In the more advanced stages the patient becomes depressed, suffers loss of reflexes, unconsciousness, and, finally, circulatory and respiratory failure.

PROPHYLAXIS. To prevent this reaction:

1. Give the patient a barbiturate as premedication.

2. When injecting the anesthetic solution into vascular areas, always add a vasoconstrictor to retard absorption of the drug by the circulation.

3. Do not use a stronger concentration of the drug than necessary to properly perform the desired task.

4. Carefully check the label of the drugs to be used immediately before use.

5. Keep a careful check on the total amount of drug used.

6. Draw back on the syringe before injecting solution to rule out the possibility of an intravascular injection.

TREATMENT. At the first evidence of an untoward reaction discontinue the injection of the drug. Have the patient inhale oxygen. If his respirations are depressed assist him by intermittently compressing the bag attached to the mask. If he becomes apneic, insert an endotracheal tube, attach it to an anesthesia machine and assist his ventilation by intermittent compression of the anesthetic bag. A face mask can be used until an endotracheal tube is procured. Insert the tube when available because this will prevent inflation of the stomach with gas and will prevent aspiration if the patient vomits. Until some type of bag is available, artificial respiration (p. 306) can be used for ventilation.

Watch the patient carefully for signs of aspiration of vomitus. Be prepared to suck out any fluid in the oropharynx. If his blood pressure is low give intravenous injections of ephedrine sulfate, 10 to 15 mg., at 3-minute intervals. If this does not help, put one ampule of neosynephrine in a liter of 5 per cent glucose in water and set up an intravenous drip. Adjust the flow to maintain a normal level of blood pressure. Intravenous atropine, gr. $1/100$, may counteract some of the effects of the anesthetic agent causing the reaction.

If the patient's heart should stop beating immediate cardiac massage should be carried out as detailed on page 308. If the patient has convulsions, small doses of intravenous Pentothal (50 mg. at a time) are indicated until the seizures stop.

Reactions Due to Vasoconstrictor Drugs

Adrenalin-like drugs, used to prolong the anesthesia, may cause reactions. These are typical adrenalin reactions consisting of pallor, tachycardia, palpitations, clammy skin, apprehension, dyspnea, rapid respiration, and hypertension.

TREATMENT. The condition is not serious; management consists of reassurance of the patient and symptomatic treatment. Until the effect of the drug has worn off have the patient breathe oxygen. Reassure him that the reaction is not serious and will disappear shortly. If he is very apprehensive, Pentothal in small doses (50 mg.) will help to calm him.

REGIONAL ANESTHESIA

Adriani* describes seven different types of regional anesthesia related to the site at which the drug is applied. The drug, coming in contact with the

---

* Adriani, J.: Nerve Blocks, A Manual of Regional Anesthesia for Practitioners of Medicine. Springfield, Ill. Charles C Thomas, 1954, p. 3.

nerve, abolishes the conduction of afferent and efferent impulses through that segment. The different types are as follows:

1. *Spinal.* The spinal nerves are blocked at the anterior and posterior roots in the subarachnoid space.

2. *Epidural.* The spinal nerves are blocked in the epidural space.

3. *Paravertebral.* The spinal nerves are blocked as they emerge from the intervertebral foramen or in the vicinity of the vertebrae.

4. *Nerve Block.* The somatic nerves are blocked at some point along their course to the periphery of the body before they divide into their terminal branches.

5. *Field Block.* The large terminal branches are blocked by injecting a wall of local anesthetic drug at the border of the area they supply, just as they branch.

6. *Infiltration.* The nerve endings are anesthetized by injecting the drug into the area they supply.

7. *Topical.* The nerve endings are anesthetized by applying the drug directly to the area they supply.

Spinal (Subarachnoid) Anesthesia

Injection of the anesthetic solution directly into the subarachnoid space of the spinal canal anesthetizes the areas innervated by all nerves from that point caudad. Spinal anesthesia is therefore satisfactory for operations on areas innervated by nerves below the third intercostal nerve. This type of anesthesia provides excellent relaxation of the abdominal muscles, thus facilitating exposure during intra-abdominal operations. Severe hemorrhage, hemorrhagic blood dyscrasias and infections in the area contraindicate the use of spinal anesthesia. It should not be used in psychotic patients or patients who are emotionally unsuited for operation while they are conscious.

Procaine (to 150 mg.), pontocaine (to 20 mg.), or metycaine (to 125 mg.) may be used.

Premedication

The majority of patients who are to have spinal anesthesia are hospitalized and premedication begins the night before operation. At bed time give the patient a barbiturate, probably 100 to 200 mg. of pentobarbital, depending upon the size and general condition of the patient. Discontinue oral feeding at bed time and repeat the barbiturate dosage on the following morning, 2 hours before the estimated time of operation. One hour before the operation give the patient morphine (10 mg.) and scopolamine (0.3 mg.).

"Single Shot" Spinal Anesthesia

Spinal anesthesia may be induced with the patient in the lateral decubitus position, in a sitting position, or in a prone position. The lateral decubitus position is used most frequently; it is easily maintained by the patient and assistance to support the patient is unnecessary. Place the patient on his side with his knees drawn up to his stomach.

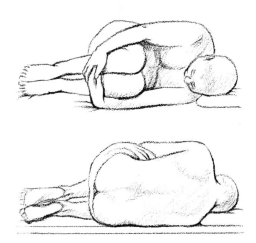

He may be placed on either side but it is preferable to have that side dependent which is to be operated. In this position the patient's spine is flexed to open up the interspace between the spinous processes of the vertebrae. Have the patient wrap his hands about his knees and attempt to pull his knees up farther. If the patient is unable to do this have him rest his upper arm across his lower chest and put his under arm under his head. Before you begin ascertain that the patient is in proper position and comfortable. A regular spinal anesthesia tray at our hospital contains:

1 stainless steel container
1 5 ml. syringe
1 2 ml. syringe
1 medicine glass
1 8.75 cm. 20 gauge spinal needle
1 8.75 cm. 22 gauge spinal needle
1 3.8 cm. 22 gauge needle
1 2 cm. 25 gauge needle
1 introducer
gauze dressings
2 towels
1 pair of gloves

An ampule of ephedrine-procaine solution and another of crystals of anesthetic drug are added to the tray after it has been opened. A separate table contains the alcohol, tincture of Zephiran, cotton sponges and a sponge-holding forceps.

Prepare the skin of the back with alcohol and tincture of Zephiran. Place a sterile towel on the table with its edge beneath the patient and a second sterile towel over his upper flank.

Place the index or middle finger of your left hand on the iliac spine and with your thumb locate the spinous process which is in line with this. The thumb will lie over the spine of the fourth lumbar or the interspace between the fourth and fifth lumbar vertebrae. Using this as a point of reference locate the desired interspace. The needle is inserted into the second, third, or fourth lumbar interspace depending upon the height of anesthesia desired. After checking your equipment to be certain that it is working properly, raise a skin wheal over the selected interspace with the short 25-gauge needle attached to a 2-ml. syringe containing the ephedrine-procaine solution. This is a mixture of 2.25 per cent ephedrine and 1 per cent procaine, intended to offset the

initial hypotensive effect of the spinal anesthesia. Change the direction of the needle to an angle of about 45 degrees with the skin and inject the interspinous ligament with the remainder of the solution. Remove the needle and insert the introducer, a largebore, short needle which is used to develop a tract through the tough interspinous ligament. This should be introduced perpendicular to all planes of the back, or slightly cephalad. It is inserted to its full length and may be either left in place, in which case the spinal needle is then introduced through it, or removed and the spinal needle inserted through the tract created by the introducer.

Using the proper obturator, which can be readily removed, introduce the spinal needle at an angle of about 45 degrees with the plane of the back; the angulation is necessary because of the caudad tilt of the spinous processes. As you advance the needle you can feel it pass through the interspinous ligament and into the epidural space, where less resistance is felt, and finally into the subarachnoid space, as evidenced by the sudden marked decrease in resistance as it pops through the dura. If the needle impinges against the spinous process, either above or below the interspace, the point of the needle should be withdrawn to the subcutaneous tissue and reinserted in a different position to keep the needle parallel with the walls of the spinous processes as it advances.

Withdraw the stylet from the spinal needle to allow fluid to flow from the needle. If no fluid appears, rotate the needle about 180 degrees without changing its position. If the needle is in proper position but against the dura or a nerve root, flow will not begin. If you feel certain that the needle is in the dural space but can obtain no fluid, attempt to aspirate fluid with a syringe. If this is unsuccessful the needle is not in the proper position and should be inserted farther until fluid is obtained.

If the fluid flowing from the spinal needle is bloody no anesthetic solution should be injected. Frequently the initial few drops will be bloody and the spinal fluid following is completely clear. Discard the first few drops and if the remainder of fluid is clear continue with the procedure. If the fluid continues to be bloody withdraw the needle and try at another level.

When a free drip of clear fluid has been obtained withdraw the desired amount of spinal fluid into a syringe. Mix the fluid with the anesthetic drug using either a liquid or crystalline preparation. You may prefer to use a solution already prepared in saline. Before injecting any of the drug withdraw the plunger of the syringe. If there is no free backflow readjust the needle before injecting. Once a free flow is established the fluid can be injected at a rate of approximately 1 ml. per second. At the completion of the injection withdraw a small amount to ascertain that the needle is still in the proper position, and replace this. The needle can then be rapidly removed.

As soon as the patient has been turned on his back, check his blood pressure. If an intravenous drip was not set up before beginning the anesthesia, it should be done at this time to provide a ready route for any medications needed subsequently. The level of analgesia should be checked and the position of the patient readjusted as necessary to arrive at the proper level of anesthesia. The anesthetic drug may be given in either hyperbaric or hypobaric solution. The hyperbaric solution has a specific gravity greater than that of the spinal fluid and will gravitate to the lower part of the space. Since the hypobaric solution has a lower specific gravity it will tend to rise. Either may be used provided proper concern is given to its specific gravity.

Complications

Spinal anesthesia may be accompanied by the following complications:

HYPOTENSION. As a result of the relaxation accomplished by spinal anesthesia, hypotension may occur about 10 minutes after the injection of the anesthetic solution. To treat this condition:

1. Give oxygen by mask. Frequently this will solve the problem.

2. Through the intravenous infusion administer ephedrine sulfate 25 mg. If this does not correct the hypotension, add 1 ml. of 1 per cent neosynephrine to the intravenous fluid. Adjust the drip to maintain blood pressure at the preoperative level. Continue the infusion until the hypotensive effect of the anesthesia has disappeared. Obviously if there was any serious blood loss this should be corrected.

NAUSEA AND VOMITING. This may be caused by hypotension, hypertension, traction on the mesentery, or reaction to the preanesthetic medication.

If due to hypotension treat the cause as recommended above.

If due to hypertension:

1. Administer oxygen.

2. If the pressure becomes alarmingly high, give intravenous Pentothal (50 mg.).

If due to traction, the analgesia should be improved:

1. By more anesthetic solution if a continuous technique is being used.

2. By a slow intravenous drip of 0.2 per cent Pentothal.

If due to a drug reaction give Dramamine 50 mg. intravenously.

RESPIRATORY ARREST. The patient complains of inability to breathe, becomes restless, and then stops breathing. The apnea is most probably due to a high spinal anesthesia with paralysis of the intercostal and phrenic nerves, but may also be caused by cerebral anemia due to hypotension.

To treat this, administer artificial respiration by bag and mask until the effect of the anesthesia is dissipated. If there is any danger that the patient will vomit, insert an endotracheal tube.

If due to hypotension treat this as outlined above. Cardiac arrest may occur and should be treated as outlined on page 308.

HEADACHE. Five to ten per cent of

patients having spinal anesthesia complain of headache, beginning anywhere from the second to the tenth day after anesthesia and lasting for a variable period of time. The pain is a severe throbbing in the occipital area which disappears when the patient is lying flat.

The simplest treatment is to have the patient lie flat until the effect disappears. Drug therapy which has been recommended includes:

1. Nicotinamide (100 mg.) and caffeine sodium (450 mg.) intravenously t.i.d. for 2 days.

2. Codeine and aspirin p.r.n. for headache. The problem is self-limited and will ultimately disappear.

Continuous Spinal Anesthesia

With continuous spinal anesthesia it is possible to use smaller amounts of drugs to complete a specific operation and also to use spinal anesthesia for prolonged operations by continuing to infuse small amounts of drug as necessary. The method of insertion of the needle is essentially the same as that described for the "single shot" type of spinal anesthesia except that a malleable needle is used. All precautions advised for the "single shot" technique should be observed here.

After the needle has been properly positioned and a satisfactory backflow obtained, the needle is attached to rubber tubing which extends to a syringe beside the head of the patient where it is readily accessible to the anesthesiologist. Before attaching fill the tubing with anesthetic solution to remove all air. Bend the external portion of the needle and tape the tubing to the patient's side. Pressure on the needle is prevented by using special thick padding on the operating table with an open area under the back. Before turning the patient have him relax but caution him that he is in no way to assist. Slowly turn the patient to the supine position in such a way that the spinal needle lies in the recess of the mattress.

After checking the backflow give an initial dose of anesthetic solution which is less than that used when a single shot spinal is given. If there is no backflow the needle should be repositioned before injecting anesthetic solution. Check the patient's blood pressure and start an intravenous drip if you have not already done so. Check the level of anesthesia and adjust it by positioning the table or giving more anesthetic solution if necessary. Reinforcing doses of anesthetic solution will be required at approximately 50- to 75-minute intervals. The first reinforcing dose should be approximately $2/3$ the original dose with subsequent doses slightly smaller. Before each injection ascertain that there is a satisfactory backflow. Complications are similar to those due to single shot spinal anesthesia.

Epidural Anesthesia

Epidural anesthesia is produced by placing the anesthetic solution in the space between the dura and the ligaments and periosteum lining the vertebral canal. This type of anesthesia has a smaller incidence of neurologic complications because the drug does not come in contact with the spinal cord. Headaches are less frequent. Since the epidural space ends at the foramen magnum, the drug cannot reach the brain. On the other hand, the extent of anesthesia produced is unpredictable and it is difficult to place the needle properly. Because of these disadvantages, epidural anesthesia in the lumbar area is not widely employed. It has its greatest applications in the caudal area.

"Single Shot" Caudal Anesthesia

This is commonly used in operations about the anus, perineum, and lower urinary tract, and for vaginal obstetrical deliveries. It is contraindicated in patients who have bleeding tendencies or who have infection at the site of injection.

Premedication is similar to that used for spinal anesthesia (p. 79).

Pontocaine (20 to 35 ml. of 0.15 to 0.25 per cent solution), procaine (20 to 35 ml. of 1.0 to 2.0 per cent solution), xylocaine (20 to 35 ml. of 1.0 to 1.5 per cent solution), and metycaine (20 to 35 ml. of 1.5 per cent solution) are the anesthetic drugs most commonly used.

Place the patient on the operating table in a prone position with the hips slightly flexed to a 35-degree angle with the table. If you are using a cart this can be accomplished by putting a large pillow under the patient's hips. If the patient is on the operating table it can be flexed. If the patient is pregnant the knee chest position should be used.

Have the patient abduct his legs and turn his toes in and his heels out. Check your equipment to be certain that the needles are patent and not likely to break. Place a gauze sponge between the gluteal folds to prevent the antiseptic solution from running down onto the perineum and burning the patient. Prepare that area over the lower back and buttocks with alcohol and tincture of Zephiran. Place a sterile towel over the lower back.

Identify the sacral cornu. The fusion of the articular processes of the five sacral bones creates a linear series of tubercles on each side of the sacrum. The most inferior of these on each side is prolonged downward and called the sacral cornu. The sacral hiatus lies midway between these. If you cannot identify the sacral cornu locate the tip of the coccyx. The sacral hiatus is usually about 5 cm. cephalad to this point.

Using a 25-gauge needle raise a skin wheal over the sacral hiatus. Replace this needle with a longer 22-gauge needle and infiltrate the subcutaneous tissue and periosteum about the sacral hiatus. Insert a standard 19-gauge spinal needle at an angle of 75 degrees with the skin, with the bevel exposed, and advance it until it reaches the sacrum. Gradually lower the angle of the needle until it is possible to advance it into the canal.

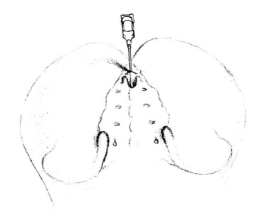

Revolve the needle until the bevel points downward, allowing advancement of the needle in the canal. Since the tilt of the female sacrum is greater than that of the male, the needle is usually at an angle of 30 to 45 degrees in the female and 10 to 20 degrees in the male.

Advance the needle into the canal about 3 cm. Ascertain the distance the needle has advanced by withdrawing the stylet and placing it on the skin overlying the needle. The needle should not be allowed to go beyond the level of the second sacral foramen.

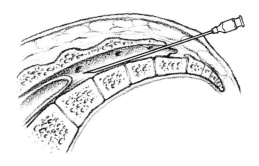

Allowing the needle to go beyond this point creates the possibility of puncturing the dura. The second sacral foramen usually lies 1.3 cm. caudal and 1.3 cm. medial to the posterior superior spines of the iliac bones.

Attach a syringe and attempt to aspirate through the needle. If no fluid is obtained, rotate the needle and reaspirate. If no fluid is obtained the needle is in the proper position for insertion of the anesthetic solution.

If spinal fluid is obtained plans to institute caudal anesthesia must be abandoned and some other type of anesthesia (preferably subarachnoid) substituted. If blood is aspirated advance the needle another 0.5 cm., reinsert the stylet and leave the needle undisturbed for 2 minutes. This advances the needle beyond the lumen of the vessel and allows the blood to clot. After 2 minutes reaspirate. If blood is again aspirated abandon the effort for caudal anesthesia and use the subarachnoid procedure.

After the needle has been properly placed in the caudal canal insert 5 ml. of anesthetic solution over a period of 10 seconds. Replace the stylet and carefully check the patient. This includes measuring the blood pressure, pulse, respirations and general state of consciousness. After 5 minutes, determine the extent of the analgesia. If there is no analgesia or if it is limited to the perianal area you know that the solution was placed outside the dura. You can now inject the additional 15 to 30 ml. of solution planned. If extensive anesthesia already exists this is because fluid has gotten inside the dura. If this occurs the caudal procedure should be discontinued and the operation performed under the anesthesia already produced. At the completion of the injection, remove the needle and turn the patient to the supine position for 15 minutes.

COMPLICATIONS. Complications of caudal anesthesia include:

1. Toxic reactions to the drugs (p. 77).

2. Intraspinal injections are dangerous only if too much drug is injected. If this occurs a dangerously high spinal anesthesia results. This must be handled as recommended on page 77.

3. Hypotension. This occurs far less commonly in epidural anesthesia than in spinal anesthesia. Management of this problem is discussed on page 81.

4. Local infection. As a result of improper aseptic technique infection may develop at the site. The typical signs of local infection should be treated as any other local infection (warm compresses, antibiotics and open drainage when localization takes place).

Continuous Caudal Anesthesia

Continuous or intermittent caudal anesthesia has been used extensively in obstetrics. The technique makes it possible to achieve satisfactory analgesia over a prolonged period of time. Any of the drugs used for "single shot" caudal anesthesia may be used. Metycaine, 1.5 per cent, has been used more often than any other drug for anesthesia in obstetrics.

The technique, including insertion of the needle, aspiration of blood or fluid, and the initial test dose of 5 ml. of fluid, is exactly as described for the single dose caudal anesthesia. However, the needle used is different. If a malleable needle is used this should be substituted for the spinal needle. If the catheter technique is to be used a 16-gauge spinal needle is used. After the needle has been properly placed, a ureteral catheter is passed through the needle which is then removed over the catheter.

Once you are satisfied that the needle or catheter is in the proper position and that neither spinal fluid nor blood can be aspirated, attach a syringe (with rubber tubing if the malleable needle is being used) and very slowly inject 20 to 30 ml. of anesthetic solution. Allow 15 minutes for the anesthesia to take effect and then determine the level. The level should be stabilized at a point between the umbilicus and the pubic bone. If necessary additional anesthetic solution can be given to achieve the proper level. Now have the patient lie on her side.

Subsequent injections, in approximately two-thirds the amount of the initial injection, should be given as soon as the patient begins to become uncomfortable, rather than after she experiences real pain. Since she is lying on her side, determine whether the pain is unilateral or bilateral. If unilateral and on the upper side it may be due to pooling of the anesthetic solution. This may be remedied by changing her position. All injections should be given by a physician. Before each additional injection aspiration of blood or fluid should be attempted.

Paravertebral Lumbar Sympathetic Ganglion Block

This procedure has no direct surgical application, but it is used extensively as a pre-operative diagnostic test to determine the effect to be expected after lumbar sympathectomy. It is also used to treat vasopastic disease of the lower extremities.

No premedication is required. The patient need not be hospitalized. After an hour of observation the patient who has had an uncomplicated block can be allowed to go on his way.

Pontocaine (10 to 100 ml. of 0.15 per cent solution), procaine (10 to 100 ml. of 1.0 per cent solution), or xylocaine (10 to 100 ml. of 0.5 to 1.0 per cent solution) may be used.

Place the patient on the table in a prone position with his arms hanging over the table. Place a pillow under his abdomen to flatten the lumbar curvature of the spine. Prepare the skin of the back with alcohol and tincture of zephiran and drape the buttocks with a sterile towel. Identify the spines of the vertebrae. A line drawn between the iliac crests crosses either the spine of the fourth lumbar vertebra or the interspace between the fourth and fifth vertebrae. The caudal portion of the transverse process of a lumbar vertebra lies opposite the cephalad edge of the spinous process of the same vertebra.

Determine by palpation the position of the vertebral spines of the ganglia to be injected. Make each injection 3 to 3.5 cm. from the midline opposite the spine.

Using a 25-gauge needle raise a wheal at the point of injection. Infiltrate deeper with a long 22-gauge needle. Insert a long needle through the wheal with the point of the needle inclined toward the head so that the shaft forms a 45-degree angle with the skin. Advance the needle until it comes in contact with the transverse process of the vertebra.

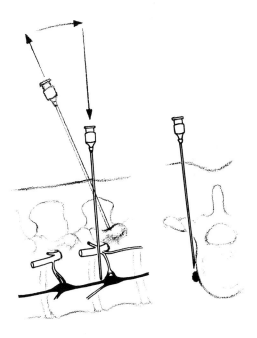

This varies from 3.5 to 5 cm. Mark on the needle a point 2.5 to 3 cm. from the skin toward the hub of the needle. This indicates the depth to which the needle should be inserted so that the point will lie near the ganglia.

Withdraw the needle to the subcutaneous tissues. Reinsert the needle, its shaft parallel with the transverse plane of the body and at an angle of 85 degrees to the skin in a sagittal plane. Rotate the needle so that its bevel surface is toward the vertebra. Insert the needle to the previously measured depth so that it just slips off the body of the vertebra; if necessary the needle may be withdrawn or reinserted until properly positioned. After aspiration for blood and spinal fluid, inject 10 ml. of anesthetic solution. Remove the needle. The injection is then repeated over any other vertebra desired, usually three or four ganglia are blocked. It is not necessary to impinge on a transverse process in subsequent injections because the depth is already known.

After a period of 20 to 30 minutes evaluate the results of the block. If vasodilation occurs it is evidenced by an increase in skin temperature, drying of skin, and some improvement in the color of the skin.

Complications

1. Toxic reactions to the drugs (p. 77).
2. Intraspinal injections (p. 77).
3. Paralysis of the lumbar nerves is manifested by motor and sensory loss in part of the lower extremity. This is due to spillover of the drug involving the lumbar nerves. No special treatment is necessary; the symptoms will disappear as the drug wears off.

NERVE BLOCKS

Preparation of the Patient

If the operation is to be a simple procedure and will not require the use of a large amount of anesthetic drug the patient needs no premedication. On the other hand, if a moderate or large amount of anesthetic is to be used, premedication with some barbiturate is advisable. The barbiturate should be used in any event if the patient is apprehensive. Withhold food for at least 4 hours prior to the time of the block. Reassure the patient before the procedure is begun; his cooperation will be required.

Place him in the most comfortable position possible. The operation should be done on an operating table or an examining table, never with the patient sitting in a chair. If the operative site is such that it is desirable to have the patient sitting, have him sit on the table so that he is in a good position to be treated if an untoward reaction should occur.

Technique

Prepare your hands as you would prepare for any minor surgical procedure. Open the tray of instruments with aseptic technique and arrange the instruments only after you have put on sterile gloves. Have your assistant pour the antiseptic solutions into the appropriate containers and the anesthetic drug into its own container after the label on the bottle has been checked by both you and your assistant. If you plan to use a vasoconstrictor, add it to the anesthetic solution at this time. Do not use a vasoconstrictor in the anesthetic solution for operations on the digits of the hands or feet, or when the patient has cardiovascular disease or peripheral vascular disease. Do not use any solutions which are discolored or cloudy.

The skin of the area on which the operation is to be performed should have been prepared as for any minor surgery with careful cleansing and shaving. Sterilize the skin with alcohol and Zephiran. Drape the operative site with sterile towels, permitting only the operative area to be exposed.

Using the small 25-gauge needle raise a small skin wheal. Before the initial wheal is made, the patient should be told that this is to occur so as not to surprise him. Insert a longer needle through the wheal and pass it down to the area of the nerve. The probing needle may or may not be attached to a syringe. When it comes in contact with the nerve the patient will experience paresthesias along the distribution of the nerve. Aspirate through the needle to ascertain whether it is within a vessel. If no blood is aspirated inject the solution into the area. If the patient complains of severe paresthesias while you are injecting the solution you are probably injecting the solution directly into the nerve. This can usually be corrected by withdrawing the needle a millimeter or two. If the block has not produced satisfactory anesthesia after 30 minutes, do not hesitate to repeat the procedure.

FIELD BLOCK

Field block anesthesia sets up a wall of anesthesia about the area of operation.

No effort is made to block individual nerves but the areas surrounding their paths are infiltrated. A knowledge of anatomy is needed in deciding which areas require the most anesthesia. Use a weak solution such as 0.5 or 1.0 per cent procaine or xylocaine.

After proper preparation of the area plan the general area of field block. At one end of the field raise a skin wheal with a 25-gauge needle. Insert a longer 22-gauge needle through this wheal and pull back on the plunger of the syringe to make certain that the needle is not in the lumen of a blood vessel. If you should happen to withdraw some blood into the syringe discard this and obtain fresh anesthetic solution before injecting. If you keep the needle in motion so that it does not remain in a vessel, you may inject the anesthetic as you move along without preliminary aspiration. Inject first the skin, then the subcutaneous tissue, and finally the deeper tissues as necessary.

A fairly large area can be injected through a single skin ostium by withdrawing the needle into the subcutaneous tissues and changing its direction before advancing it again into the deeper tissues.

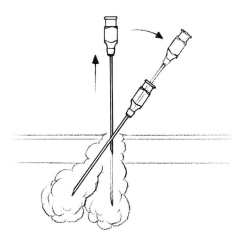

Where possible, when multiple skin injections are required the subsequent injections should be begun through skin which has already been anesthetized.

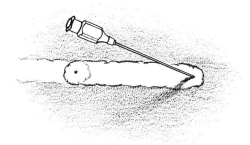

Never insert any needle to the hub. This is the weakest point in the needle and the place where it is most likely to break. If this should happen the broken needle would be buried in the tissues. This can be prevented if you use a beaded needle.

Should any signs or symptoms of toxic reaction appear during the injection, discontinue the injection immediately.

LOCAL INFILTRATION

Local infiltration diffuses anesthetic solution throughout the area where you plan to work. Weaker solutions of drug are used for this procedure, the commonest being 0.5 and 1.0 per cent procaine or xylocaine. After proper preparation raise a skin wheal with a 25-gauge needle. To infiltrate the area desired, insert a longer 22-gauge needle through the wheal to infiltrate the area desired. Keeping the needle in motion, inject carefully and systematically the skin, subcutaneous tissues, and deeper tissues as indicated. The drug is placed in and about the immediate area to be operated on. Injection of too much anesthetic solution is a common error. Since weak concentrations of the drug are used there is a tendency to be careless as to the total amount of agent injected. Have your assistant place only a measured amount of drug on the tray. She should add more only at your request and at the same time she should remind you of the total quantity put on the table.

APPLICATIONS OF REGIONAL BLOCK

BLOCK OF THE SCALP

For localized lesions of the scalp, field block or local infiltration provide adequate anesthesia, but a block of the entire scalp is needed for extensive work on the scalp or the brain. Because the nerve supply to the scalp emerges from below the cranium and runs superiorly, a wall of anesthesia is set up at the base of the skull. Pontocaine (to 100 ml. of 0.15 per cent solution), procaine (to 100 ml. of 1.0 per cent solution, or xylocaine (to 100 ml. of 1.0 per cent solution) may be used. The patient is given premedication as for any major procedure (p. 79).

Place the patient on the operating table in a comfortable position with his head supported and facing forward. Because of the extreme vascularity of the scalp, it is advisable to add a vasoconstrictor to the anesthetic solution (0.1 ml. 1:1000 epinephrine to 100 ml. anesthetic solution). Raise a wheal at the occiput and at the glabella with a 25-gauge needle. Insert a longer 22-gauge needle through the wheal and proceed to make a ring of anesthesia about the base of the skull, infiltrating first the skin and then the subcutaneous tissues, and finally the fascial and muscular layers down to the skull. One is usually surprised to find how much muscle is in the area of the temporal fossa. Repeat this until a ring of anesthesia is complete. This will afford anesthesia for the whole top of the skull in a skull-cap type of distribution.

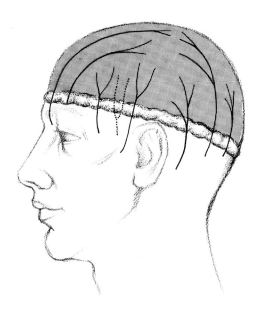

Complications in this area usually are related to the general toxic reactions to the drugs employed (p. 77).

BLOCK OF SUPRATROCHLEAR AND SUPRAORBITAL NERVE

The supratrochlear and supraorbital nerves are blocked for minor surgical procedure on the forehead and for relief of neuralgias. Routine preoperative medication (p. 79) may be given or omitted. Place the patient on the operating table in a supine position and stand at the head of the table. Palpate the supraorbital nerve where it emerges from the supraorbital foramen approximately one inch (2.5 cm.) from the midline at the inferior edge of the supraorbital ridge. The nerve emerges at this point and curves superiorly onto the forehead. The supratrochlear nerve is medial to this and also curves onto the forehead. Raise a skin wheal directly over the foramen. Use 1 to 2 per cent procaine or its equivalent. If you are planning to inject only the nerve, probe with the needle until it comes in contact with the nerve. At this point the patient will experience paresthesias over the forehead. Then inject 2 ml. of the anesthetic solution. On the other hand, if you wish to accomplish analgesia of the area for a minor operation, infiltrate a linear wall of local anesthetic solution through the skin, subcutaneous tissues, and fat down to the bone at the level of the supraorbital ridge, extending from the midline laterally to the outer edge of the orbit.

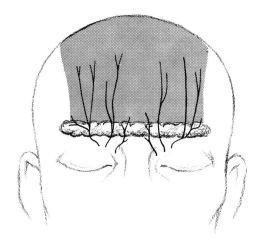

Five to six milliliters of anesthetic solution are adequate for each side.

Complications

In addition to toxic reactions to the drugs (p. 77), injection of the drug in this area may cause swelling of the eyelid. This occurs either because an excessive amount of anesthetic solution is injected or because of hemorrhage. It can be prevented by limiting the amount of solution injected and maintaining pressure over the eyelid with a cotton sponge during the infiltration. If the swelling is due to hemorrhage, apply pressure to the area until the hemorrhage stops.

Once the bleeding has stopped, warm, moist compresses will hasten the absorption of the blood or anesthetic solution from the eyelid. The patient will be unable to open his eyes for a few hours, but reassurance is all that is necessary and, with time, the fluid is absorbed without sequelae.

BLOCK OF THE INFRAORBITAL NERVE

The infraorbital nerve is blocked for operations beneath the eye and for relief of neuralgia. This is a very satisfactory method of supplying superficial anesthesia for work in this area. On the other hand, if one is planning a procedure that is quite tedious it is unfair to ask a conscious patient to remain for a long time in an abnormal position covered with drapes. Under such circumstances, it is better to have the patient asleep and under endotracheal anesthesia.

The infraorbital nerve innervates the lower eyelid, the side of the nose, the mobile portion of the nasal septum, the upper lip, the mucous membrane of the mouth under the lips and the upper incisor and bicuspid teeth. The last portions are supplied by the anterior superior alveolar nerve which branches from the infraorbital nerve in the canal before the nerve comes out onto the face. Have the patient lie in a supine position facing forward with his arms at his side. Stand on the patient's right side facing his head. Palpate the infraorbital foramen. This lies approximately 1 inch (2.5 cm.) from the midline in the infraorbital ridge of the maxillary bone. Make a skin wheal approximately ¼ inch (0.6 cm.) below this, using 2 per cent procaine solution or its equivalent. Infiltrate the subcutaneous tissues along the line leading up to the infraorbital foramen, using approximately 2 ml. of the solution. Direct the needle outward, upward and backward to the infraorbital foramen. The patient will experience paresthesias when the needle comes in contact with the nerve. When the opening of the foramen is located, inject 1 ml. of anesthetic solution. This should anesthetize the infraorbital nerve. Advance the needle slowly into the infraorbital canal, all the while injecting small amounts of the anesthetic solution. After the needle is approximately ¼ inch inside the canal, inject another milliliter of anesthetic solution to anesthetize the anterior superior alveolar nerve.

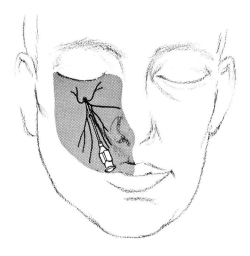

As the needle is withdrawn inject 1 more ml. of anesthetic solution. If the lesion is near the midline, a bilateral block may be necessary because of the crossover of fibers on each side. When it is difficult to palpate the infraorbital foramen you can locate it by taking advantage of the fact that the supraorbital foramen, the infraorbital foramen, and the mental foramen all lie in a straight line approximately 1 inch (2.5 cm.) from the midline of the face; therefore, locating any two should make it possible to line up the third. Do not inject more than 6 ml. for the entire block because excess of the drug will cause swelling of the eyelids.

Complications

1. Reaction to the drugs (p. 77).
2. Swelling of the tissue about the orbit due to the injection of too much anesthetic solution or a hemorrhage within the tissues (p. 89).

3. Disturbances due to the introduction of the anesthetic solution or hemorrhage into the orbit. Blurred vision, diplopia, loss of vision, and pain in the eyeball may result from inserting the needle too far up into the canal and either puncturing a blood vessel or injecting a large amount of anesthetic solution into the orbit. The signs and symptoms will usually disappear as the anesthetic wears off and no specific treatment is indicated.

BLOCK OF THE MENTAL NERVE

The mental nerve is blocked for operations on the lower lip, lower jaw, and skin about the anterior portion of the chin leading up to the lower lip. The patient is placed on the operating table in a supine position with his arms at his side; his head is turned away from the side which is to be blocked. If you have difficulty palpating the mental foramen, you can use either the second bicuspid or a line running through the supraorbital and infraorbital nerves to approximate its position. To do this you should be standing at the head of the patient. Make a skin wheal approximately 0.5 cm. superior and posterior to the nerve, using 2 per cent procaine solution or its equivalent. Introduce the needle through the skin at this point and direct it toward the foramen.

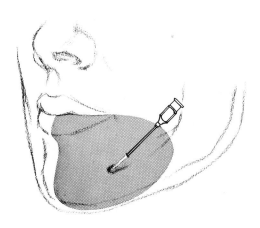

Infiltrate the subcutaneous tissue with approximately 1 ml. of solution as you advance the needle to the foramen. When the patient feels paresthesias, the needle has reached the mental canal. At this point inject 2 ml. of anesthetic solution; then introduce the needle into the canal, injecting small amounts as you advance it. When the tip of the needle is a quarter of an inch (0.6 cm.) inside the canal inject 2 more ml. As you withdraw the needle inject another 1 to 3 ml. of solution. You should use no more than 10 ml. of solution in all.

There are usually no complications related to this specific block other than those caused by reactions to the drug (p. 77).

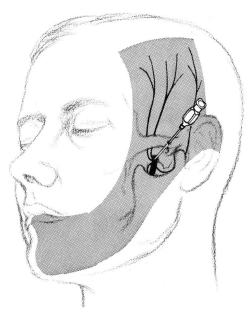

BLOCK OF THE MANDIBULAR NERVE

The mandibular nerve is blocked for operations on the lower jaw, including the teeth, the gums, the mandible, the lower lip and the anterior two-thirds of the tongue. Place the patient in a supine position on the operating table with his head facing forward. Stand at the head of the table for a right mandibular block and at the left side of the table for a left mandibular block. Locate the zygomatic arch and palpate the mandibular notch between the coronoid and condyloid process of the mandibular bone. This is done by exerting gentle pressure with the index finger, just anterior to the temporamandibular articulation, while the patient opens and closes his mouth. Raise a skin wheal at the mid portion of the mandibular notch. Use 2 per cent procaine solution or its equivalent. Insert a longer 22-gauge needle through the wheal toward the nerve until the patient experiences paresthesias over the distribution of the mandibular nerve when the needle comes in contact with the nerve. This usually occurs after the needle has penetrated about 4 or 5 cm.

At this point inject 5 to 10 ml. of the anesthetic solution. Because of the great vascularity of this area, the usual practice of injecting solution as the needle is withdrawn or inserted is not permitted here. The injection should be made only when it is known that the needle is in direct contact with the nerve and that there is no blood vessel at this point. This will avoid an intravascular injection of the anesthetic drug.

Complications

1. The usual reactions to the drug may occur (p. 77).
2. Intradural injections are extremely rare. If this happens the patient will have a high spinal anesthesia and respiration must be supported and the patient ventilated until the effect of the drug disappears (p. 77).
3. Hemorrhage into the cheek may occur. Pressure over the site of the bleeding vessel prevents a hematoma. If a large hematoma develops, warm compresses will encourage resorption.
4. A facial nerve block, characterized by the inability to close the eye or by an

expressionless face and sagging of the face muscles, may result. This is not serious but interferes with the ability of the patient to cooperate by moving his facial muscles during the operation. It will clear without treatment within 24 hours as the drug is absorbed. Primarily all the patient requires is reassurance.

Block of the Stellate Ganglion

Block of the stellate ganglion has no specific surgical application; it is used to relieve discomfort of the arm and in deciding whether or not a sympathectomy would relieve pain due to interference with the blood supply to the upper extremity. It also is used to relieve the associated vasospasm of the cerebral vessels after cerebrovascular accidents. The stellate ganglion is formed by the fusion of the inferior cervical and the first thoracic sympathetic ganglia, and is situated between the base of the transverse process of the last or the seventh cervical vertebra and the neck of the first rib.

Place the patient on the operating table in a supine position with his arms at his side and his head tilted back so that his neck is in full extension. Warn the patient that he is to hold his head still and not to talk or cough during the actual injection. It is well to repeat these instructions as you begin. Stand facing the table on the side on which the injection is to be made. The point of injection is 1 inch (2.5 cm.) lateral to the middle of the jugular notch of the sternum and the same distance above the clavicle. This should lie over the transverse process of the seventh cervical vertebra and along the medial border of the sternocleidomastoid muscle. Raise a wheal at that point with a 25-gauge needle. Pick up a 10 ml. Luer-Lok syringe filled with anesthetic solution with a 22-gauge needle attached. Using the index and middle finger of your left hand, straddle the

wheal and with downward and lateral pressure retract the sternocleidomastoid muscle and the carotid sheath laterally. Maintain this pressure throughout the procedure. When the retracting fingers are in a proper position, the pulsation of the carotid artery should be felt on the lateral side of the fingers. Insert the needle through the skin wheal perpendicular to the surface of the skin. This should be pushed slowly posteriorly until it impinges on the transverse process of the 7th cervical vertebra. This is rarely deeper than 1½ inches (3.8 cm.). If the patient experiences paresthesias, the needle has probably come down on the brachial plexus and should be withdrawn and reinserted. After it impinges on the transverse process it should be withdrawn about ¹⁄₁₆ of an inch (0.15 cm.) to free it from the muscles which lie over the transverse process. Aspirate to be certain that the needle does not lie within a blood vessel. If no blood is obtained, insert the entire contents of the syringe at this point and withdraw the needle.

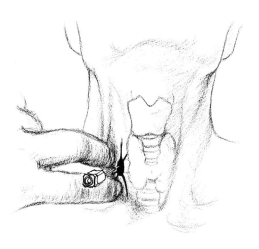

If a successful block has been accomplished the patient should show evidence of a Horner's syndrome and evidence of sympathetic block to the extremity. The Horner's syndrome occurs rapidly but the sympathetic block to the extremity may not become evident for 15 to 30 minutes. A Horner's syndrome is characterized by ptosis of the eyelid, a constricted pupil, and enophthalmus. A satisfactory block of the arm will result in an increased temperature and anhydrosis of the arm and face. It is possible to produce a Horner's syndrome without having adequately blocked the upper extremity. If there is evidence of sympathetic activity in the arm after at least 30 minutes, more medication should be injected in order to insure blocking of the upper extremity.

Complications

1. Reactions to the drug (p. 77).
2. Intraspinal injection (p. 77).
3. Pneumothorax. This results when the needle perforates the lung where it extends up into the neck. The majority of these accidents are serious only because they are unrecognized. After completion of the block, examine the chest with a stethoscope. If there is a pneumothorax, the breath sounds will be diminished or absent. If the patient is dyspneic, immediate thoracentesis (p. 242) is indicated. If the sounds are diminished but the patient is comfortable, order an x-ray of the chest. If the pneumothorax is minimal the patient should be re-examined in a few hours to ascertain that it is not increasing and to avoid the development of a tension pneumothorax (p. 234).
4. Paralysis of the recurrent laryngeal nerve, as evidenced by hoarseness and difficulty in swallowing, is due to overflow of the anesthetic solution. No particular treatment is needed. The situation will clear when the effect of the drug has worn off.
5. Paralysis of part or all of the brachial plexus may occur as a result of overflow of the drug. The symptoms will disappear as soon as the effect of the drug has been dissipated.

BRACHIAL PLEXUS BLOCK

The brachial plexus is blocked for operations on the upper extremity. Pontocaine (30 to 50 ml. of 0.25 per cent solution), procaine (30 to 50 ml. 1.0 per cent solution), or xylocaine (20 to 50 ml. 1.0 per cent solution) is used. Routine premedication (p. 79) is given.

Place the patient on the operating table in a supine position with his arms at his side. His head, lying flat on the table, is turned to the side opposite to the one being blocked.

Ask the patient to raise his head from the table to put tension on the muscles of the neck. This will enable you to identify the sternocleidomastoid muscle and the anterior scalenus which is lateral to the sternocleidomastoid. The brachial plexus emerges from the lateral border of the anterior scalenus. The patient can now lower his head. Make a skin wheal at the lateral edge of the anterior scalenus muscle $3/8$ inch (1 cm.) above the clavicle. Palpate the subclavian artery with the middle finger of the left hand and retract it medially. Instruct the patient to tell you as soon as he feels paresthesias in his arm or hand. Attach a longer 22-gauge needle to the filled syringe and advance it slowly downward, inward and backward at a 90 degree angle with the skin, toward the transverse process of the third thoracic vertebra. If the patient feels paresthesias, stop inserting the needle, aspirate for blood, and inject 5 ml. of solution. Rotate the needle 180 degrees, reaspirate, and inject the remainder. The needle should make contact with the first rib. If the rib is not reached withdraw the needle and reinsert it, advancing it cautiously until it does reach the rib. The needle should never be inserted any deeper or a pneumothorax may develop.

After you reach the first rib "walk" the needle by gentle tapping along the rib until paresthesias are elicited.

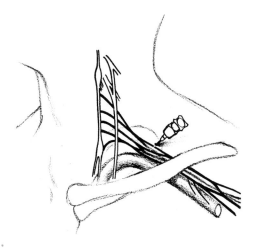

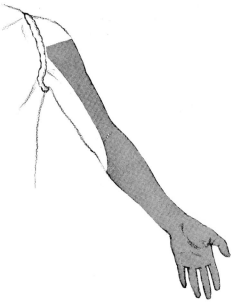

Maneuver along the length of the rib and not across the width of it; otherwise the pleura will be punctured. Aspirate after each change of position. If blood is obtained the needle is in the subclavian artery; withdraw the needle and reinsert it at a point ⅛ inch (0.35 cm.) lateral to the artery. Paresthesias will be elicited. Aspirate and inject 5 ml. of solution, turn the needle 180 degrees, aspirate again and inject another 5 ml. Advance the needle until it is against the rib. Remove the syringe leaving the needle in place; refill the syringe and as you withdraw the needle toward the skin inject 10 ml. of solution. Advance the needle again to a point ½ inch (1.3 cm.) lateral to the previous point and inject the solution as you withdraw the needle. Repeat this again but insert the needle to a point ½ inch (1.3 cm.) medial to the original point.

This will produce satisfactory anesthesia for operations on the lower arm, hands, fingers and upper outer arms to the insertion of the deltoid. Dislocations of the shoulder may be reduced under this block. Skin anesthesia exists over the upper outer arm, the forearm, and the hand. When brachial plexus block is used for operations on the elbow, on the inner upper arm, or on the shoulder, additional anesthesia must be obtained by intradermal and subcutaneous infiltration.

The shaded area diagrams the area of anesthesia accomplished by the brachial plexus block.

Complications

1. Horner's syndrome (p. 93). No special treatment is required; merely reassure the patient. Symptoms will disappear as the effect of the block is dissipated.
2. Pneumothorax (p. 93).
3. Block of phrenic nerve. The patient may be unaware of the block. There will be uneven motion of the chest due to paralysis of the diaphragm. This is dangerous only if the block is bilateral. Under such circumstances the patient's respiration must be assisted until the effect disappears.
4. Reactions to the drugs (p. 77).
5. Intraspinal injection (rare) (p. 77).

DIGITAL BLOCK

The digits are blocked for operations on the fingers or toes. Pontocaine (0.25 percent), procaine (2.0 per cent), or xylocaine (1.0 per cent) may be used. Premedication is rarely necessary.

Prepare the hand with alcohol and tincture of Zephiran. Raise skin wheals on the dorsolateral aspect of the finger near its base. Create a ring of anesthesia about the digit from the bone to the skin.

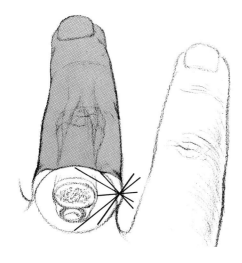

Complications

1. Gangrene has on occasion resulted from digital block. In order to eliminate the possibility, do not add a vasoconstrictor and do not use more than 10 ml. of solution for each finger or toe.

2. Those related to toxic reactions (p. 77).

BLOCK OF THE INTERCOSTAL NERVES

The intercostal nerves may be blocked for surgical procedures of the thoracic wall or to relieve the pain of fractured ribs. Bilateral intercostal nerve block provides satisfactory anesthesia for operations on the upper portion of the abdominal wall. When combined with celiac plexus block it provides satisfactory anesthesia for working within the abdomen. Many simple abdominal procedures, such as a colostomy or gastrostomy, can be done under intercostal block alone.

Pontocaine (up to 100 ml. of 0.1 per cent solution), procaine (up to 80 ml. of a 1.0 percent solution) or xylocaine (up to 80 ml. of a 0.5 per cent solution) may be used. For intra-abdominal procedures routine premedication (p. 79) is used.

The most satisfactory point for injecting intercostal nerves is at the posterior angle of the rib; at a point farther anterior, the lateral cutaneous branches of the nerves may be missed. The nerves are injected at the angle in the last 7 or 8 ribs; owing to the interference of the scapula this is not possible on the upper ribs. The bilateral block can be performed at the angle of the ribs most satisfactorily and with the least motion on the part of the patient if he is in a prone position. If you plan to include a celiac plexus block, this can also be done in this position before the patient is turned onto his back. It is simpler to stay on one side of the patient and reach across the midline to anesthetize the other side. The lower margin of the rib is palpated at this angle and a skin wheal is raised at this point. A 22-gauge needle attached to a filled 10 ml. Luer-Lok syringe is inserted through this wheal and aimed at impingement upon the lower portion of the rib. Advance the needle until it touches the rib; withdraw the needle and advance it again at an angle which will allow it to slip under the edge of the rib and into the upper portion of the interspace.

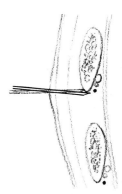

Advance the needle about ⅛ of an inch (0.3 cm.). The patient may experience some paresthesias. Aspirate through the needle at this point to be certain that it is not in the lumen of an intercostal vessel. If no blood is aspirated, inject 5 ml. of the anesthetic solution. Repeat this method of injection to whatever other nerves you plan to inject.

If you want to inject nerves above the seventh and eighth intercostal spaces, you must turn the patient on his back and inject the higher intercostal nerves in the posterior axillary line. If you are injecting the nerves for a localized procedure on the thoracic wall or to relieve the discomfort of fractured ribs, the injection need only include the two nerves above and two below the area of involvement, as well as the nerves going to the involved area itself. When the intercostal block is to be unilateral, the patient can be placed in a lateral decubitus position.

CELIAC PLEXUS BLOCK

Block of the celiac plexus relieves pain originating in the abdominal viscera. It is combined with intercostal nerve block for intra-abdominal operations done under local anesthesia.

Pontocaine (50 ml. of 0.05 per cent solution), procaine (50 ml. of 0.5 per cent solution), or xylocaine (50 ml. of 0.25 per cent solution) may be used. Routine premedication (p. 79) is used.

The patient is in the prone position as for the blocking of lower intercostal nerves bilaterally. Stand on the side to be blocked. Make a skin wheal at the lower edge of the 12th rib. Insert a 10 or 12.5 cm. 20-gauge needle at a 45 degree angle to the skin and direct it slightly cephalad and medial. Advance it until it comes in contact with the body of the first lumbar vertebra. After noting the depth of the needle, withdraw it until the angle can be changed to 60 degrees and repeat the maneuver. Continue to advance the needle until it is felt to slip off the body of the vertebra. Advance it another half inch (1.3 cm.). This should now put it in the prevertebral areolar tissue in the vicinity of the celiac plexus.

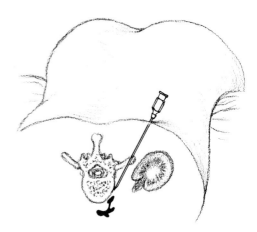

Aspirate to be certain that the needle is not lying in the lumen of the vessel and inject 25 ml. of anesthetic solution.

Complications

1. Reactions to the drugs (p. 77).
2. Intraspinal injections (p. 77).
3. Low blood pressure. There is usually a drop in blood pressure with the systolic drop greater than the diastolic. It is usually successfully treated with vasopressors, the most satisfactory being neosynephrine, 1 ml. added to a liter of fluid and dripped intravenously at whatever rate is necessary to maintain a satisfactory blood pressure. After the abdomen has been closed, there is usually no further need to support the pressure artificially.

BLOCK OF THE PENIS

The penis is blocked for operations on the superficial portion, such as circumcision, and for working within the urethra. The patient is placed on the operating table in a supine position. Three points of reference are identified. One is 0.5 inch (1.3 cm.) caudal and another 0.5 inch (1.3 cm.) medial to the spine of the pubic bones bilaterally, and the third is the median raphe of the scrotum at the base of the penis. Raise a skin wheal at these points and, using a longer 22-gauge needle, join the three points by slow careful intradermal and subcutaneous infiltration with the anesthetic solution. While the penis is held elevated by an assistant, deposit anesthetic solution fanwise from this area into the base of the penis.

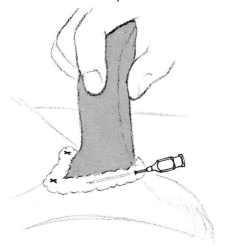

The complications are the reactions due to the drug (p. 77).

PUDENDAL BLOCK

The pudendal nerve is sometimes blocked for rectal operations, but its most common application is in anesthesia of the female perineum for uncomplicated obstetrical procedures. The block is satisfactory for an episiotomy and outlet forceps delivery, but any higher procedures require a more elaborate type of anesthesia. A pudendal block does not relieve the pain associated with uterine contractions, but merely the local pain related to injury to the perineum. Pontocaine (50 to 100 ml. of 0.15 per cent solution), procaine (50 to 100 ml. of 1.0 per cent solution), or xylocaine (50 to 100 ml. of 0.5 per cent solution) may be used.

Place the patient in the lithotomy position. Locate the ischial tuberosity by palpation. The pudendal nerve lies medial to the ischial tuberosity. Raise a skin wheal over the medial inferior border of the tuberosity. Using a 10 ml. syringe of anesthetic solution, insert a 7.5 or 10 cm. 22-gauge needle through the wheal perpendicular to the skin. Insert the index finger of your left hand into the rectum to guide the needle point to the tuberosity. As the needle is advanced inject small amounts of anesthetic solution. Inject 5 to 10 ml. of solution around the anterior side of the tuberosity and under the tuberosity. Guide the needle point to the medial side of it and insert 10 ml. of solution. Inject an additional 10 ml. as you advance the needle approximately 1 cm. beyond the point of the ischial tuberosity on its medial surface. Now guide the point of the needle underneath the spine of the ischium with the index finger in the rectum. This is done so that the needle does not enter the rectum. Guide the needle into the sacrospinous ligament. The ligament can be palpated by the finger in the rectum. Advance the needle ¼ inch (0.6 cm.) beyond the ligament and inject another 10 ml. of solution. This portion of the block is accomplished by the needle on the right.

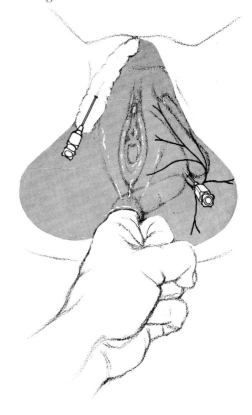

Change your gloves and infiltrate the area ½ inch (1.3 cm.) lateral and parallel to the labia majora from the middle of the labia majora to the mons pubis. This anesthetizes the iliohypogastric, ilioinguinal and genitocrural nerves which innervate the skin over the mons pubis and the labia. This block must be done bilaterally for satisfactory anesthesia. Do not begin the block until the head is on the perineum. Allow at least five minutes after completion of the block before beginning the operation. This will provide satisfactory anesthesia of the anus, the perineum, the labia and the vagina. Since no systemic medication is given this type of anesthesia will have no depressing effect on the newborn infant. The complications possible are reactions to the drugs (p. 77).

Chapter Seven

Trauma

GENERAL MEASURES

Trauma may be minor and localized, or it may be severe and generalized. Before discussing trauma to a local area it seems appropriate to discuss trauma to the whole individual. Special care should be taken not to injure the patient further by injudicious handling after he reaches the accident room. The simplest and safest method of removing his clothes is to cut them off. Any moving of the patient (as for instance, for x-ray studies) should be supervised by the physician in charge. To avoid further contamination of the wound it should be examined under aseptic precautions by masked personnel. In order to insure a dependable intravenous route for subsequent therapy, a venipuncture should be done as soon as a seriously injured patient is seen. Blood should be drawn for base line studies, and a needle or catheter left in the veins and kept open with a slow drip of solution. When the patient goes into frank shock this is much more difficult to set up.

Make a rapid estimate of the extent of the trauma. Quickly check his state of consciousness, the adequacy of his airway and respirations, his pulse, any evidence of bleeding, and state of shock without evidence of bleeding. When multiple injuries are present priority of care must be established. Wounds which interfere with ventilation must be dealt with first, hemorrhage next.

After you are satisfied that the state of consciousness of the patient requires no immediate care, that there is no interference with ventilation, that cardiorespiratory function is not embarrassed, that hemorrhage is under control and that appropriate supportive measures have been undertaken, a rapid examination of the patient must be made.

The whole body should be inspected, noting the presence and degree of any superficial trauma (bruises, lacerations, etc.), paralysis of any muscles, anesthesia of any parts, or asymmetry of chest motion. All joints should be manipulated through a full range of function, passively at first and then actively if the patient is able. All bony prominences should be palpated and pressure exerted over the rib cage and the pelvis to rule out fractures. Careful palpation and percussion of the abdomen must be made. If there is any suggestion of a fracture of the pelvis, a catheter should be passed into the bladder at once and left in place. It is far simpler to do this early than after edema has set in.

Serious trauma may be either the result of a single severe injury or the cumulative effect of moderate or minor trauma to multiple areas. The measures necessary for effective treatment of severe trauma may be summarized in order of importance as follows:

1. Assure adequate ventilation.
2. Control hemorrhage.
3. Treat shock.
4. Prevent infection.
5. Prevent tetanus.
6. Repair the wound.

Adequate Ventilation

In most cases of trauma ventilation is not impaired, but it is important to bear the possibility in mind when the chest, head or neck are injured. Furthermore, signs of interference with ventilation may suddenly appear and become increasingly dangerous in a person originally without symptoms. Interference with ventilation can kill the patient in 6 to 10 minutes; maintenance of an adequate airway is the most important measure. The airway may be occluded by aspirated blood, mucus, or vomitus. If the patient is unconscious the tongue may drop back and occlude the pharynx. In all instances of trauma about the head and face, if the patient is unconscious, fluids should be aspirated from the posterior pharynx, the tongue pulled forward, and an airway inserted. If it does not seem possible to prevent spillage into the trachea, perform a tracheostomy (p. 202). The spillage can then be aspirated.

Trauma to the neck may destroy the cartilaginous support of the trachea. A patient so injured is able to exhale, but when he tries to inhale the trachea collapses. He will obviously be short of breath and there will be external evidence of trauma to the neck or chest. Treatment is immediate tracheostomy.

Another serious problem is tension pneumothorax. This may not be immediately apparent because the patient may show very little external evidence of injury. The patient with tension pneumothorax is short of breath and his respiratory excursions are limited. Air is accumulating under tension in one pleural cavity. The trachea is shifted away from the affected side. There is little motion of the affected hemithorax. The percussion note is hyperresonant and there are no breath sounds on auscultation. Treatment is immediate thoracentesis (p. 242), followed by intercostal tube drainage (p. 244). This situation represents a truly acute emergency; delay can be fatal. You must manage the situation yourself as there is not time to call a consultant. The procedure is not difficult.

Trauma to the chest is discussed in more detail on page 232.

Hemorrhage

Uncontrolled hemorrhage can be rapidly fatal and even moderate bleeding can be most upsetting to the patient. The best method of stopping either arterial or venous hemorrhage is direct pressure to the area involved. Classically, arterial bleeding is bright red and spurting, whereas venous bleeding is darker and does not spurt. Unfortunately, the differentiation is not always so clear cut. It is common practice, particularly outside professional circles, to apply a tourniquet when serious bleeding occurs. However, surgeons who treat a great deal of trauma feel that tourniquets have, over the years, done far more harm than good. Many an overzealous individual has applied a tourniquet so tightly as to cause permanent damage to either the blood vessels or the nerves of the extremity. An improperly applied tourniquet may interfere with venous return without compressing the arterial blood supply, and hence may not control bleeding. It is a dramatic experience to watch a wise surgeon remove the tourniquet, thereby lowering the venous pressure and stop the bleeding. A tourniquet need never be applied within a hospital except in case of a disaster when there are many emergencies at the same time. If individual attention can be given to a single patient, pressure directly over the area will control the bleeding until it can be definitively managed. Fist pressure directly over the aorta can control severe bleeding distal to the point of pressure but is difficult to maintain for long. In such a situation preparation for operation must be prompt.

It is inadvisable to stab deeply (and blindly) at a bloody area with hemostats. Often, the hemostats may do more damage than the original injury. However, if the bleeding point can be seen it should be grasped with a hemostat. If it cannot be visualized, the bleeding should be controlled with pressure, the patient prepared for operation, and, under appropriate anesthesia, the source of bleeding isolated. If the area cannot be properly visualized, the wound should be extended under anesthesia. The bleeding areas can then be treated as indicated. If serious bleeding has occurred, or is likely to occur, matched blood should be obtained.

Severe hemorrhage may not be obvious but may occur in the thoracic or abdominal cavity as a result of trauma. These are discussed in the chapters dealing with these areas (chest, p. 241, abdomen, p. 257).

SHOCK

When the systolic blood pressure is less than 100 mm. of mercury, the pulse rate is more than 100 per minute, the extremities are cold, and the patient is pale, he is in shock. In the first few hours after trauma, shock is far more likely to be due to blood loss than to reflex vasodilatation or to bacterial toxins. Hypoxia or cranial trauma are the only other circumstances which cause early shock. Cardiac tamponade or respiratory embarrassment are easily diagnosed and should be treated immediately. Trauma to the brain does not cause shock as frequently as was once thought. If there is no evidence of cardiorespiratory embarrassment and nothing to suggest head injury, it should be assumed that shock occurring after trauma is due to blood loss.

Hemorrhagic Shock

More blood is lost during trauma than is generally appreciated. A closed fracture of the femur in an adult may cause the loss of 800 to 1400 ml. of blood into the soft tissues. The Committee on Trauma of the American College of Surgeons* suggests that, disregarding amputated parts, one can estimate that approximately 10 per cent of the patient's blood volume is lost per volume of badly contused tissue equivalent to the mass of the patient's fist. In a normal young adult, injuries which cause a loss of 30 per cent or more of the normal blood volume will produce shock. The estimated blood volume of a normal male weighing 70 kg. is 5 liters. Thus when a previously healthy young man weighing 70 kg. has lost 30 per cent of his blood volume, or 1500 ml. of blood over a period of hours, he will be in shock. The physician must remember that a patient who has lost a substantial amount of blood may still be normotensive or even hypertensive. Loss of only a small additional amount may throw him

* The Management of Fractures and Soft Tissue Injuries, 2nd ed. By the Committee on Trauma, American College of Surgeons. W. B. Saunders Co., 1965.

into shock; the usual signs and symptoms can therefore not be relied upon as indices of the danger. The safest procedure is to estimate the blood loss. Hematocrit and hemoglobin determinations are of no value early because time is necessary for hemodilution after blood loss.

When you see a patient in whom shock is a possibility insert a needle into a vein immediately. One of the most accessible veins is the long saphenous; it is located in the same position in almost all individuals and can be found readily. If you cannot palpate the vein do not hesitate to cut down on it and insert a cannula (p. 298). Keep the vein open with intravenous fluids until blood is available for replacement.

Plasma or plasma volume expanders are not as useful as blood in hemorrhagic shock. They restore the blood volume but they do not replace the red cells lost. They should be considered as nothing more than a temporary expedient until whole blood can be obtained. It must be remembered that 50 per cent of most plasma volume expanders is lost from the vascular tree in 10 hours. Consequently, it is necessary to restore the volume within that time. If the patient's need of blood is sufficiently severe you can give him "O" negative blood without cross-matching while his blood is being typed and cross-matched. Rules concerning the proper rate of flow of blood transfusions do not apply when you are replacing blood just lost. There is no need for concern about overloading the circulation. If the blood pressure is down, infuse the blood as fast as possible until the pressure comes back up. All blood lost need not be immediately replaced but enough should be given to eliminate shock and an extra 500 ml. to assure against its reappearance. If the patient is to undergo operation, he will need an additional 500 to 1000 ml. blood. Any blood lost during operation should immediately be replaced, volume for volume. The longer the patient is in shock the larger the amount of blood required to treat the shock. After each 1000 ml. of blood is transfused the patient should be given 10 ml. of 10 per cent calcium gluconate in a separate vein. This will counteract the citrate he received in the blood.

All patients in shock should have an indwelling urinary catheter inserted (p. 285) because urinary output is a good indicator of the severity of shock. The urinary output should be 25 to 50 ml. per hour. A smaller volume is probably due to an inadequate blood pressure or to dehydration. If a diminished urinary output persists for 6 to 8 hours, in spite of seemingly adequate blood and fluid administration, the possibility of kidney damage must be considered.

Many patients in shock do not require narcotics; those who do rarely require dosages as heavy as those needed by the normotensive individual. If morphine is necessary to relieve pain, give it intravenously, slowly, 4 to 8 mg. at a time. Do not remove the needle from the vein; if the pain is not relieved in 5 minutes give additional small doses as needed. Narcotics should not be given subcutaneously to patients in shock because in the presence of peripheral vascular collapse the circulation may be incapable of absorbing the drug. When the collapse is corrected multiple doses, which may have been given periodically, will be absorbed simultaneously with a resultant overdose. The same reasoning applies to oral medication because gastrointestinal absorption is poor when a patient is in shock. Body heat should be conserved by using blankets under the patient and to cover him. Applying external heat could be harmful because patients in shock are more sensitive to heat than normotensive individuals.

While the patient's blood pressure is low the foot of the bed should be elevated about 12 inches. This is contraindicated only if the head-down position seems to interfere with ventilation. In such cases the patient should be put in whatever position permits the most adequate respiration. Oxygen is not usually required in the treatment of shock but should be used if there is dyspnea or cyanosis. Vasopressor drugs are of no value in hemorrhagic shock and they may delude the physician concerning the adequacy of blood replacement. Results of recent experimental work suggest that the use of vasopressors in these cases may actually be harmful. Steroids are of no value in hemorrhagic shock unless the patient is known to have adrenal insufficiency, in which case they must be used.

Hypotension from Adrenal Insufficiency

Trauma or operation may cause hypotension from adrenal insufficiency in patients who have received cortisone or one of its derivatives in the previous two or three months, or in adrenalectomized patients. Give such a patient 100 mg. of hydrocortisone intravenously immediately, and repeat this every 4 hours until he is out of shock. After shock has been relieved give two additional intravenous doses and begin treatment with intramuscular hydrocortisone (50 mg. q.6h.). Continue this for three days, then decrease the dose by 50 mg. every 2 days. The drug can be given orally as soon as the gastrointestinal tract is functioning properly.

Hypotension from Tranquilizing and Antihypertensive Agents

Operation or trauma may cause hypotension in patients who are taking tranquilizers. Preoperative workup should include questioning the patient about such drugs. The effect is counteracted by norepinephrine; place one or two ampules of the drug in a liter of 5 per cent glucose in water or physiologic salt solution and administer intravenously. The flow rate must be carefully adjusted according to the response of the patient's blood pressure.

The patient who has had reserpine as recently as two weeks prior to operation or trauma may develop hypotension. Atropine in large amounts will counteract this.

INFECTION

Care of the Wound

Traumatic wounds are produced under unsterile conditions and all are contaminated to some degree when they are first seen; many of them are grossly contaminated. After an adequate airway has been assured and bleeding has been controlled, attention can be directed to the wound. The first aim should be to prevent infection. The specific reparative measures should be carried out under anesthesia, local or general, as dictated by the nature of the wound and the general condition of the patient. The entire area about the wound should be cleansed with a bland soap solution. If the skin is intact but the contaminating material is imbedded in the skin, more vigorous scrubbing with a brush is permissible. Continue the cleansing until the wound seems clean or until no more material can be removed by scrubbing. Particles which cannot be removed by brushing should be picked out with forceps. This is particularly important about the face. Obviously, devitalized tissue should be cut away and deeply imbedded material removed with a scalpel if necessary. Removal of all nonviable tissue is the best prophylaxis against gas gangrene. The next step is debridement, which means excision of all tissue of questionable viability. The edges of most traumatic wounds are jagged and discolored. These should be revised so as to leave no tissue containing imbedded material and to develop more satisfactory wound edges for closure. This means excising sufficient tissue to insure a sharp clean wound edge.

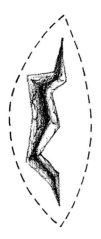
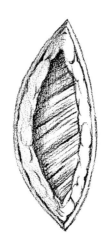

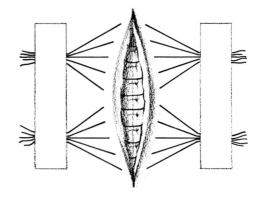

Use #30 braided wire and hold down the free ends with adhesive plaster. Pack the wound open with gauze over a single layer of nonadherent material. In four to seven days when the condition of the wound is satisfactory, it can be closed in the patient's room. Do not uncover the wound until you are ready to close it. Give the patient morphine or Demerol 30 minutes prior to closing the wound. Under sterile conditions, using sterile gloves, remove the packing and tie the sutures. If there are associated fractures, they are taken care of as soon as the soft tissues have been treated and the patient's condition permits.

It is particularly important to remove damaged muscle of questionable viability. A reasonable assurance of viability can be obtained from (1) the color, (2) evidence of bleeding, and (3) contraction of the muscle when it is pinched. In military service, where extensive contusion of muscle is often seen, much more extensive debridement is necessary than in civilian practice, where most wounds are lacerations rather than extensive contusions.

After thorough debridement establish hemostasis by ligating all bleeding points. Cleanse the wound by irrigation with copious amounts of saline. Any structures which have been divided should be repaired (p. 111). The wound must be closed so as to leave no free or "dead" space deep in the wound. Serum pockets are the breeding places of infection. If it appears that there will be considerable oozing, put a soft rubber tissue drain in the area and bring it out to the surface. If you are satisfied that no contamination to the subcutaneous tissues remains you may close the entire wound in layers, including the skin; otherwise it is best to leave the subcutaneous tissue open. Close the wound to the fascia. Insert the sutures for closing the subcutaneous tissues and skin, but do not tie them.

Antibiotics

Since most traumatic wounds are contaminated, the advisability of antibiotic therapy should be considered. The following types of injured patients should receive antibiotics:

1. Those with extensive wounds.
2. Those with diabetes or vascular disease.
3. Those with visceral injuries of the abdomen and chest.
4. Those with bite wounds.
5. Those who have been exposed to excessive radiation.
6. Those with coexistent infections.

The patient should be questioned concerning known sensitivity to particular antibiotics. Penicillin is the favorite antibiotic for prophylaxis of infection in wounds. If the patient is receiving intravenous fluid or is in shock, the penicillin should be given intravenously at the rate of 500,000 units of aqueous penicillin G to the liter. This is followed by intramuscular administration of 600,000 units every 6 to 8 hours. The dosage can be doubled if the injury or contamination is very extensive. Less seriously injured patients can be given antibiotics orally: 200,000 to 500,000 units of penicillin or 250 mg. of chloramphenicol, chlortetracycline, or oxytetracycline every 6 hours. If there is contamination by fecal bacteria, or if there are extensive wounds of the mouth, 0.5 gm. streptomycin intramuscularly is added to the penicillin regimen. An alternate choice is one of the cycline derivatives, given slowly in 5 per cent dextrose and water in a dosage of 500 mg. twice a day.

If infection develops, it should be cultured, the antibiotic sensitivity of the offending organism established and treatment prescribed accordingly.

TETANUS

If the wound is dirty (almost all are), or has been caused by firearms or fireworks, the patient should be given prophylactic treatment against tetanus. The importance of proper debridement of all devitalized tissue from contused wounds cannot be overemphasized, but even this is no assurance against the development of tetanus. Tetanus infection requires less traumatized tissue than gas bacilli infection. Puncture wounds are the common route of entry. The safest prophylaxis against tetanus is immunization; this is highly recommended.

Prophylaxis

A high percentage of our population, including all who have been in the armed forces, has been immunized against tetanus. The usual adult course consists of three doses of alum-precipitated toxoid subcutaneously. The second dose is given one month after the first; the third is given six to twelve months later. Boosters should be given every few years.

In infants and children tetanus toxoid is combined with diphtheria toxoid and pertussis vaccine. Three doses are given at monthly intervals and a fourth one year later. Boosters of tetanus and diphtheria toxoids are given every four years.

Patients sustaining dirty wounds should be immunized as follows: If they have had tetanus toxoid within four years they should receive alum-precipitated or fluid toxoid subcutaneously. A similar booster dose of 0.5 ml. of toxoid is usually sufficient for patients originally immunized with toxoid but who have not had a booster within four years. However, if the wound is badly contaminated it is safer to increase the protection with tetanus antitoxin. Give 5000 units of tetanus antitoxin in one arm and, with a separate syringe and needle, give 0.5 ml. of alum-precipitated tetanus toxoid in the other arm.

Patients who have never been immunized and who have a contaminated wound should receive 5000 units of tetanus antitoxin (see section on sensitivity to serum, below). It is a good idea to begin a course of tetanus toxoid at the same time, giving 0.5 ml. of the alum-precipitated tetanus toxoid in a different extremity with a separate syringe and needle.

Sensitivity Tests

Before giving the antitoxin the possibility of sensitivity should be investigated. Ask the patient whether he has ever had injections of any type of serum and if so whether he had a reaction. Also inquire whether there is any history of allergic disorders. Finally, even if there is no history, check the patient for sensitivity to the serum. Draw 0.1 ml. of the serum into a tuberculin syringe; dilute this with 1 ml. sterile saline (making a 1:10 dilution). Inject a small wheal intracutaneously on the volar surface of the forearm. Read in 30 minutes.

A positive reading consists of a central blanched wheal surrounded by a zone of erythema. More severe reactions cause pseudopod formation. If the skin reaction is positive, the ophthalmic test must be made. Place a drop of 1:10 dilution of the serum in the lower conjunctival sac of one eye. A positive reaction produces congestion, lacrimation, and burning within ten minutes. This can be relieved by a drop of 1:1000 dilution epinephrine in the conjunctival sac. If the tests are positive, some other type of serum should be obtained. If only the skin test is positive, the patient should be desensitized. If there is no reaction to the sensitivity test, the entire dose of 5000 units can be given subcutaneously.

Desensitization

Give 0.01 ml. of the 1:10 dilution of serum subcutaneously. Each 30 minutes thereafter give doses of 0.02 ml., 0.02 ml., 0.5 ml., 1 ml., and 2 ml. Then administer undiluted serum in dosages of 0.05 ml. followed by 0.1 ml. at half hour intervals until the desired amount is given. If a mild reaction occurs, the same dose should be repeated at the end of the half hour instead of increasing it. Reactions can be treated with 0.03 ml. epinephrine in 1:1000 dilution.

If the patient has a clear-cut history of severe reaction to both equine and bovine serum, or if a reaction occurs with the 0.1 ml. of antitoxin, do not give more antitoxin. Human hyperimmune serum may be given if available. In urgent cases transfused blood from a donor who has received a booster dose of tetanus toxoid one month previously may be considered. Give penicillin or tetracycline derivatives promptly in large doses over the estimated incubation period of tetanus which is a minimum of 10 days. In all instances start immunization with alum-precipitated tetanus toxoid.

INTRACRANIAL DAMAGE

The possibility of intracranial trauma in an injured patient should be considered. It is uncommon, but not unheard of, for intracranial trauma to be the cause of shock. Shock is far more likely to be due to bleeding. Many cases of intracranial trauma require no specific emergency treatment but proper assessment by a physician may make a considerable difference to the ultimate result. The state of consciousness is the most important index of the patient's condition. The patient should be asked to speak. His ability to follow commands should be measured by some simple request such as asking him to protrude his tongue. If he does not respond readily, painful stimuli, such as pinching the skin or compressing the supraorbital nerve, should be employed. Normal purposeful movements are encouraging, whereas uneven, delayed and unpurposeful movements are a bad sign.

Hypoxia of the brain is the most likely cause of death from brain injury. First one should ascertain that the airway is not obstructed. Relief of such obstructions takes precedence over anything else because of danger of direct cerebral damage. The second cause of hypoxia is intracranial pressure on the brain structure. If the patient's condition begins to deteriorate one suspects a gradually spreading lesion which probably requires decompression. When there is a rise in the intracranial pressure the pulse slows, the respirations decrease, the blood pressure rises, and the temperature is elevated. Since some of these changes are the direct opposite of signs of serious damage elsewhere in the body, the picture can be confusing, especially during the period of compensation. Ultimately, when the intracranial pressure becomes sufficiently high, decompensation ensues. The signs are then reversed, the pulse becomes very rapid, the respiratory rate increases, the blood pressure may or may not fall, the temperature remains elevated. Such changes are indication for immediate surgical intervention.

Psychological Trauma

One must appreciate that injury usually includes psychological as well as physical trauma. It is important to recognize the impact of this on normal reactions. Some seem depressed while others appear excited. With overanxious individuals one must be careful not to administer excessive amounts of narcotics.

The patient often overestimates the magnitude of his injury, especially if he notes any indecision or discouragement on the part of the surgeon. He should be sedated with a barbiturate and reassured by a calm and confident appraisal of his injuries and a brief outline of treatment. A quiet, depressed patient needs this every bit as much as a hysterical individual.

Indifferent attitudes by the house staff and injudicious discussion of the patient's condition within his earshot are very disturbing. Hysterical relatives add little solace and should be sent out of the treatment room. These people also need sympathy and understanding.

SPECIFIC TYPES OF WOUNDS

Contusion

Contusion, or bruise, is a non-penetrating wound created by blunt force. If the skin is intact, very little treatment is indicated unless there is a large hematoma which should be evacuated. He-matomas which are not particularly bothersome can be left alone; they will be absorbed. If ecchymosis is considerable its absorption can be accelerated by the use of a systemic anti-inflammatory enzyme (tab. i b.i.d.). If the hematoma requires evacuation, cleanse the area properly and inject a small amount of 1 percent procaine into the skin. Attach an 18-gauge needle to a syringe and insert it through the anesthetized area into the hematoma. Draw out the blood and apply a small dry dressing. Apply a pressure dressing if there is possibility of recurrence of the hematoma (p. 69).

Abrasion

Abrasions are, in essence, multiple superficial scratches or brush burns. They often involve a fairly extensive surface and, since they occur at a skin level which contains many nerve endings, they may be quite painful. Dirt is frequently ground into them and it should be removed completely, by scrubbing if necessary. Imbedded particles can be picked out with a forceps. If the abrasion occurs on a weight-bearing area a nonadherent dressing should be applied covered by a thick gauze dressing. Abrasions elsewhere should be left uncovered and exposed to the air; an eschar will form which will provide proper protection.

Laceration

A laceration is made by a sharp object and is the commonest type of wound which the physician is asked to treat. The laceration may be deep enough to injure nerves, tendons, or blood vessels, as well as skin. In the main, lacerations are deep, have sharp clean edges, bleed freely and can be properly cleaned and repaired as primary procedures. Bleeding should be controlled, any raw edges excised, the entire area irrigated, and the wound closed in layers so that no dead space is left. Local or general anesthesia may be necessary, depending upon the extent and the location of the wound.

PENETRATING WOUNDS

There are two types of penetrating wounds: puncture wounds, made by sharp long objects such as ice picks, nails, or knives, and those produced by firearms. Penetrating wounds may damage deep structures in the chest or the abdomen. A wound penetrating deep into the chest may not require operative intervention if it is possible to expand the lung and remove any blood by thoracentesis or tube drainage (p. 242). On the other hand, any wound which might conceivably have penetrated the peritoneal cavity requires laparotomy to rule out injury to the abdominal viscera. Puncture wounds are the most common means of entry of tetanus and all patients who have sustained these wounds should have either tetanus antitoxin or a booster dose of tetanus toxoid (p. 105). Firearm injuries are often more serious because the force of the missile may be expended in several directions within the body; the site and nature of the wound of entry may therefore be deceptive as regards the extent of the injury. The decision as to operative intervention must be individualized. Clothing, wood or dirt buried in the body are a source of infection and should be removed. On the other hand, a metal missile need not necessarily be removed unless it is in a position to cause some difficulty of itself. The wound should be debrided; it should not be closed, but rather left open to drain.

FOREIGN BODIES

Foreign bodies which should always be removed include those which pro-trude through the skin, those that cause symptoms, wooden splinters, dirt and cloth, or any object which causes a wound to continue to drain.

Dirt

This is the most common of all foreign bodies. All visible dirt should be removed; that which can be seen and cannot be scrubbed out should be removed by sharp dissection. Badly traumatized tissue impregnated with much dirt is best excised. Copious amounts of water are very helpful in cleaning dirt from a wound.

Wooden Splinters

These are usually easy to see; they travel a straight line and are usually superficial. Usually the splinter can be pulled out by grasping the end; if this should be very painful, infiltrating the area with procaine will help. A splinter under a nail is a common circumstance. This is painful and should be removed to prevent infection. Remove a V-shaped segment from the nail with the point overlying the splinter.

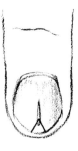

Grasp the base of the splinter and pull it out. If necessary, the pain of the procedure may be relieved by a nerve block at the base of the finger (p. 95).

Needles

Hypodermic injections are the commonest cause of imbedded broken needles. They may be difficult to locate and if not bothersome are probably best left alone. On the other hand, if they are symptomatic they should be removed. An x-ray of the area made beforehand, and fluoroscopic guidance during the course of removal are both helpful in finding the needle. Such an operation may be time consuming.

Cloth

This is usually introduced into the wound as a result of a penetrating injury. At the time of the injury, every effort should be made to remove imbedded cloth. If cloth is not seen in the wound but drainage continues the wound should be opened and the sinus tract followed down until the offending material is found and can be removed. The wound will then usually heal. Do not close the wound; it will granulate.

Glass

Following injury the patient is often uncertain whether glass actually entered the body. If there is any question, the part should be x-rayed. Since much glass contains lead it is frequently possible to locate the foreign body in this way. If x-ray demonstrates glass in the wound it should be explored; the glass can be recognized by the grating sensation as the probing instrument comes in contact with it.

Fish Hooks

If a fish hook becomes imbedded in the skin beyond the barb push the hook on out through a wound of exit until the barb is clear.

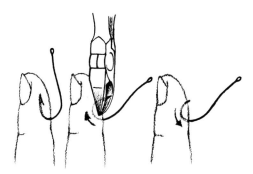

With a sharp shears cut off the barb and remove the remainder of the hook by pulling it back through the original site of entrance.

BITES

Bite wounds create special problems. For purposes of discussion they may be divided into human bites, animal bites, and snake bites.

Human Bites

The human mouth contains a variety of bacteria to which the subcutaneous tissues are vulnerable. Consequently, a human bite is a contaminated wound. The majority of human bite wounds involve the fingers and the most serious are those involving the joints. These commonly occur during a fight when in reality the patient wounds himself by smashing his fist into the teeth of his opponent. This causes a penetrating wound which frequently extends into a joint space and represents a serious problem. Immediate intensive treatment is required to preserve the function of the joint. The infected joint should be drained and the hand immobilized in a position to allow continuous drainage.

Since the injury occurred when the fist was clenched, the hand must be immobilized in this position so that the defect in the skin will overlie the defect in the joint capsule.

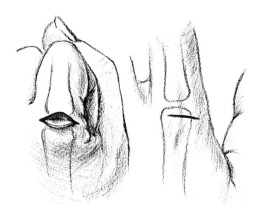

The patient should receive antibiotics as indicated by sensitivity studies of the joint fluid.

TREATMENT. The tendency to treat bites by chemical or thermal cauterization is to be condemned; cauterization adds nothing to the efficacy of the treatment and only compounds the injury by doing further damage to the tissues. The wound should be cleansed thoroughly by scrubbing and copious irrigations. All contaminated or necrotic tissues must be excised (excepting, of course, extensive areas of cellulitis). Bite wounds should never be closed primarily. If the wound is gaping, it may be narrowed with loose sutures after it has been properly debrided.

Animal Bites

The greatest danger of animal bites lies in the possibility of contamination of the wound with rabies. In this country, dogs are the commonest vectors of the disease, although almost any animal, either wild or domestic, may be rabid. This includes cats, foxes, coyotes, skunks, and even bats. Consequently, a bite by any of these animals should be considered a potential source of trouble. The best means of ascertaining whether the animal is rabid is to keep it quarantined for two weeks under observation for the development of rabies symptoms. If the animal is killed before the two weeks have elapsed, his head should be sent to a qualified laboratory to be examined for rabies. If the animal escapes, a considered judgment must be made as to whether or not vaccine is necessary.

TREATMENT. The wound should be thoroughly cleansed. The age-old habit of cauterizing the wound chemically or thermally should be avoided. In the main, the incubation period is sufficiently long that the decision concerning vaccination is not urgent. However, when the head or neck is bitten the incubation period may be shorter and an immediate decision with regard to vaccination should be made.

MATERIALS AVAILABLE. The standard Pasteur vaccination consists of phenol inactivated virus which is given daily over a period of fourteen days in the dosage recommended by the particular manufacturer. The treatment occasionally produces distressing neurological side effects and the vaccine should not be given indiscriminately. There is also an antiserum available which is used in a dosage of 0.5 ml. per kilogram of body weight. Since it produces a high antibody titer rapidly it is particularly useful in urgent situations. However, since this involves the injection of a large amount of horse serum it must be preceded by the usual tests for serum sensitivity (p. 105). The U.S. Public Health Service suggests: (1) In multiple wounds and those involving the face, head or neck give the antiserum immediately and determine later the need for vaccine by proof of rabies in the animal held under observation or by a strong suspicion of the disease if the animal has escaped. (2) In less urgent situations, when the animal has symptoms of rabies while under observation, or when the animal appears to have been rabid at the time of contact but further observations are impossible, omit the antiserum and proceed with the administration of vaccine.

Snake Bites

A snake bite should be treated as follows: Apply a tourniquet immediately to the extremity proximal to the bite, tight enough to obstruct only the superficial venous and lymphatic circulation. Make multiple, short, circumferential incisions through the skin in the area of the bite and attempt to suck out venom by bulb suction or by mouth if necessary. There is available a polyvalent serum which neutralizes the venom of pit vipers. The smaller the victim the larger should be the dose, because in a small person a given amount of venom is more concentrated. From one to five 10-ml. vials should be given as the initial dose, a portion being injected directly into the tissues in the vicinity of the bite and the remainder distributed subcutaneously or intramuscularly in the affected part. Additional antivenom may be given every one-half hour to two hours. A comatose patient should be given intravenous injections. Since this is a horse serum the customary precaution against sensitivity must be taken. One must remember that the fangs of the snake may be contaminated with tetanus or clostridium. Clostridium infection should not be a problem since there will be little devitalized tissue. However, tetanus immunization should be started. Snake bite victims should be admitted to the hospital and blood typing and cross-matching done immediately, since late hemolysis may interfere with the typing and cross-matching done at a later time.

INJURY TO STRUCTURES

NERVES

If a nerve is only partially divided, the area should be carefully cleaned, any devitalized tissue debrided, and the partially divided nerve sutured together. Use sutures of fine, interrupted silk which pass through only the nerve sheath and should be approximated without tension.

Usually the nerves are completely divided and the ends are jagged. Before attempting to debride the end of the

nerve place a stay suture in each segment so that it can be properly apposed. Grasp each jagged end with a hemostat. Cut off the jagged area, making a clean perpendicular cut at the end of the nerve so as to provide two fresh smooth surfaces. Align the two ends of the nerve so that the stay sutures previously inserted are properly apposed. With a fine silk suture, which only penetrates the sheath, sew the nerve together.

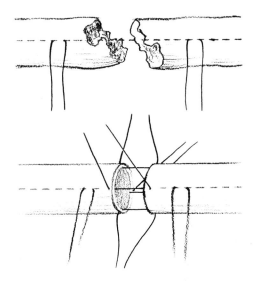

Initially insert such a suture in each quadrant of the nerve. Frequently this is adequate, but if more sutures are indicated they can be added.

If the ends cannot be readily brought together, joints should be flexed. Three-fourths of an inch can be gained by flexing the proximal finger joint; flexing the wrist and elbow may overcome a 3½ inch gap. If more length is required it can be achieved by dissecting the nerve from behind to in front of the elbow. The repaired nerve must be covered. If adequate tissue is not available use a skin graft. The repaired nerve must be immobilized for three weeks.

After the operation is completed the tendons and joints must be protected until they are ready to resume function.

Every muscle has an antagonistic muscle. When a muscle becomes paralyzed its antagonist is free to act without resistance from the injured muscle. This causes deformities which can be permanent if not treated. The deformity should be corrected by a splint which brings the muscles and joints back to a position of function, but with attention to the possibility of overcorrection.

The patient should be warned of the danger of trauma to a paresthetic extremity. He should never use an anesthetized hand to smoke because of the danger of burns. He should always check the temperature of hot water with the normal extremity before immersing the paresthetic one.

Blood Vessels

If there is a rent in the blood vessels, an atraumatic clamp should be applied at both sides of the opening to control the hemorrhage. The area should be cleaned and any clot removed. A solution of saline containing a small amount of heparin (10 mg./L.) is very satisfactory for irrigating the area. After the wound has been cleaned the rent can usually be closed with either an interrupted or a continuous suture, using (4-0) arterial silk. If the wound is quite jagged and involves most of the vessel, or if the vessel is divided, the jagged ends should be removed at right angles to the direction of the vessel, and the vessel segments approximated, using either interrupted silk or a running silk suture.

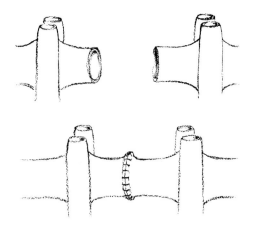

The commonest method is to insert two continuous sutures posteriorly and then carry one suture around each side of the vessel. If there is bleeding from the suture holes, a few moments of digital pressure over the bleeding points will usually stop it. If a portion of the wound in the vessel continues to bleed, an interrupted suture will control it.

Tendons

Lacerations anywhere in the body may divide tendons. The two ends should be identified and sutured together. Since the tendon is under considerable tension it must be sutured securely and firmly. Simple over-and-over sutures are not adequate. Most tendon injuries occur in the upper extremity and are discussed in detail in that section (p. 212). The principles described can be applied to any part of the body.

Chapter Eight

Infection

GENERAL DEVELOPMENT OF INFECTION

When bacteria invade a superficial area of the human body, the first reaction noted is *cellulitis*. The patient complains of pain. The pain is more severe in sensitive areas, such as the tips of the fingers, and where the skin is thick and subcutaneous tissue sparse, such as the back of the neck. In such areas swelling causes a rapid increase in tissue tension. In looser tissues, the pain may be less severe but the swelling more pronounced. There is frequently a throbbing which is aggravated if the inflamed part is in a dependent position. The area has a fiery red center which gradually fades out at the periphery to normal skin. The erythematous area is quite tender. This stage is called cellulitis.

Occasionally, there may be an associated erysipeloid reaction of the skin. An erythematous edema of the skin with palpable borders extends for a considerable distance from the obvious area of cellulitis. The erythema is bright red and blanches completely on pressure.

The infection may spread along the lymphatics. If the lymphatic channels become inflamed, one sees red streaks extending from the infected area toward the regional lymph nodes. The lymphatic channels are edematous and are readily palpable as tender, thickened cords. This is *lymphangitis.*

Most infections spread early to the regional lymph nodes causing the nodes to become enlarged and tender. This is *lymphadenitis.* It may or may not be accompanied by lymphangitis. It occurs more frequently than lymphangitis.

Many inflammations resolve promptly and without residual. On the other hand, some inflammatory processes go on to localized *suppuration* and abscess formation. Necrotic material, liquefied bacteria, dead leucocytes, and exudate make up a localized mass of pus. This is usually softer than the surrounding tissues, and fluctuation, which is evidence of abscess formation, can be elicited by the palpating fingers. If the abscess is under considerable tension, fluctuation is not evident but the area will show point tenderness.

The proper treatment of suppuration is surgical drainage which is frequently all that is necessary. In an occasional case where the tissues surrounding the abscess remain inflamed, or there is lymphadenitis and lymphadenopathy, antibiotics may be helpful. Antibiotics, whether administered parenterally or orally, cannot reach bacteria within an abscess in sufficient concentration. Consequently, the antibiotics may control the systemic reaction and systemic spread of an infection, but they cannot eliminate localized suppuration. They merely give the surgeon a false sense of security by masking the general symptoms and the infection may ultimately supersede the antibiotic therapy and become further advanced because its presence was not appreciated early.

Cellulitis, lymphangitis, lymphadenitis, and erysipeloid reaction are treated by local rest, warm, moist applications, and antibiotics. The involved part should be put at rest and when this does not seem adequate the patient should be put to bed. Warm compresses should be applied (p. 69). Do not keep the compress in place continuously, Apply it for about 30 minutes; remove the wet dressing and allow the skin to dry thoroughly before you apply the next compress. The skin can be protected during the compress by applying a thin coating of vaseline before putting on the compress. Compresses can be applied every two hours and should be used at least four times a day.

CHOICE OF ANTIMICROBIAL DRUGS

All infections should be treated by specific antibiotics. There is a delay of at least 48 hours before the identity and antibiotic sensitivity of the offending organism is known. In severe infections antibiotic treatment should not be delayed until the final laboratory report is available. Before this report arrives, therapy should be started on an empirical basis. The experienced clinician can often make an accurate guess as to the identity of the offending organism on the basis of clinical evidence. A gram stain of sputum, urine, wound exudate, or spiral fluid often yields a clue to the identity of the infecting organism and aids in the choice of a drug for initial therapy before positive identification of the organism and determination of its sensitivity to antibiotics. The most common offenders are the Staphylococcus and the B hemolytic Streptococcus, Lancefield-Group A. If the offending organism is the Streptococcus it will be sensitive to penicillin. If it is a Staphylococcus and was acquired outside the hospital environment, in 66 per cent of cases it will be sensitive to all antibiotics, but the remainder will be resistant to penicillin, streptomycin and tetracycline. If the organism was acquired in a hospital in most cases it will be a resistant variety. The immediate choice of antibiotics will depend upon the physician's knowledge of the type of organism present within his community or hospital.

The table, "Bacteria, Fungi and Viruses Most Likely to Cause Acute Infections," beginning on page 123, lists the common pathogens encountered in various infections together with the antimicrobial agents that are likely to be most effective. This table can be used to choose the drug of choice for preliminary treatment while awaiting the results of sensitivity tests.

COMPLICATIONS OF ANTIMICROBIAL THERAPY

Superinfections

Most antimicrobials, whether administered orally or parenterally, can predispose to superinfection in the alimentary tract and other organs, but superinfections are most frequent with broad spectrum drugs such as the tetracyclines. Enterocolitis and pneumonia caused by Staphylococcus aureus (usually strains resistant to penicillin G) are among the most serious superinfections. Anal itching and vulvovaginitis, frequent side effects of oral antimicrobials, are generally attributed to superinfection by fungi, especially Candida species.

Use in Renal Insufficiency

Most antimicrobial agents and their metabolites are excreted mainly in the urine with some excretion by way of the biliary tract. A few (Erythromycin, Novabiocin, Chlortetracycline, Troleandoxmycin, and probably Lincomycin) are excreted mainly through the biliary tract. During the first 24 hours of therapy most patients with impaired kidney function can tolerate the usual doses of antimicrobial drugs that are excreted mainly by the kidneys. Subsequent doses should, however, be reduced to minimize the risks that renal insufficiency will increase drug concentrations in blood and tissues to toxic levels. Maintenance doses of all agents excreted largely by the kidney should also be reduced if the patient is dehydrated. Where laboratory facilities are available, measurement of antibiotic blood levels by chemical analysis or bio-assay is occasionally helpful in guiding the adjustment of dosage and minimizing toxicity.

Some of the antimicrobials excreted mainly by the kidneys are themselves capable of causing renal damage; these include Amphotericin B, Bacitracin, Neomycin, Kanamycin, the Polymyxins, Viomycin, Vancomycin, Cephaloridine, and the Sulfonamides. Griseofulvin, Methenamine mandelate, Hippurate and Methicillin have rarely been known to cause renal damage. Since the injurious effects of these agents are dose-dependent, doses must be carefully regulated to avoid toxic damage to the kidneys and other organs.

Use in Pregnant Women and in the Newborn

Parenterally administered tetracycline has caused severe liver damage in pregnant women. The tetracyclines can also cause bone lesions and staining and deformity of teeth in children up to about eight years of age and in the newborn when the drug is given to pregnant women after the fourth month of gestation. Chloramphenicol and the Sulfonamides should be administered cautiously to pregnant women near term and premature and newborn infants, since mechanisms for detoxifying these drugs are not fully developed until later infancy. Although there is no convincing evidence that administration of any antimicrobial to pregnant women produces teratogenic effects, these drugs, like drugs generally, should be prescribed for pregnant women with special caution.

The chart entitled "Adverse Effects of Antimicrobial Drugs," on page 132, outlines the principal adverse effects of the common antimicrobial agents. In general adverse effects are dose-related and serious effects are more common with parenteral than with oral administration. Gastrointestinal disturbances, including malabsorption states, are more frequent with oral than with parenteral administration.

The widespread discussion of hospital infections has tended to create a separate problem. Bacteria acquired in a hospital atmosphere are more likely to be resistant to many of the older or more commonly used antibiotics. Except for this point the problem is the same from a surgical standpoint. The infections probably occur as a result of a break in technique, and cannot be prevented by prophylactic administration of antibiotics. Treatment consists of local heat, rest and antibiotics; when the infection is localized open surgical drainage is necessary. The problem may be more difficult than with other infections because fewer antibiotics are helpful in controlling the infection.

LOCALIZED SUPPURATION

STITCH ABSCESS

Purulent material may collect about a single skin suture, and occasionally about many sutures. Unless the offending sutures are removed the infection may spread and cause a generalized wound infection.

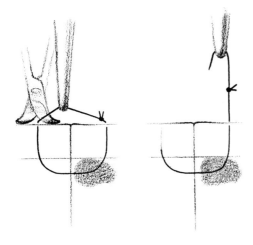

Grasp a free end of the suture with a forceps. Lift the suture so that the point of the scissors can be passed between the knot and the skin. Divide the suture at the skin level on the uninfected side. Pull the portion of the suture within the abscess through the infected, not the uninfected, part of the wound. The abscess will usually clear up after the suture is removed.

Warm compresses (page 69) will accelerate the resolution of the associated cellulitis.

Stitch Granuloma

Another type of stitch abscess is the granulomatous reaction which sometimes occurs about buried, nonabsorbable suture material. This first appears as a small, elevated, erythematous, nontender, fluctuant area which periodically drains. Following drainage, the lesion will clear and then recur. The su-

ture acts as a foreign body and the sequence will persist until the suture is removed or sloughs out. It may be removed by blindly probing deep in the wound with a pointed hemostat. A crocheting needle will allow one to probe deeply in the wound without enlarging the opening in the skin. If this is not successful, infiltrate the area with procaine and extend the incision sufficiently so that you can find the suture. After removing the suture, make no effort to close the wound; it will granulate satisfactorily.

FURUNCLE

A furuncle is a collection of pus in a *single chamber* about a single hair follicle. Commonly called a boil, it begins as an elevated, markedly tender, erythematous area. After it localizes, the center becomes yellowish or black. When the center exhibits point tenderness and then fluctuation it is ready for surgical drainage. Prepare the operative area by shaving a wide margin. This is important because most reinfections arise from the surface as the bacteria follow a hair follicle beneath the skin.

After anesthetizing the area, drive the point of a bayonet-type blade deep into the fluctuant area. Bring the blade out in a wide sweeping motion to open the entire width of the pocket of pus.

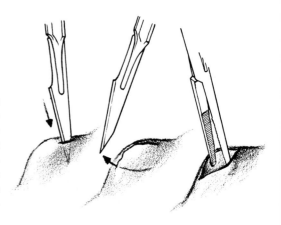

Next, insert a closed hemostat deep into the wound and open it to spread the edges of the incision. Frequently, the pus is quite thick. Pick out as much as possible with a hemostat, but do not try to express the purulent material by pressing on the wound. Send a specimen of the pus to the laboratory for smear, culture and determination of antibiotic sensitivity. Insert a small rubber tissue drain to keep the edges apart. A dry dressing is satisfactory. Have the patient treat the wound with wet compresses for thirty minutes four times daily until drainage ceases. After each compress he should cleanse the area with 70 per cent alcohol, and apply a bactericidal ointment (such as bacitracin, triclobisonium chloride, betadine or neomycin) and a clean dry dressing. He should wash his hands carefully after each application. Antibiotics are not routinely needed, but are sometimes of value or necessary in reducing and containing the surrounding inflammation.

Furunculosis

Occasionally, you will be consulted by a patient who has been bothered by multiple furuncles over a prolonged period of time. At any one time he may have from one to twenty furuncles in various stages of development. The most common areas of involvement are the axillae, the buttocks, and the back of the neck, but any part of the body may be attacked. Since this is a chronic problem it is wise to advise the patient that it may be some time before he is free of furuncles. Systemic antibiotics are of little value except in containing the associated inflammation at the high point of an individual furuncle. Some surgeons recommend making a vaccine from a culture of the pus from the furuncle, and vaccinating the patient to build up his resistance to the offending bacteria. While this may be helpful, it is

rarely necessary. The condition is treated as follows:*

The patient must practice strict personal hygiene and carry out meticulous and painstaking local measures. He must shower two to four times daily with hexachlorophene soap starting with his head and working caudad, being careful to avoid returning to already washed areas. To avoid minor skin abrasions the use of wash cloths is not permitted and the skin is dried by patting. Tub baths are prohibited. All clothes should be laundered or cleaned to remove the offending bacteria before they are reworn. All bedding should be covered with plastic and disinfected daily. Bed clothing should be changed daily and underclothing changed twice daily to avoid recontamination of the skin. All clothing should be washed as soon as possible and rinsed in a solution containing a phenolic germicide (Lysol). The local lesions should be compressed for 30 minutes four times daily, until they either disappear or become fluctuant. If fluctuation occurs, they are drained (p. 116). A wide area of skin surrounding each lesion should be cleansed with hexachlorophene soap and rinsed with generous amounts of 70 per cent alcohol. The skin is allowed to air dry and then is covered with a thin layer of a local antibacterial ointment (such as triclobisonium chloride, Triburon [Roche]; bacitracin, Bacitracin Ointment [Pfizer]; or neomycin, Myciguent Ointment [Upjohn]). The area is covered with a dry dressing held in place with cellulose tape. Adhesive plaster is avoided because of its irritating and abrading characteristics.

This routine must be continued for a period of at least 3 to 6 months after all lesions have disappeared. Antibiotics are given only to those patients with severe toxic manifestations, with lesions

_____

* Sweeney, F. J., Bell, T. G., and Wise, R. I.: The Hygienic Treatment of Persistent Staphylococcal Furunculosis. Exhibit. Annual Meeting, A.M.A., 1961.

above the upper lip, or with a large area of cellulitis or lymphangitis surrounding the lesion which appears to be increasing in size. The antibiotic used depends on the physician's knowledge of strains present at the time.

CARBUNCLE

Occasionally, an infection will migrate and become multilocular, causing a carbuncle. In this case a simple incision is not adequate treatment because all pockets will not be opened. Such patients should always receive appropriate antibiotic therapy. A carbuncle is best treated surgically under general anesthesia. After proper preparation of the skin (shaving, alcohol and an iodophor solution) make a cruciate incision, which extends back to normal tissue in all directions, through the full thickness of the skin. Cut back the skin flaps and excise the infected area.

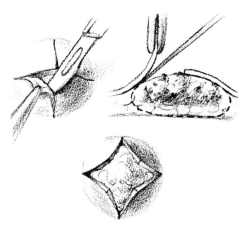

Pack the wound open with gauze. Culture the pus from the wound, determine antibiotic sensitivity, and adjust the antibiotics if necessary. Remove the gauze pack after a few days and allow the wound to granulate. It may be necessary to place skin grafts on the area or revise the scar at a later date. One should not be concerned with cosmetic result at the time of treating the carbuncle; nothing should interfere with adequate excision.

ABSCESS

An abscess is a circumscribed collection of pus of any size in any location. The abscess may be directly under the skin or may be situated deep within the body. Antibiotics cannot reach bacteria within an abscess. Regardless of its position or size, the treatment of choice is adequate surgical drainage, which means that the abscess should be opened to the full width of the cavity.

Most abscesses are loculated; incision into the cavity will not provide adequate drainage. Using some form of anesthesia, incise the cavity, pass a finger into the incision and break down the loculation to convert the space into a single cavity. Drainage to the exterior should be maintained by keeping the wound open with a gauze wick or a rubber drain. The exterior wound should be kept open until the cavity granulates from within. Antibiotics are usually unnecessary once the abscess has been adequately drained and usually they are discontinued at this time. This prevents the antibiotics from obscuring the effects of an undrained collection. If the patient is afebrile and is not receiving antibiotics the collection has been properly drained. In the occasional case where considerable inflammatory reaction surrounds the abscess antibiotics are helpful. Anatomic relationships must be considered during the drainage of an abscess; adequate hygienic care of the surrounding skin is necessary to prevent satellite infections.

GANGRENE

In early gangrene there is loss of circulation, there is no pulsation in local arteries, and vessels do not empty on pressure. The area is cold and has no sensation. Motor function is lost and the area gradually becomes darker. If these changes are confined to a small area the situation may reverse itself, otherwise it goes on to frank gangrene. The gangrene may be dry or wet; dry gangrene is due to the interference with arterial blood supply while wet gangrene is due to interference with venous return as well as arterial supply. It is important to differentiate between the two types.

Dry Gangrene

Dry gangrene is really mummification. The tissues become dry, hard and shriveled from loss of fluid. The liberated hemoglobin turns the tissues black. There is a sharp line of demarcation and little tendency to spread unless the blood supply to the proximal tissues is affected. This type of gangrene is frequently painful. The severity of the pain is the only reason for urgency in removing the gangrenous area.

Wet Gangrene

Wet gangrene occurs when the venous return as well as the arterial supply is impaired. It may turn to dry gangrene if the wound remains aseptic until evaporation of fluid in the area takes place. Unfortunately, this happens only rarely and, in most instances, full blown wet gangrene and infection ensue. The area becomes purplish and edematous. The superficial tissues become raised in blisters and the deeper tissues are swollen. There is marked inflammation of the adjacent living tissues and the condition rapidly spreads up the extremity. There is an associated, severe, febrile, systemic reaction with marked toxemia which will be rapidly fatal if the limb is not removed.

Ice Anesthesia

Unfortunately, gangrene often develops in a desperately ill patient with other serious complications. Typical is a person whose diabetes is out of control and in whom operation may be considered too hazardous. The toxemia can be controlled and the condition of the patient improved for operation by placing the extremity in ice. However, it must be appreciated that this move commits the extremity to amputation just as certainly as does the scalpel. The anesthesia produced by the cold is sufficient for the subsequent amputation. The leg is packed in ice as follows: Make a wooden trough to fit about the extremity. Line the trough with heavy rubber sheeting. Put a layer of chopped ice in the bottom of the trough. Lay in a rubber tourniquet at the point where you plan to apply it later. This must be above the level of involvement but below the planned level of the amputation. Set the leg in the trough. Fill the trough with ice. After about thirty minutes, tighten the tourniquet. Cover the ice with a rubber sheet. Maintain this condition until amputation.

ULCER

The commonest ulcers of the leg are varicose ulcers. These are not due to infection but rather to tissue anoxia secondary to varicose veins. They most commonly occur on the medial aspect of the leg and have associated varicosities. This subject is discussed in detail on p. 280.

Undermining Ulcers

Occasionally, when an anaerobic organism is responsible for the infection, the ulcer may be of the undermining type. Instead of shallow sloping edges, the ulcer edges will be punched out and undermined. A culture of organisms from the ulcer, including an anaerobic culture of the edge of the ulcer, should be made and specific antibiotic therapy instituted. Zinc peroxide dressings should be applied. For this treatment every part of the infected surface must be made accessible to the zinc peroxide. The entire area should be widely opened and all the necrotic tissue debrided. The zinc peroxide must be properly activated. It can be obtained as finely divided, white powder and must be heated to 140° C. for four hours to sterilize it and to mobilize the oxygen. The zinc peroxide is then made into a thick cream or paste with sterile distilled water or physiologic salt solution. Make a dam about the ulcer area with petrolatum gauze and work the paste into every niche of the wound, taking particular care to get it into any undermined area. Next, fill the entire space within the dam. Cover the pool of paste with wax paper or petrolatum gauze. This keeps the paste moist and favors the liberation of oxygen; the free oxygen will be kept in contact with the wound. The application should be repeated every 24 hours.

SPECIFIC INFECTIONS

GAS GANGRENE

Badly traumatized wounds are frequently infected with bacteria of the clostridium group. The clostridium organisms can be found in the soil of gardens and in dirt in many areas. In North Africa in World War II, clostridia were grown from approximately 80 per cent of all wounds cultured. Fortunately, less than one per cent of these became clinically active. A clostridium is a highly virulent, anaerobic, gas-forming organism by virtue of its peptonizing action. It takes hold in infected, devitalized, or avascular areas or in areas of hematoma. In reality, three different types of infection may occur: clostridium myositis, or gas gangrene, which may be either wet or dry; and clostridium cellulitis, or gas abscess.

Clostridium Myositis

The *dry type* of clostridium myositis usually is characterized by the production of much gas, and the offending organism is usually Clostridium welchii. Clostridium oedematiens predominates in the wet type in which swelling and exudate are most prominent. Dry gas gangrene usually begins a day or two after the wound is made. The first symptom is sudden pain in the wound. The patient is apprehensive and has a tachycardia out of proportion to his temperature rise. He is anemic and rapidly becomes hypotensive. Some of these wounds have a meat market odor, but this is not necessarily characteristic. Crepitus can be felt in the wound and also beyond the area of trauma. X-ray will demonstrate gas in the fascial planes and in the muscle bundles.

In *wet gas gangrene,* the first symptom is usually a new feeling of heaviness in a wound. The patient has a marked systemic reaction; he may be apathetic and occasionally delirious. Again, he has a tachycardia without any marked elevation in temperature and the blood pressure is low. The tissues are markedly edematous and there is considerable exudate from the wound; characteristic odor may or may not be present. There is very little if any crepitus in the wound. Considerably less gas forms than with the dry type and it may only appear late in the course of the disease.

Clostridium Cellulitis

The main complaint is the foul odor from the wound. There is rarely any pain. There may be some elevation of temperature and pulse rate but these usually are proportional to each other and the patient's blood pressure is normal and the sensorium is clear. There is a profuse, brownish, seropurulent, foul discharge from the wound. Gas bubbles escape from the wound and crepitus can be palpated both within the wound and beyond the edges of the traumatized area. X-ray will show gas within the wound but will not show gas in the tissues beyond the area of trauma. Exploration of the wound will show devitalized muscle with necrotic raised slough. However, once the devitalized muscle has been removed, the remaining muscle is found to be normal. It will bleed when cut and contract when pinched.

The muscle tissue in dry gas gangrene is markedly edematous, firm, and dark, and bulges from within the wound. When the muscle is cut it will not contract but will ooze serosanguineous fluid and the involvement extends well beyond the area of trauma.

Treatment

The most important point in the treatment of this disease is to establish the proper diagnosis. The demonstration of the microorganism and gas are not of themselves sufficient. As a matter of fact, these can be present in relatively benign wounds. The most satisfactory means of making a diagnosis is surgical exploration of the wound and determination of the extent of the involvement. The most significant point is whether the bacteria have involved fresh muscle beyond the area of trauma. A diagnosis of gas gangrene is made if nontraumatized muscle is invaded. The most important part of the treatment is to excise all the involved muscle. If it is possible to do this with a local excision, this is satisfactory. However, in most cases of gas gangrene it is not possible and a guillotine type of amputation, leaving the wound open, is required. When tissue above the highest practical point of amputation is involved the incision must be carried above the amputation, all the involved muscle excised and the entire area left open. In addition to the wide local surgical extirpation the patient must be treated generally. The profound anemia which is always present must be corrected. Large doses of antibiotics (penicillin, chloramphenicol, chlortetracycline, or oxytetracycline) are helpful. A polyvalent serum is available which contains antitoxin for Clostridium welchii, Clostridium novyi and Clostridium histolyticum. Of itself this is incapable of curing any case but some believe that it is of value in combating toxemia.

When it is found by exploration that muscle involvement is confined to the area of trauma, one knows that one is dealing with clostridium cellulitis, or an anaerobic cellulitis. In this case complete excision of all of the devitalized muscle, with the entire area laid open, is usually adequate. The wound is left open and treated with an oxidizing solution such as hydrogen peroxide.

Tetanus

The early clinical manifestations of tetanus are temperature elevation, muscle tenderness or tetanic spasm, and stiffness or locking of the jaw. The area near the wound may sometimes be markedly tender with deep induration, and possibly suppuration. However, in a significant number of cases the original site of entrance is not known. One of the early subjective signs is spasm and tenderness in the muscles of the abdomen. The abdominal muscles become as rigid as a board. The organism may often be identified directly from wound secretions, but if there is a reasonable probability of the disease, treatment should be begun without waiting for laboratory confirmation.

Treatment

Proper treatment requires a team consisting of a surgeon, an anesthesiologist, an internist and a neurologist. The important agent in treatment is tetanus antitoxin. The rules concerning testing for sensitivity (p. 105) should be followed. After the possibility of sensitivity has been ruled out, treatment is as follows: (1) Give 50,000 units of tetanus antitoxin intravenously as the first dose. This can be augmented by an intramuscular injection of an additional 40,000 units. If the site of injury is known the tissues surrounding it should be infiltrated with multiple injections to a total of 10,000 units of antitoxin. The treatment should be continued with daily injections of 5,000 units of antitoxin until the disease is under control. The relative degree of abdominal tenderness and spasm is considered a fairly good test of effectiveness of the treatment. If there is any question whatsoever of respiratory difficulty a tracheostomy should be performed immediately. These patients tend to develop respiratory arrest or depression and they should be guarded against this possibility and if necessary have proper treatment instituted immediately (p. 77). Convulsive seizures may be controlled by either barbiturates or paraldehyde administered orally, rectally or intramuscularly. A dilute solution of Pen-tothal sodium (0.5 gm. to 1 liter of physiologic salt solution) given intravenously, 20 to 25 drops a minute, is very effective in reducing the frequency and severity of convulsions. A stronger (2.5 per cent) solution of Pentothal sodium should be prepared for emergency injection of a few ml. in the event of convulsive respiratory arrest. Curare-like drugs may be given to aid in the control of the convulsive seizures. Myanesin in a 1 to 2 per cent solution may be given in amounts sufficient to meet the requirements of the patients. Massive doses of aqueous penicillin, 10,000,000 to 20,000,000 units per day is considered worthwhile. The severity of the disease varies with individual patients and specific measures mentioned must be adjusted to the particular circumstances.

Table 1. Bacteria, Fungi and Viruses Most Likely to Cause Acute Infections

INFECTING ORGANISM	DRUG OF FIRST CHOICE†	ALTERNATIVE DRUGS†

Skin and Subcutaneous Tissues

Skin Infections

INFECTING ORGANISM	DRUG OF FIRST CHOICE†	ALTERNATIVE DRUGS†
* Staphylococcus aureus		
non-penicillinase-producing	a penicillin[1]	an erythromycin; lincomycin
penicillinase-producing	a penicillinase-resistant penicillin[1]	an erythromycin; lincomycin; a cephalosporin;[3] vancomycin[4]
Streptococcus pyogenes (Group A)	a penicillin[1]	an erythromycin;[2] lincomycin
Dermatophytes and Candida albicans	griseofulvin[25] amphotericin B[4,23]	none nystatin
Gram-negative bacilli	(see page 129)	
Treponema pallidum	penicillin G (P)	an erythromycin (P); a tetracycline (P)[4,5]

Burns

* Staphylococcus aureus		
non-penicillinase-producing	a penicillin[1]	an erythromycin; lincomycin
penicillinase-producing	a penicillinase-resistant penicillin[1]	an erythromycin; lincomycin; a cephalosporin;[3] vancomycin[4]
Streptococcus pyogenes (Group A)	a penicillin[1]	an erythromycin;[2] lincomycin
Pseudomonas aeruginosa and other gram-negative bacilli	a polymyxin (P) (see page 129)	gentamicin (P); carbenicillin (P)

Decubitus Wound Infections

* Staphylococcus aureus		
non-penicillinase-producing	a penicillin[1]	an erythromycin; lincomycin
penicillinase-producing	a penicillinase-resistant penicillin[1]	an erythromycin; lincomycin; a cephalosporin;[3] vancomycin[4]
Escherichia coli[12] other gram-negative bacilli	kanamycin[14] (see page 129)	ampicillin; a tetracycline[5]
Streptococcus pyogenes (Group A)	a penicillin[1]	an erythromycin;[2] lincomycin
* Streptococcus anaerobius	penicillin G (P)	a tetracycline
Clostridium	penicillin G (P)	a tetracycline (P)[4,5]

Traumatic and Surgical Wounds

* Staphylococcus aureus		
non-penicillinase-producing	a penicillin[1]	an erythromycin; lincomycin
penicillinase-producing	a penicillinase-resistant penicillin[1]	an erythromycin; lincomycin; a cephalosporin;[3] vancomycin[4]
Streptococcus anaerobius	penicillin G (P)	a tetracycline[5]
Gram-negative bacilli	(see page 129)	
Clostridium	penicillin G (P)	a tetracycline (P)[4,5]

Eyes

Cornea and Conjunctiva

Herpes	idoxuridine (topical)	none
Neisseria gonorrhoeae	a penicillin[1]	an erythromycin; a tetracycline[5]
Staphylococcus aureus		
non-penicillinase-producing	a penicillin[1]	an erythromycin; lincomycin
penicillinase-producing	a penicillinase-resistant penicillin[1]	an erythromycin; lincomycin; a cephalosporin;[3] vancomycin[4]
Pseudomonas aeruginosa	a polymyxin (P)	gentamicin (P); carbenicillin (P)
Diplococcus pneumoniae	a penicillin[1]	an erythromycin;[2] lincomycin
Coliform bacilli	(see page 128)	
Haemophilus influenzae	ampicillin	a tetracycline;[5] a cephalosporin[3]
Fungi	(see page 129)	

* Because resistance may be a problem, susceptibility tests should be performed.

† (P) Although both parenteral and oral formulations are available, parenteral administration is preferred for this infection.

See footnotes on page 130.

Table 1. (*Continued*)

Infecting Organism	Drug of First Choice†	Alternative Drugs†
Para-Nasal Sinuses		
Diplococcus pneumoniae	a penicillin[1]	an erythromycin;[2] lincomycin
Streptococcus pyogenes (Group A)	a penicillin[1]	an erythromycin;[2] lincomycin
* Staphylococcus aureus		
non-penicillinase-producing	a penicillin[1]	an erythromycin; lincomycin
penicillinase producing	a penicillinase-resistant penicillin[1]	an erythromycin; lincomycin; a cephalosporin;[3] vancomycin[4]
Haemophilus influenzae (in children)	ampicillin	a tetracycline;[5] a cephalosporin[3]
meningitis	ampicillin (P)	chloramphenicol (P),[4] with or without streptomycin[4]
Klebsiella and other gram-negative bacilli	(see page 129)	
Mucor	amphotericin B[4]	no dependable alternative
Mouth		
Herpes viruses	idoxuridine (topical)	none
Candida albicans	amphotericin B[4,23]	nystatin[23] (oral or topical)
Fusobacterium fusiforme (Vincent's infection)	a penicillin[1]	a tetracycline;[5] an erythromycin
Bacteroides	a tetracycline[5]	ampicillin; chloramphenicol[4]
Treponema pallidum	penicillin G (P)	an erythromycin (P); a tetra-cycline (P)[4,5]
Throat		
		a tetracycline[5]
Respiratory viruses	an erythromycin	
Streptococcus pyogenes (Group A)	a penicillin[1]	an erythromycin;[2] lincomycin
Diplococcus pneumoniae	a penicillin[1]	an erythromycin;[2] lincomycin
Haemophilus influenzae	ampicillin	a tetracycline;[5] a cephalosporin[3]
Neisseria meningitidis	penicillin G (P)	a sulfonamide (P),[4,5] a tetra-cycline[4,5]
Fusobacterium fusiforme (Vincent's infection)	a penicillin	a tetracycline; an erythromycin
Candida albicans	amphotericin B[4,23]	nystatin (oral or topical)
Corynebacterium diphtheriae	an erythromycin	a penicillin[1]
Bordetella pertussis	ampicillin	a tetracycline[5]
Ear		
Auditory Canal		
* Staphylococcus aureus		
non-penicillinase-producing	a penicillin[1]	an erythromycin; lincomycin
penicillinase-producing	a penicillinase-resistant penicillin[1]	an erythromycin; lincomycin; a cephalosporin;[3] vancomycin[4]
Streptococcus pyogenes (Group A)	a penicillin[1]	an erythromycin;[2] lincomycin
Diplococcus pneumoniae	a penicillin[1]	an erythromycin;[2] lincomycin
Pseudomonas aeruginosa (mostly chronic)	gentamicin (P);[4] carbenicillin (P)	a polymyxin (P)[4]
Haemophilus influenzae (in children)	ampicillin	a tetracycline,[5] a cephalosporin[3]
Fungi	(see page 129)	
Middle Ear		
Respiratory viruses	an erythromycin	a tetracycline[5]
Diplococcus pneumoniae	a penicillin[1]	an erythromycin;[2] lincomycin
Haemophilus influenzae (in children)	ampicillin	a tetracycline;[5] a cephalosporin[3]

Table 1. (*Continued*)

Infecting Organism	Drug of First Choice†	Alternative Drugs†
Ear, Middle Ear (Continued)		
* Staphylococcus aureus		
non-penicillinase-producing	a penicillin[1]	an erythromycin; lincomycin
penicillinase-producing	a penicillinase-resistant penicillin[1]	an erythromycin; lincomycin; a cephalosporin;[3] vancomycin[4]
Streptococcus pyogenes (Group A)	a penicillin[1]	an erythromycin;[2] lincomycin
Pseudomonas aeruginosa	gentamicin (P);[4] carbenicillin (P)	a polymyxin (P)[4]
Larynx, Trachea and Bronchi		
Respiratory viruses	an erythromycin	a tetracycline[5]
Diplococcus pneumoniae	a penicillin[1]	an erythromycin;[2] lincomycin
Haemophilus influenzae	ampicillin	a tetracycline;[5] a cephalosporin[3]
Streptococcus pyogenes (Group A)	a penicillin[1]	an erythromycin;[2] lincomycin
Pleura		
* Staphylococcus aureus (in children)		
non-penicillinase-producing	a penicillin[1]	an erythromycin; lincomycin
penicillinase-producing	a penicillinase-resistant penicillin[1]	an erythromycin; lincomycin; a cephalosporin;[3] vancomycin[4]
Diplococcus pneumoniae	a penicillin[1]	an erythromycin;[2] lincomycin
Streptococcus pyogenes (Group A)	a penicillin[1]	an erythromycin;[2] lincomycin
* Streptococcus anaerobius	penicillin G (P)	a tetracycline[5]
Lungs		
Pneumonia		
Diplococcus pneumoniae	a penicillin[1]	an erythromycin;[2] lincomycin
Mycoplasma pneumoniae (a typical pneumoniae)	an erythromycin	a tetracycline[5]
Respiratory viruses	an erythromycin	a tetracycline[5]
Haemophilus influenzae	ampicillin	a tetracycline;[5] cephalosporin[3]
Streptococcus pyogenes (Group A)	a penicillin[1]	an erythromycin;[2] lincomycin
* Staphylococcus aureus		
non-penicillinase-producing	a penicillin[1]	an erythromycin; lincomycin
penicillinase-producing	a penicillinase-resistant penicillin[1]	an erythromycin; lincomycin; a cephalosporin;[3] vancomycin[4]
Klebsiella and other gram-negative bacilli	(see page 129)	
Rickettsia	a tetracycline[5]	chloramphenicol[4]
Agent of psittacosis	a tetracycline[5]	chloramphenicol[4]
Mycobacterium tuberculosis (in children)	isoniazid combined with either aminosalicylic acid or ethambutol, with or without streptomycin	pyrazinamide;[4] cycloserine;[4] ethionamide;[4] viomycin;[4] kanamycin (P);[4] apreomycin;[4,18] an erythromycin
Pasteurella pestis (bubonic plague)	a tetracycline (P)[4,5]	streptomycin[4]
Systemic fungi	(see page 129)	(see page 130)
Abscess		
* Streptococcus anaerobius	penicillin G (P)	a tetracycline[5]
* Bacteroides	a tetracycline[5]	ampicillin, chloramphenicol[4]
* Staphylococcus aureus		
non-penicillinase-producing	a penicillin[1]	an erythromycin; lincomycin
penicillinase-producing	a penicillinase-resistant penicillin[1]	an erythromycin; lincomycin; a cephalosporin;[3] vancomycin[4]
Klebsiella[12]	gentamicin[4] with or without a cephalosporin[4]	Kanamycin (P);[4,14] a polymyxin (P);[4] chloramphenicol[4]

Table 1. (*Continued*)

INFECTING ORGANISM	DRUG OF FIRST CHOICE†	ALTERNATIVE DRUGS†
Abscess (*Continued*)		
Enterobacter (Aerobacter)	gentamicin[4]	a tetracycline,[5] with or without streptomycin,[4] a polymyxin (P)[4] kanamycin[4]
Gastrointestinal Tract		
* Salmonella	chloramphenicol[4]	ampicillin
* Escherichia coli (especially in infants)	kanamycin (oral)[4]	ampicillin; a tetracycline[5]
* Shigella	ampicillin	a tetracycline[5]
* Staphylococcus aureus (enterocolitis)		
non-penicillinase-producing	a penicillin[1]	
penicillinase-producing	a penicillinase-resistant penicillin[1]	an erythromycin; lincomycin; a cephalosporin,[3] vancomycin[4]
Vibrio cholerae (cholera)[13]	a tetracycline[5]	an erythromycin
Treponema pallidum (anus)	penicillin G (P)	an erythromycin (P); a tetracycline (P)[4,5]
Female Genital Tract		
Vagina		
Candida albicans	amphotericin B[4,23]	nystatin[23] (oral or topical)
Neisseria gonorrhoeae	a penicillin[1]	an erythromycin; a tetracycline[5]
Streptococcus pyogenes (Group A)	a penicillin[1]	an erythromycin;[2] lincomycin
Coliform bacilli (see page 128)		
Treponema pallidum	penicillin G (P)	an erythromycin (P); a tetracycline (P)[4,5]
Uterus		
* Streptococcus anaerobius	penicillin G (P)	a tetracycline[5]
* Clostridium[9]	penicillin G (P)	a tetracycline (P)[4,5]
Escherichia coli (or other gram-negative bacilli)	kanamycin (see page 129)	ampicillin; a tetracycline
Streptococcus pyogenes (Groups A, B, C, and E)	a penicillin[1]	an erythromycin;[2] lincomycin
* Bacteroides	a tetracycline[4]	ampicillin; chloramphenicol[4]
* Neisseria gonorrhoeae	a penicillin[1]	an erythromycin; a tetracycline[5]
Treponema pallidum	penicillin G (P)	an erythromycin (P); a tetracycline (P)[4,5]
Fallopian Tubes		
* Neisseria gonorrhoeae	a penicillin[1]	an erythromycin; a tetracycline[5]
Escherichia coli (or other gram-negative bacilli)	kanamycin[14] (see page 129)	ampicillin; a tetracycline[5]
* Streptococcus anaerobius	penicillin G (P)	a tetracycline[5]
Urinary Tract		
Neisseria gonorrhoeae (urethra)	a penicillin[1]	an erythromycin; a tetracycline[5]
Escherichia coli (or other gram-negative bacilli)	kanamycin[14] (see page 130)	ampicillin; a tetracycline[5]
Staphylococcus aureus (after surgery)		
non-penicillinase-producing	a penicillin[1]	an erythromycin; lincomycin
penicillinase-producing	a penicillinase-resistant penicillin[1]	an erythromycin; lincomycin; a cephalosporin,[3] vancomycin[4]

Table 1. (*Continued*)

Infecting Organism	Drug of First Choice†	Alternative Drugs†
Urinary tract (Continued)		
Enterococcus	penicillin G (P) with strepto-mycin[4]	vancomycin[4] with streptomycin[4]
Candida albicans	amphotericin B[4,23]	nystatin[23] (oral or topical)
Treponema pallidum (urethra)	penicillin G (P)	an erythromycin (P); a tetra-cycline (P)[4,5]
* Mima (urethra)	kanamycin (P)[4]	a polymyxin (P);[4] a sulfonamide gentamicin[4]
Meninges		
Neisseria meningitidis	penicillin G (P)	a sulfonamide (P);[4,6] a tetra-cycline[4,5]
Haemophilus influenzae[17] (in children under 5 years old)	ampicillin (P)	chloramphenicol[4] with or without streptomycin
Diplococcus pneumoniae	a penicillin[1]	an erythromycin,[2] lincomycin
Streptococcus pyogenes (Group A)	a penicillin[1]	an erythromycin;[2] lincomycin
Escherichia coli (or other gram-negative bacilli)	ampicillin (see page 128)	kanamycin (P);[4,14] a polymyxin (P);[4] a tetracycline (P);[4,5] carboni-cillin, gentamicin[4]
* Staphylococcus aureus (after surgery)		
non-penicillinase-producing	a penicillin[1]	an erythromycin; lincomycin
penicillinase-producing	a penicillinase-resistant penicillin[1]	an erythromycin; lincomycin; a cephalosporin;[3] vancomycin[4]
Mycobacterium tuberculosis	isoniazid combined with either aminosalicylic acid or etham-butol, with or without strepto-mycin[4]	pyrazinamide;[4] cycloserine;[4] ethionamide;[4] viomycin;[4] kana-mycin[4] (P); capreomycin; an ery-thromycin; rafampin
Cryptococcus neoformans	amphotericin B[4]	no dependable alternative
* Listeria monocytogenes	an erythromycin	a penicillin,[1] a tetracycline[5]
Bones (Osteomyelitis)		
* Staphylococcus aureus		
non-penicillinase-producing	a penicillin[1]	an erythromycin; lincomycin
penicillinase-producing	a penicillinase-resistant penicillin[1]	an erythromycin; lincomycin; a cephalosporin,[3] vancomycin[4]
* Salmonella[11] (or other gram-negative bacilli)	chloramphenicol[4] (see page 129)	ampicillin
Streptococcus pyogenes (Group A)	a penicillin[1]	an erythromycin;[2] lincomycin
Joints		
* Staphylococcus aureus		
non-penicillinase-producing	a penicillin[1]	an erythromycin; lincomycin
penicillinase-producing	a penicillinase-resistant penicillin[1]	an erythromycin; lincomycin; a cephalosporin;[3] vancomycin[4]
Streptococcus pyogenes (Group A)	a penicillin[1]	an erythromycin;[2] lincomycin
* Neisseria gonorrhoeae[7]	a penicillin[1]	an erythromycin; a tetracycline[5]
Gram-negative bacilli	a penicillin[1] (see page 129)	
Diplococcus pneumoniae	a penicillin[1]	an erythromycin;[2] lincomycin
Neisseria meningitidis (in epidemics)	penicillin G (P)	a sulfonamide (P); a tetracycline
Endocardium		
Viridans group of Strepto-coccus	a penicillin[1] with or without streptomycin[4]	vancomycin[4] with or without streptomycin[4]

Table 1. (*Continued*)

INFECTING ORGANISM	DRUG OF FIRST CHOICE†	ALTERNATIVE DRUGS†
Endocardium (*Continued*)		
Enterococcus	penicillin G (P) with strepto-mycin	vancomycin with streptomycin
* Staphylococcus aureus		
non-penicillinase-producing	a penicillin[1]	an erythromycin; lincomycin
penicillinase-producing	a penicillinase-resistant penicillin[1]	an erythromycin; lincomycin; a cephalosporin;[3] vancomycin[4]
* Streptococcus anaerobius	penicillin G (P)	a tetracycline[5]
Streptococcus pyogenes (Group A)	a penicillin[1]	an erythromycin;[2] lincomycin
Gram-negative bacilli	(see page 129)	
Diplococcus pneumoniae	a penicillin[1]	a erythromycin; lincomycin
Candida albicans	amphotericin B[4,23]	nystatin[23] (oral or topical)
Blood (*Septicemia*)		
Newborn Infants		
* Escherichia coli (or other gram-negative bacilli)	kanamycin[14] (see page 129)	ampicillin; a tetracycline[5]
* Straphylococcus aureus		
non-penicillinase-producing	a penicillin[1]	an erythromycin; lincomycin
penicillinase-producing	a penicillinase-resistant penicillin[1]	an erythromycin; lincomycin; a cephalosporin;[3] vancomycin[4]
Streptococcus pyogenes (Group A)	a penicillin[1]	an erythromycin;[2] lincomycin
Children		
Neisseria meningitidis	penicillin G (P)	a sulfonamide (P);[4,6] a tetracycline (P)[4,5]
Haemophilus influenzae	ampicillin	a tetracycline;[5] a cephalosporin[3]
Diplococcus pneumoniae	a penicillin[1]	an erythromycin;[2] lincomycin
Escherichia coli (or other gram-negative bacilli)	kanamycin[14] (see page 129)	ampicillin; a tetracycline[5]
* Staphylococcus aureus		
non-penicillinase-producing	a penicillin[1]	an erythromycin; lincomycin
penicillinase-producing	a penicillinase-resistant penicillin[1]	an erythromycin; lincomycin; a cephalosporin;[3] vancomycin[4]
Streptococcus pyogenes (Group A)	a penicillin[1]	an erythromycin;[2] lincomycin
Adults		
* Staphylococcus aureus		
non-penicillinase-producing	a penicillin[1]	an erythromycin; lincomycin
penicillinase-producing	a penicillinase-resistant penicillin[1]	an erythromycin; lincomycin; a cephalosporin;[3] vancomycin[4]
Diplococcus pneumoniae	a penicillin[1]	an erythromycin;[2] lincomycin
Escherichia coli	kanamycin[4]	ampicillin; a tetracycline[5]
Salmonella (or other gram-negative bacilli)	chloramphenicol[4] (see page 129)	ampicillin
Streptococcus pyogenes (Group A)	a penicillin[1]	an erythromycin;[2] lincomycin
Neisseria meningitidis	penicillin G (P)	a sulfonamide (P);[4,6] a tetracycline (P)[4,5]
* Bacteroides	a tetracycline[5]	ampicillin; chloramphenicol[4]
Candida albicans	amphotericin B[4,23]	nystatin[23] (oral or topical)
Peritoneum		
Escherichia coli	kanamycin[4]	ampicillin; a tetracycline[5]
Enterococcus	penicillin G (P) with strepto-mycin[4]	vancomycin with streptomycin[1]
* Bacteroides (or other gram-negative bacilli)	a tetracycline[5] (see page 129)	ampicillin; chloramphenicol[4]
* Streptococcus anaerobius	penicillin G (P)	an erythromycin (P); a tetracycline (P)[5]

Table 1. (*Continued*)

Infecting Organism	Drug of First Choice†	Alternative Drugs†
Peritoneum (Continued)		
* Clostridium[9]	penicillin G (P)	a tetracycline[4,5]
Diplococcus pneumoniae	a penicillin[1]	an erythromycin,[2] lincomycin
Gram-negative bacilli		
* Salmonella[11]	chloramphenicol[4]	ampicillin
* Shigella	ampicillin	a tetracycline[5]
* Escherichia coli[12]		
enteropathogenic[13]	kanamycin (oral)[14]	ampicillin; a tetracycline[5]
sepsis	ampicillin (P)	kanamycin (P); a polymyxin (P); a tetracycline (P)
* Enterobacter (Aerobacter)[12]	gentamicin[4]	a tetracycline[5] with or without streptomycin;[4] a polymyxin (P);[4] kanamycin[4]
* Klebsiella pneumoniae[12]	gentamicin[4] with or without a cephalosporin[3]	kanamycin (P);[4,14] a polymyxin (P);[4] chloramphenicol[4]
Gram-negative bacilli		
* Proteus mirabilis[12,15]	ampicillin	kanamycin (P);[4,14] a cephalosporin;[3] gentamicin[4]
other Proteus[12,15]	kanamycin (P)[4,14]	
* Pseudomonas aeruginosa[12]	gentamicin[4] (P); carbenicillin (P)	nalidixic acid; a tetracycline;[5] gentamicin;[4] corbenicillin
Actinobacillus mallei (glanders)	streptomycin[4] with a tetracycline[5]	a polymyxin (P)[4] streptomycin[4] with chloramphenicol[4]
* Pseudomonas pseudomallei (melioidosis)	a tetracycline[5] with or without a sulfonamide	chloramphenicol[4] with or without a sulfonamide; kanamycin (P)[4,14]
* Brucella (brucellosis)	a tetracycline[5]	
* Francisella (Pasteurella) tularensis (tularemia)	streptomycin[4]	a tetracycline[5]
Pasteurella pestis (bubonic plague)	a tetracycline (P)[4,5]	streptomycin[4]
Haemophilus influenzae respiratory infections	ampicillin	a tetracycline;[5] a cephalosporin[3]
* meningitis[17]	ampicillin (P)	chloramphenicol (P)[4] with or without streptomycin[4]
* Bacteroides	a tetracycline[5]	ampicillin; chloramphenicol[4]
Haemophilus ducreyi (chancroid)	a tetracycline[5]	a sulfonamide; streptomycin[4]
Bordetella (Haemophilus) pertussis (whooping cough)	ampicillin	a tetracycline[5]
* Mima, Herellea	kanamycin (P)[4]	a polymyxin (P);[4] a sulfonamide, gentamicin[4]
Fusobacterium fusiforme (Vincent's infection)	a penicillin[1]	a tetracycline;[5] an erythromycin
Calymmatobacterium granulomatis (granuloma inguinale)	ampicillin	a tetracycline;[5] streptomycin[4]
Vibrio cholerae (cholera)[13]	a tetracycline[5]	an erythromycin
Fungi		
Histoplasma capsulatum	amphotericin B[4]	no dependable alternative
Candida albicans	amphotericin B[4,23]	nystatin[23] (oral or topical)
Aspergillus	amphotericin B[4]	no dependable alternative
Cryptococcus neoformans	amphotericin B[4]	no dependable alternative
Mucor	amphotericin B[4]	no dependable alternative
Coccidioides immitis	amphotericin B[4]	no dependable alternative
Blastomyces dermatitidis (N. Amer.)	amphotericin B[4]	2-hydroxystilbamidine[4]
Blastomyces brasiliensis (S. Amer.)	amphotericin B[4]	a sulfonamide
Sporotrichum schenckii	an iodide	amphotericin B;[4] griseofulvin
Fonsecaea (chromoblastomycosis)	amphotericin B[4,24]	no dependable alternative
Dermatophytes (tinea, etc.)	griseofulvin[25]	no alternative systemic drug

[1] Penicillins should always be used with awareness of the possibility of hypersensitivity reactions. Potassium penicillin G, penicillin V, or phenethicillin can be used for oral treatment of infections by non-penicillinase-producing staphylococci and other cocci. Although penicillin G is more susceptible to gastric acid degradation than is penicillin V or phenethicillin, adequate amounts are absorbed if it is taken on an empty stomach. For initial therapy of severe infections, crystalline penicillin G, administered parenterally, is first choice. For somewhat longer action in less severe infections, procaine penicillin G aqueous, an intramuscular formulation, is administered once or twice daily. Benzathine penicillin G, a longer-acting intramuscular preparation, is used for treatment at intervals of a week or 10 days, and for prophylaxis against rheumatic fever, at intervals of a month. For oral use against penicillinase-producing staphylococci, cloxacillin or dicloxacillin is preferred; for severe infections, a parenteral formulation of nafcillin, methicillin, or oxacillin should be used. Penicillinase-resistant penicillins should be used only against penicillinase-producing staphylococci. Ampicillin is not effective against penicillinase-producing staphylococci. Carbenicillin is available for treatment of Pseudomonas infections.

[2] Some strains of Group A streptococci and pneumococci are resistant to erythromycin.

[3] The cephalosporins—cephalothin and cephaloridine—are effective against many coccal and some gram-negative bacillary infections. Both are administered only parenterally. Cephalothin is more effective than cephaloridine against penicillinase-producing staphylococci. Renal toxicity restricts the usefulness of cephaloridine in patients with impaired renal function. Except against Klebsiella, for which a cephalosporin is the drug of choice, these drugs have been used chiefly as alternatives to penicillins in patients with severe infections who are allergic to penicillins. The cephalosporins can also induce hypersensitivity reactions, and cross-sensitivity with penicillins occurs.

[4] Because of the frequency of serious adverse effects, the drug should be used only in severe infections or when less hazardous drugs are ineffective.

[5] Many different systemic tetracycline drugs are now available. Tetracycline hydrochloride and phosphate complex, chlortetracycline, and oxytetracycline are available in both oral and parenteral formulations; tetracycline base, demeclocycline, methacycline, and doxycycline are available only for oral use and rolitetracycline only for parenteral use. (See page 132 for adverse effects of tetracyclines, which are sometimes serious.)

[6] Sulfonamide-resistant strains are not frequent at present in the civilian population of the United States, but susceptibility should be established either by susceptibility tests or by clinical experience in the community. A soluble sulfonamide such as sulfisoxazole diolamine or sodium sulfadiazine should be administered intravenously. An oral soluble sulfonamide can be used for prophylaxis in contacts of patients with meningococcemia or meningitis.

[7] Some strains of gonococci are relatively resistant to penicillin G, penicillin V, and phenethicillin, and very large doses may be required.

[8] Débridement is primary; the value of antitoxin is not certain; large doses (at least 30 million units daily) of penicillin G are required. Hyperbaric oxygen therapy may be needed.

[9] For prophylaxis, proper débridement and a fluid toxoid booster dose are primary. If the patient has not received previous toxoid immunization, tetanus immunoglobulin (human) in doses of at least 3000 units should be administered. Clinicians disagree over the usefulness of including penicillin G for prophylaxis or therapy.

[10] Antitoxin is primary; antibiotics are used only to halt further toxin production and prevent the carrier state.

[11] Chloramphenicol, oral or parenteral, is the first choice for Salmonella typhi; either chloramphenicol or parenteral ampicillin can be used for other severe systemic Salmonella infections. Most cases of Salmonella gastroenteritis subside spontaneously without antimicrobial therapy. The drug of choice for S. typhi carriers is ampicillin.

[12] If the organism is responsible for an acute uncomplicated lower urinary tract infection, the drug of first choice is one of the oral soluble sulfonamides, such as sulfisoxazole, sulfisomidine, sulfamethizole, or trisulfapyrimidines, with oral ampicillin or an oral tetracycline as an alternative. If there is no improvement after 48 hours, or if the urinary tract infection is chronic, recurrent, severe, or if it involves the kidneys, cultures and susceptibility tests should be used in selecting an effective drug. Among other drugs useful for urinary tract infections are nitrofurantoin, methenamine mandelate, and methenamine hippurate.

[13] Antibiotic therapy is an adjunct to and not a substitute for prompt fluid and electrolyte replacement.

[14] Neomycin can be used as the therapeutic equivalent or kanamycin, although there is some evidence that kanamycin is a little less hazardous than neomycin.

[15] Ampicillin is often the most active drug (as determined by susceptibility tests) against Proteus mirabilis, but large doses (6 Gm or more daily) are usually necessary. Large doses (about 20 million units) of penicillin G have also been effective.

[16] Carbenicillin has recently been approved by the FDA.

[17] Consultants are divided as to the first-choice drug; most prefer ampicillin administered intravenously until the results of susceptibility tests are known.

Table 1. *(Continued)* **131**

[18] Not yet (January, 1971) approved for marketing in the United States.

[19] In spite of frequently encountered resistance of atypical mycobacteria to most antituberculosis drugs, intense vigorous chemotherapy with combinations of drugs (guided by drug susceptibility tests) can be effective.

[20] Acetosulfone, dapsone, sulfoxone sodium, or glucosulfone sodium.

[21] A clear-cut choice is difficult because of paucity of data.

[22] Methisazone is an investigational drug not yet approved for marketing by the FDA in the United States, but it can be obtained by application to the manufacturer, Burroughs Wellcome, Tuckahoe, New York.

[23] Amphotericin B administered intravenously is first choice for systemic Candida infections; where oral or topical therapy is indicated, nystatin is preferable to amphotericin B.

[24] Amphotericin B administered subcutaneously beneath lesions.

[25] Oral griseofulvin (micronized) should be used when topical drugs are ineffective.

Table 2. Adverse Effects of Antimicrobial Drugs*

	Lupus-like Syndrome	Depression of Oral Anticoagulate Activity	Elevated Serum Uric Acid	Vestibular Damage	Vasculitis	Urticaria	Thrombophlebitis	Thyroid Enlargement	Stomatitis	Staining of Teeth	Renal Damage	Rash	Psychosis	Interference with Protein Metabolism	Photosensitivity	Peripheral Neuropathy	Optic Neuritis	Neonatal Hyperbilirubinemia	Malabsorption	Liver Damage	Jaundice
p-Aminosalicylic Acid (PAS)								O			O	O							O	O	
Amphotericin B (P)							F				F	R				R				R	
Bacitracin (P)											F										
Cephaloridine (Loridine)							R				O										
Cephalothin (Keflin)							O														
Chloramphenicol																R	R				
Colistimethate (Coly-Mycin) (P)											O					O					
Cycloserine (Seromycin)													R			O			O	O	
Erythromycin									O												O
Ethambutol											R					R	O				
Ethionamide																O				O	
Gentamicin (P)				O							O	O									
Griseofulvin	R	F									R				O						
Isoniazid												R	R			O	R			O	
Kanamycin (Kantrex) (P)											O					R					
Lincomycin (Lincocin)																					
Methenamine Mandelate (Mandelamine)																					
Nalidixic Acid (gram neg.)													F		F						R
Neomycin (P)											O					R					
Nitrofurantoin (Furadantin)																O					R
Novobiocin (Albamycin)																				F	F
Nystatin (Mycostatin)																					
Paromomycin											F(P)								R		
Penicillin											R	F									R
Polymyxin (P)											O					O					
Pyrazinamide			R													R				O	
Streptomycin (P)				F																	
Sulfonamides					O						O	F			F					O	F
Tetracyclines														R	O					O	O(P)
Traleandomycin (Cyclamycin)									O												O
Vancomycin (Vancocin) (P)						O					O					R					
Viomycin											O	O									

F—Frequent
O—Occasional
R—Rare
(P)—Generally occurs with parenteral administration

Table 2. (*Continued*)

Hypotension	Hypomagnesemia	Hypokalemia	Hyperkalemia	Hyperglycemia	Gynecomastia	Gray Syndrome in Infants	Glossitis	GI Disturbances	Febrile Reactions	Enterocolitis	Eighth Nerve Damage	Dysuria	Diabetes Out of Control	Crystalluria	Coomb's Test	Convulsions	Confusion	Coma	CNS Disturbance	Bone Lesions	Blurred Vision	Blood Dyscrasia	Apnea	Anemia	Anaphylaxis	Allergic Reactions	Acidosis	Abnormalities in Porphyrin Metabolism
		R						F														O				O	R	
R	O	F						R	F						R						R	R			O	R		F
																						O						
																						R		O	O			
														F								R		O	O			
						O		O	R													O		O		R		
																									R	R		
																F	F							O				
								O																		R		
																										R		
					O			F					O													O		
								O											R			R				O		O
			R					O	O						R							R				R		
											F											R	R			R		
								O														O				O		
								O			O	O																
								F								R		O				R						
								F														R	R			R		
								F														O				O		
								F														O				F		
								O																		O		
								F			O(P)															R		
			R													O	R		R						R	O	F	
																							R			R		
			R																			R	R			O		
									F													O				F		
								F		O									R	F		R				R		
								O																		R		
									O		F																	
		O									F																	

Chapter Nine

Burns

By RONALD N. OLLSTEIN, M.D.

Assistant Attending Surgeon, Section of Plastic Surgery,
St. Vincent's Hospital and Medical Center of New York, New York.

Burn injury is fundamentally a heat-transfer phenomenon. While the source of the heat may vary, the end result is always tissue destruction, most obvious in the skin, but with significant multisystem injury that can critically affect lung, kidney and liver. The systemic effects and mortality following burn injury are directly related to the extent and depth of skin destruction. Most burns are caused by flame or by scalding with hot liquid. Determining the heat source, i.e., the agent which caused the burn, will aid in predicting the usual extent and depth of injury. These determinations are of value in planning proper intravenous fluid therapy.

CAUSES AND SEVERITY OF BURNS

CAUSE	EXTENT	DEPTH
Flame	Great	Deep
Scald	Moderate	Superfical and/or deep
Flash	Limited to exposed parts	Superficial
Contact	Limited	Superficial
Electrical	Limited	Deep
Chemical	Limited	Deep

EXTENT OF BURN

The *"rule of nines,"* while only approximate, remains a reasonable guide to assessment of extent of burns: head, 7 per cent and neck, 2 per cent for a total of 9 per cent; each upper extremity, 9 per cent; the anterior trunk, 2 × 9 or 18 per cent; the posterior trunk, 13 per cent, buttocks, 5 per cent, for a total of 18 per cent; each lower extremity, 2 × 9, 18 per cent; and the genitalia, 1 per cent.

For scattered areas of burn, one may estimate on the basis that the area of the patient's hand and fingers with fingers adducted is equal to about 1 per cent of his total body surface.

There is a difference in relative body surface areas in the *child*, who in general has a much greater proportion of *head* surface to lower extremities than the adult. The head area is 19 per cent at birth (10 per cent more than in the adult); this occurs at the expense of the two lower extremities, which would then be 13 per cent each. With each year of age up to ten, 1 per cent is subtracted from the head area and added in equal amounts to each lower limb. After ten years of age, adult percentages are used.

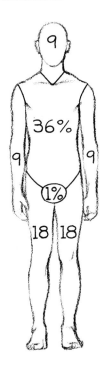

DEPTH OF BURN

First degree burn is a superficial injury with destruction of the outer layer of epidermis. Clinically it presents with erythema. The most usual cause is sunburn. Within several days following exposure, the dead outer epidermis "peels," and a complete epithelial layer is regenerated from the underlying intact epidermis.

Second degree burn is the destruction of the entire epidermis and part of the underlying dermis. Secondary skin appendages, which are epithelial structures (sweat glands, sebaceous glands, hair follicles), persist in the deeper part of this wound, which therefore qualifies as a *partial thickness* burn. The second degree burn is characterized by *pain*, a *moist* pink-red mottled coloration and *blister* formation. Scald, flash and contact exposures usually inflict superficial burns. Within three to four days, the burn surface dries to a thin tan-brown parchment-like crust. Within the next several weeks, separation of the crust occurs as regeneration of a new but thinner epithelium occurs from the

deeply placed, unburned bases of the epithelial skin appendages. Spontaneous healing, therefore, is the rule in this superficial or partial-thickness burn.

Third degree burn usually involves the destruction of the *entire skin thickness.* Even if the entire skin is not destroyed, however, a burn is considered third degree if all the secondary skin appendages are destroyed and no capacity for spontaneous skin regeneration (re-epithelialization) remains. This full thickness or deep burn, usually caused by flame, electricity or chemicals, may be *pearly-white* and is usually *non-blistered, dry* and relatively anesthetic. Within several days, the deep burn wound develops a thick, tight, leathery black eschar.

CRITERIA FOR HOSPITALIZATION

1. Any suspicion of respiratory tract injury—a history of flame burn, particularly one which occurred indoors, smoke inhalation, loss of consciousness, together with coughing, voice change, labored breathing or disorientation—is an indication for admission.

2. Any superficial burn greater than 9 per cent of body surface area.

3. Any deep burn greater than 3 per cent of body surface area.

4. Burn of critical part: burns so located that they induce significant pain, obvious inability to render self-care, or threaten critical disability—such as in instances of damage to eyes, ears, face in general, hands, feet or genitalia—require hospitalization.

5. Associated injury; the lesser burn, when compounded by other injury such as fracture, extensive laceration or blunt trauma to chest or abdomen, also require hospitalization.

INITIAL EVALUATION

The sequence of emergency treatments will depend on an initial over-all evaluation of the patient, which should include the following:

A. Respiratory function

B. Mental status—confusion, agitation, delirium, stupor or coma can be indicative of hypoxia on the basis of respiratory tract injury and/or burn shock

C. Extent of burn, expressed in per cent of body surface area

D. Depth of burn: third degree burns (deep, full thickness) have far greater significance than second degree burns (superficial, partial thickness injury)

E. Site of burns; note particularly face and head area, eyes, ears, hands, feet and genitalia

F. Age of patient

G. Any pre-existing disease states

H. Associated injuries

IMMEDIATE TREATMENT

Attention is then directed to instituting prompt therapy. The following is an outline of such care:

A. Airway—oxygenation

B. Intravenous fluid therapy

C. Urinary bladder catheter

D. Analgesia

E. Flow sheet

F. Gastrointestinal decompression

G. Tetanus prophylaxis

H. Antibiotics

I. Vitamins

J. Digitalis

K. Laboratory analyses:
1. Blood: hematocrit, type and cross match, urea nitrogen, electrolytes, pH, gases (pO_2, pCO_2)
2. Urine: analysis, including specific gravity and hemoglobin determinations
3. X-rays: chest and others as dictated by associated injuries
4. Electrocardiogram

L. Burn wound care

AIRWAY

A secure airway must be provided immediately. Respiratory tract injury is caused mainly by the inhalation of superheated, noxious, particulate products of combustion, which results in rapidly progressive respiratory tract *edema, hemorrhage* and *alveolar-capillary membrane disruption.*

Tracheostomy is indicated in the patient with depressed mental status, frank respiratory tract injury, extensive flame-burn injury with deep neck, face or head burns, or in one in whom progressive respiratory insufficiency with labored breathing, rapid respiratory rate or chemical (blood gas) deterioration is apparent. It is essential that humidified oxygen be administered by nasal catheter or mask with suction as required.

Oxygen can be administered by bubbling it through a wetting solution containing the mucolytic heparin, as well as antibiotics and steroids in a saline base. Detergent agents and topical bronchodilators may also be used. Systemic steroids administered intravenously in high doses (hydrocortisone 1000 mg.) have been used on a single dose basis to relieve bronchospasm as often as every four to six hours around-the-clock.

INTRAVENOUS FLUID THERAPY

The basic pathophysiologic change occurring after a burn is local blood vessel damage with increased capillary permeability and massive and immediate loss of fluid into burned tissues. This vast leakage and shift of fluid and electrolytes, particularly sodium, results in a circulating volume deficit, or *hypovolemic* shock. Further fluid losses by evaporative water loss through the burn-damaged body surface worsen the hypovolemic state.

Rapid intravenous infusion of large amounts of electrolyte-containing fluid, e.g., lactated Ringer's solution, is the basis for *burn shock resuscitation.* A secure intravenous line is required by cutdown if necessary, and the insertion of a long, preferably radio-opaque, catheter into the central venous spaces near the right atrium is recommended. Fluid therapy should be started with lactated Ringer's solution at a *rapid rate until a urine flow is established;* thereafter, more specific intravenous fluid titration is indicated, using essentially lactated Ringer's or a similar crystalloid solution based in part on formula calculations and more importantly on hourly re-evaluations of patient response. The Brook formula, introduced in 1953, offers a reasonable quantitative approach to the first 48 hours of fluid therapy; it is restated here not as an infallible rule, but as a rough *guide.*

First 24 hours—1.5 ml. electrolyte solution and 0.5 ml. colloid for each 1 per cent body surface area burn per kilogram of body weight plus 2000 ml. non-electrolyte-containing fluid.

Second 24 Hours—one-half of the first day's electrolyte and colloid requirements plus 2000 ml. non-electrolyte-containing fluid.

Electrolyte solution stresses sodium and indicates its administration in a balanced (plasma electrolyte pattern) form, as in lactated Ringer's solution. Higher sodium concentration solutions, e.g., 225 mEq. per liter, may permit adequate electrolyte replacement in a smaller total volume with less risk of overhydration. This might be of advantage among the very young, the very elderly and those with pulmonary damage.

Colloid refers to Dextran or Plasmanate, both high molecular weight products in electrolyte solutions. Whole blood is not indicated in the early postburn period when high hematocrit values and small vessel sludging and thrombosis are common. Should hematocrit values below 32 per cent be repeatedly verified, blood replacement would be necessary.

The suggestion of 2000 cc. of non-electrolyte-containing fluid (5 per cent dextrose in water) per day is based on the usual daily adult requirement for water. Estimates of daily water needs in children based on age are: birth to three

months, 700 cc; four to six months, 1000 cc; seven to 12 months, 1200 cc; and a subsequent gradual climb to the adult daily water requirement of 2000 cc. at age 14 years.

The "rule of 50" must be considered in all formulas based on per cent of body surface area burned. *Fifty per cent* is the maximum figure for the purpose of calculating fluid needs regardless of the per cent of body surface area burned beyond 50 per cent.

As an example of fluid calculation, consider a 50 per cent body surface area burn in a man weighing 70 Kg.:

First 24 hours:

Lactated Ringer's solution	$1.5 \times 50 \times 70 = 5250$ ml.
Plasmanate	$0.5 \times 50 \times 70 = 1750$
5 per cent dextrose in water	2000
Total	9000 ml.

Second 24 hours:

Lactated Ringer's solution	$5250/2 = 2625$ ml.
Plasmanate	$1750/2 = 875$
5 per cent dextrose in water	2000
Total	5500 ml.

The quantity and rate of administration of electrolyte-containing fluid with prompt establishment of urine flow is probably more important than more detailed calculations, since no formula will supersede clinical and chemical monitoring of the patient's response to treatment.

Central venous pressure is monitored in the vena cava via a long catheter. If pressure is not significantly elevated and not rapidly rising, fluid therapy is probably not excessive.

URINARY BLADDER CATHETER

Urine output provides the single best objective guide to the adequacy of fluid replacement. Preferred urine flows would be as follows: children under age one year, 8 to 20 cc. per hour; children, ages one to six years, 20 to 30 cc. per hour; children, ages 7 to 14 years, 30 to 50 cc. per hour; adults, 50 to 70 cc.

per hour. If a low urine output persists despite usual fluid infusions and if this is *not* associated with obvious signs of overhydration such as progressive edema, pulmonary rales and a rising central venous pressure, a *fluid challenge* is indicated to differentiate between inadequate fluid therapy and renal failure. The rapid infusion of 1500 cc. of lactated Ringer's solution is effected. A clear-cut rise in urine flow would indicate the need for additional fluid, while no change in flow would demand a reduction in infusion rate and suggest a diagnosis of renal damage. If a low urine flow is noted and total fluid volume replacement seems adequate, the use of Mannitol is indicated. Mannitol may be used in 25 gram doses intravenously every 4 to 6 hours, depending upon the patient's response. Such therapy is particularly important if hemoglobinuria occurs, especially if adequate urine flows are not being achieved with apparently large amounts of electrolyte infusion.

Analgesia

Analgesia is best provided by *Demerol* administered *intravenously* (our dose 0.5 mg./Kg.). This can be repeated every 2 to 4 hours as necessary.

Flow Sheet

A flow sheet normally lists the following observations:
1. *Mental status* remains clear if adequate oxygenation and circulating volume are maintained and electrolyte pattern is relatively normal.
2. *Respiratory status,* recording the ease and rate of respirations, complements the same considerations of oxygenation and circulating volume as noted in (1). Auscultation may reveal rales and other adventitious sounds if overhydration or inhalation injury produces tracheobronchial exudation,

bronchospasm or progressive pulmonary edema.
3. *Vital signs,* most specifically pulse and respiratory rates, are general indices of compensated well-being in burn shock with or without respiratory tract injury.
4. *Hourly intake and output.*
5. *Daily weight.*

Gastrointestinal and Nutritional Factors

Adequate nutritional support constitutes one of the most significant factors in the successful care of the burned patient. In the early phase after injury, intravenous feeding is indicated. The frequent occurrence of paralytic ileus and gastric dilatation contraindicates oral feeding in cases of severe burns. In lesser burn injuries, such as those covering 15 per cent of body surface area, oral electrolyte-rich fluid will be tolerated as a basis for burn shock resuscitation. The oral salt-soda solution is prepared by mixing one-half teaspoon salt and one-half teaspoon sodium bicarbonate in one quart of cold water flavored with lemon or a fruit syrup to make it more palatable. In most burn cases and in all instances of burns in excess of 15 per cent of body area, intravenous therapy becomes necessary. With clinical stabilization at three to five days after injury, intravenous fluid volumes can be decreased, and with the expression of hunger, the confirmation of active bowel sounds and hopefully a bowel movement, gradually increased oral intake can ensue. By seven to ten days after injury most adequately resuscitated victims will tolerate a large oral intake. It is essential that this great amount of food be offered when the patient is hungry in the form of appetizing meals that cater to the patient's tastes. There is an additional absolute need for increased amounts of vitamins after burns.

Curling's ulcer and gastrointestinal

ulceration, primarily in the *duodenum, stomach* and *esophagus*, may occur following burn injuries. Essential causes are hemoconcentration and postburn hyperadrenalism and sepsis. *Prophylactic antacid treatment* is necessary in all cases of major burns. Surgical intervention may be indicated, such as with bleeding or perforation; use clinical criteria similar to those in unburned patients.

TETANUS PROPHYLAXIS

This procedure is carried out as described on page 105.

ANTIBIOTICS

Systemic antibiotics are given as described on page 140.

VITAMINS

Therapeutic vitamins including at least 1 Gm. of vitamin C are given daily.

DIGITALIS

While not used routinely, digitalis should be considered in cases of massive burn (greater than 35 per cent of body surface area) particularly in the elderly and particularly when large quantities of intravenous infusions are planned.

LABORATORY ANALYSES

Hematocrit

This serves as a crude over-all guide to hydration and blood oxygen-carrying capacity. The hematocrit, usually elevated for several days following major burn trauma, will gradually decline to more normal or low values as fluid therapy progresses, volume expansion occurs and heat-damaged red blood cells die. If the hematocrit decreases to 32 per cent or less, whole blood or packed cell replacement is indicated to improve the ability of perfusion fluid—i.e., circulating medium—to oxygenate cells.

Serum Electrolytes

Serum electrolyte determination, particularly of sodium, will often indicate the need for a change in the construction of fluids administered. If serum sodium is persistently high, more sodium-free water (5 per cent dextrose in water) may be indicated. If serum sodium is low, there may be a relative increase in total body water, recommending administration of only electrolyte solution. Should a relatively satisfactory sodium concentration, in association with a high serum chloride and low serum carbon dioxide, be determined, the use of intravenous sodium bicarbonate should be considered.

Blood pH, Oxygen and Carbon Dioxide

These are indicators of critical acid-base balance and respiratory adequacy. The early chemical recognition of abnormal values may dictate the use of bicarbonate solution and force essential measures to rapidly correct an often unsuspected deteriorating respiratory state by means of techniques noted under *Airway Oxygenation* (page 136).

BURN WOUND CARE

Infection can be considered the single greatest hazard to the burned patient who survives the shock period. Burn wound infection can increase the extent of tissue destruction to a wider and deeper zone beyond that originally caused by the physical thermal trauma. Pseudomonas aeruginosa and Staphylococcus aureus are the predominant organisms in the vast majority of significant burn wound infections, while streptococci and Proteus are less frequent. Effective suppression of bacterial activity in burn wounds requires both topical antimicrobial agents and systemic antibiotics.

Topical Agents

Numerous topical drugs have been employed, all with the theoretical aim of suppressing bacterial growth in the dead tissue pablum of the burn wound. Topical therapy of burn wounds has *significant benefit*. No one topical drug has been accepted by all, and the development of new topical agents can be expected in the future. Proper technique, meticulous and intensive wound care and systemic patient support remain the keystones of care.

SILVER NITRATE. A 0.5 per cent solution has been used to continuously saturate gauze dressings applied to the burn wound. The solution is poured onto the dressings every four hours, and complete dressing changes, with or without tub baths, are performed daily. This technique has proved reasonably effective in suppressing some forms of bacterial growth. Among its impressive disadvantages are: a narrow therapeutic range, argyria of limited magnitude, formation of a *non*-antiseptic silver proteinate on the wound surface, formation of methemoglobin by the action of surface bacteria on the nitrate fraction, relative ineffectiveness of the agent to control already established infection, and incompatibility with other local physical features, such as the presence of grease and dead epidermis. *Most significant,* however, are the certain significant *electrolyte losses* into the *hypotonic silver nitrate dressings* and the marked intolerance to such shifts in burned children.

MAFENIDE ACETATE (SULFAMYLON). When applied as a 10 per cent cream, three to four times daily, directly to the otherwise exposed burn wound, mafenide acetate has proved effective in combating burn wound sepsis, especially that based on invasive Pseudomonas aeruginosa infection. The hydroscopic nature of the cream promotes the development of a clean, dry wound. Daily tubbing complements this form of topical therapy. Significant pain on application, a local allergic response in approximately 8 per cent of those treated and a metabolic acidosis, often further compromising an already burdened pulmonary oxygenation-acid-base buffer mechanism, have posed real problems in its use.

GENTAMICIN SULFATE. Particularly effective against gram-negative bacteria, gentamicin sulfate, which is also available in parenteral form, has proved satisfactory in the control of Pseudomonas burn wound sepsis, but has demonstrated toxic effects on the eighth nerve (vestibular division) and kidney tissue. It can be used in a gentamicin-impregnated gauze dressing that is changed daily with tubbing.

SILVER SULFADIAZINE. This has been used in both a "butter-on" manner similar to Sulfamylon and in an impregnated-gauze technique similar to gentamicin. It has proved painless on application to the burn wound, and while appearing to permit the development of a wetter, sloppier wound surface, it has been relatively effective in suppressing bacterial growth.

Systemic Antibiotics

Despite the obvious advances in topical burn wound antisepsis, systemic antibiotic protection remains necessary in the care of the severely burned patient. If initial prophylactic therapy is elected, penicillin appears the logical choice because of its ability to destroy most skin staphylococcal and streptococcal organisms. Subsequent antibiotic therapy should be based on bacteriologic studies.

Local Care

It is the *healing* of the burn wound that constitutes the *cure* of the disease.

The key to successful treatment of the severely burned patient rests with separation of the burned tissue and the provision of viable skin cover as early after injury as possible.

EXPOSURE. Exposure of the burned part to usual room air comprises the most practical, efficient and effective means of yielding a cool, dry and clean wound environment. Exposure may be complemented by the use of a topical antibacterial cream or ointment, the application of which generally follows an initial gentle cleansing with a dilute solution of soap and water, rinsing-irrigation of the burned surface with water and gentle drying with sterile cotton-free gauze pads or lint-free towels. Such gentle washing may be done daily in a limited manner or by whole body tubbing; exposure with or without topical agents should be permitted at all other times. Crust formation may be anticipated in the superficial injury, and crust separation and spontaneous healing may be completed within two to four weeks after injury. Eschar development, accompanied later by curling, cracking and separation with thick drainage, occurs in deep wounds. At this point, usually two to four weeks following injury, exposure may be abandoned and daily surgical débridements, tubbings and dressing procedures are instituted. Frequent changes (every four hours) of dry, sterile cotton-free gauze dressings or frequent changes of saline-soaked gauze dressings can be used to maintain free drainage of infected material and promote eschar separation. This process is continued until satisfactory granulation of tissue is achieved.

Granulations of deep red color that are flat, clean and not grossly purulent and showing initial epithelialization at the edges constitute the bed on which split-thickness skin grafts taken from another part of the body can be applied.

The *split-thickness skin graft (autograft) is the fundamental operative method of achieving burn wound closure.* The transplanted skin provides the essential epithelial cover for the granulating surface from which no spontaneous re-epithelialization is possible. The *size and thickness of a skin graft should be directly proportional to the perfection of the wound;* therefore, one would favor a smaller, thinner graft on the surface of the less ideal, granulating burn wound surface that is invariably contaminated.

Causes of a poor graft "take" are as follows: (1) poor timing of the grafting procedure—the grafts are placed on a pale, friable, edematous granulating bed; (2) hematoma formation beneath the graft; (3) failure of immobilization, with resultant distraction of the graft from the recipient bed; and (4) purulent exudation from the granulating bed secondary to excessive wound contamination.

If functional splinting or positioning of a burned part is required, skeletal traction can be used, favoring the calcaneous and tibial tubercle in the lower limb and the bases of the second and third metacarpals of the upper limb is the preferred sites for pin insertion. Such a technique could be employed with the exposure plan outlined earlier. If plaster splints are used for neck or extremity positioning, dressing of the part would be indicated and can be composed simply of an inner greased-gauze dressing. This can be an outer layer with dry sterile gauze changed in the sterile soap and water cleansing, as wound conditions require, i.e., as often as necessary to maintain a cleansed state.

HOMOGRAFTS AND HETEROGRAFTS. The use of foreign skin as temporary cover for the granulating burn wound has been effective in reducing water, electrolyte, protein and blood losses from the wound surface and in decreasing bacterial burn wound sepsis. Both the homograft (skin from another member of the same species, e.g., another human) and the heterograft (skin from a member of another species, e.g., pig or dog) have been used with similar effectiveness.

INDICATIONS. These include the following:

1. *massive burn excision in children,* with immediate postexcisional homografting; autografting is delayed until two to four days later.

2. *inadequate autograft donor sites* at a time when granulating wounds may be receptive to grafting. Homografts have been used to maintain the receptive quality of burn wounds and reduce fluid losses and sepsis while new donor sites are prepared.

3. tide patient over a *complicating intercurrent illness,* such as severe pneumonia, congestive heart failure and gastrointestinal hemorrhage by promoting the same effects as noted under (2) without the need for the additional trauma of autografting at the time.

4. *accelerate the healing of partial thickness burns.* Clinically and by histologic analysis, improved healing of second degree burn wounds has been noted to occur beneath homografts.

5. *testing of the recipient sites* prior to autografts, particularly if the certainty of graft "take" is questioned and autograft donor sites limited. If early homograft "take" is noted, immediate removal of homograft and replacement by autograft can be accomplished with greater likelihood of success.

SPECIAL CONSIDERATIONS.

1. *The electrical burn:* The electrical burn most frequently involves (a) the lip-mouth-intraoral area, (b) the hand and (c) the scalp and skull. A conservative approach is mandatory in cases of electrical burns about the oral area, permitting gradual separation of eschar, care regarding delayed bleeding and healing by split thickness skin grafts or by scar contracture. Secondary reconstructive plastic surgery is much preferred over attempts at early wound excision and complex tissue transfer repair. Head burns assume an intermediate station inasmuch as slow separation of a full thickness burn of scalp and

skull can be allowed to occur over several months, with subsequent skin-grafting to exposed dura and granulations, or radical excision of non-viable scalp and skull with immediate scalp flap reconstruction can be effected. The hand burn, usually on the palmar surface, is best treated by early excision and abdominal pedicle flap resurfacing if one is to achieve maximum salvage of nerves and tendons.

Aside from these specific anatomic, functional and cosmetic considerations peculiar to the electrical burn, the fundamentals of burn wound care as previously discussed can be applied in these instances with the more common forms of burn trauma.

2. *The chemical burn:* Most important in early chemical burn wound care is immediate, continuous and prolonged water irrigation. As in electrical burns, the destruction is usually deep, separation of slough required and skin grafting obligatory. Conservative wound management, as opposed to early excision, is generally preferred, particularly in the facial or scalp regions where assault-lye injuries are most frequent and regenerative powers great.

ICE-WATER TREATMENT. Ice-water cooling of the injured part in burns of lesser surface area (less than 20 per cent) seen shortly after injury, hopefully within the hour, can afford prompt relief of pain and prompt reduction in the temperature of the burned part with ultimate decrease in total amount of skin destruction. Compresses of ice-cold water at temperatures of 5 to 15° C., renewed every 20 minutes and continued until pain is relieved or approximately six hours have passed, are recommended.

Outpatient Care of the Lesser Burn

In the lesser burn in which hospitalization is not indicated, gentle cleansing of the burned part with dilute soap and water, rinsing and gentle drying with gauze pads are advised. Blisters may be gently debrided with sterile forceps and scissors and the entire burned area dressed with small segments of a lightly greased gauze (e.g., Adaptic or Xeroform) molded in a single layer to the wound. Cotton-free gauze roll (e.g., Kling or Kerlix) may then be applied as an outer absorbent and protective dressing. Tetanus prophylaxis is required and antibiotic therapy may be considered.

The patient is instructed to keep the burned part at rest, the dressing clean and dry, and to return for care in three to five days, or sooner if pain or fever develops or if odorous drainage on the dressing occurs. At this time the initial dressing is inspected, and if intact, clean and dry and without significant patient complaints, it may be left undisturbed. If any of the problems noted earlier are present, the outer gauze roll is removed down to the basic layer of non-adherent gauze. This innermost layer should not be disturbed if it is dry and encrusted, since it may be presumed that islands of epithelial regeneration are developing in intimate contact with it and removal would serve only to tear them away. A fresh outer cotton-free gauze roll may be reapplied. If the wound surface is wet with exudate, the innermost gauze layer will come away readily, the wound surface may be washed as initially and the basic dressing structure reapplied. This process is repeated every three to five days until healing of the superficial burn wound is complete, usually at 14 to 28 days. In this time the epithelial regeneration from deeply placed viable skin appendages will have provided a new epidermal surface and permitted the crust and innermost gauze layer to separate readily and come away as a "peel" with the dressing.

Protection of the newly healed thin, pink, sensitive surface is essential and may be provided in the form of topical lubricants such as lanolin, cocoa butter, cold cream, baby oil or lotion. Direct mechanical trauma and excessive exposure to sun should be avoided.

Chapter Ten

Minor Surgery of Skin and Superficial Tissues

EQUIPMENT

Most minor surgery requires only simple equipment. However, as a precaution, some hospitals insist that all operative procedures be done in the regular hospital operating rooms where all instruments will be available if needed. If the operating room is not used the following are needed:

FURNITURE

1. A separate room through which there is no traffic.

2. A comfortable table on which the patient can recline.

3. A tray or additional table to hold the instruments.

4. Adequate lighting—a goose neck lamp on a stand with a 100-watt bulb is satisfactory.

5. A wash basin to wash one's hands.

6. A receptacle for discarded materials.

INSTRUMENTS

The makeup of the instrument tray will vary depending upon the procedure; the average tray will consist of:

Hemostatic forceps
  Two 6-inch forceps
  Six mosquito hemostats (3 straight and 3 curved)

Scissors
  Mayo scissors, 5½-inch, either curved or straight
  1 suture scissors
  1 bandage scissors (this need not be on the sterile tray)

Scalpels
  1 Bard-Parker scalpel handle #3
  2 scalpel blades #10, #11 or #15

Retractors
  2 rake retractors, small, 3 pronged
  (A self retaining mastoid retractor is very useful.)

Forceps
  1 plain thumb forceps, dressing, 4½-inch
  1 tissue forceps, 4½-inch
  2 Allis forceps
  4 towel clips
  1 needle holder

Needles
  1 straight skin needle
  1 medium curved cutting edge needle
  1 medium curved taper point needle
Suture material (subject to preference of surgeon)
Miscellaneous
  1 culture tube
  4 sterile towels
  12 4x4 gauze squares
  2 small metal containers ⎫ This
  1 pack of cotton balls   ⎪ material
  1 10-ml. Luer-Lok syringe ⎬ is for local
    with handles   ⎪ anesthesia.
  3 needles, hypodermic #23, ⎪
    #21, and #20   ⎪
  2 medicine glasses   ⎭

PREPARATION

PATIENT

For most minor surgical procedures no preoperative medication is used. In the rare case when it seems necessary, give the medication at least 30 minutes before beginning the operation. The amount and type of sedation vary with the individual. Either a barbiturate or Demerol in appropriate dosage is satisfactory. If sedation is used the patient should be detained after operation until the effect has worn off.

Plan your schedule so that the patient will not have to wait. Make him as comfortable as possible as soon as he arrives. Have him remove clothing as necessary to provide adequate exposure of the field of operation. The most satisfactory arrangement is to have the patient disrobe and put on a hospital gown. If blood should stain his clothes advise him to remove it by soaking the garment in cold water before conventional washing.

Before the patient lies on the table ask him to scrub the operative area with generous amounts of soap and water. If the area is not readily accessible you can scrub it after it has been shaved.

Get the patient settled in a comfortable position on the table and try to put him at ease. If the patient is uncomfort-

able he will become restless during the procedure.

Remove any hair from the area to be operated upon. The short hair on relatively hairless areas, as well as the usually well endowed hairy areas, should be shaved. This can usually be done without lather by using a fresh, sharp razor blade. If the hair is long, cut it short with a scissors before shaving it. A wide area should be shaved except when the lesion is on the head where a smaller area should be shaved to avoid an unsightly postoperative appearance. The loose hairs must be removed; brushing will seldom remove all of them but they may be conveniently picked up with the adhesive side of a two inch strip of adhesive plaster.

OPERATING TEAM

The ideal team consists of the surgeon, an assistant, a nurse, and an anesthetist if necessary. Most often in practice only the surgeon and a nurse are available. The nurse is needed to get supplies for the surgeon. After all is in readiness she may also scrub and join him at the table. If she does not scrub, she can sometimes help the surgeon by holding instruments such as retractors through the sterile drapes without contaminating the field.

Don a cap and mask. Then scrub your hands and arms exactly as you would in the operating room (p. 26). Proper attire includes a sterile gown although in many hospitals a gown is not worn for minor surgery. After a routine scrub the gown and gloves are put on as described on page 29.

INSTRUMENT TRAY

The instruments should be laid out neatly on the tray. After you gown and glove, sort the instruments, grouping the various types together. Have the nurse pass you the suture material.

Open this as described on page 3. If the suture is a continuous one, cut several proper lengths and thread an appropriate needle if you alone are to scrub. If the nurse plans to scrub later, she can take care of the suture material at that time. Use quarter lengths of material for sutures. Roll an entire suture length on another tube of suture material for ties. You can hold this in your hand and tie multiple vessels. Long sutures already on a spool are available commercially.

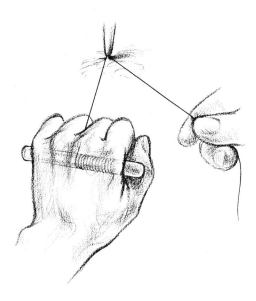

Separate the containers. Have the nurse pour alcohol into one container, the antiseptic solution into the other, and the local anesthetic solution into a medicine glass.

OPERATIVE SITE

Grasp a cotton ball with a large hemostat, soak the cotton with alcohol and use this to vigorously cleanse the operative area. Begin cleaning the skin at the point of the intended incision and gradually widen the area. Keep the skin saturated with alcohol for five minutes. Discard the cotton ball and repeat the cleansing using antiseptic solution. Repeat this once. Hand the two containers

to the nurse to allow more room on the tray.

Some institutions supply a single drape with a small opening in the center. This type of drape is applied with the opening directly over the operative area. However, more versatility is possible if four towels or rectangular drapes are applied, one on each side of the wound. They are clipped together with towel clips where

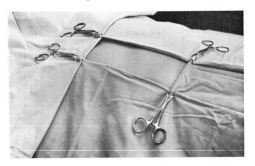

they cross, with care taken not to catch the patient's skin in the clips. If the nurse is to scrub, she can now do so and join you.

GENERAL CONSIDERATIONS

Since the patient is conscious, restrict talking to a minimum. Depend heavily on signals (p. 34) in asking for instruments. Do not cover the patient's mouth and nose with the drapes. If you are working near the patient's head place a Mayo stand or its equivalent over the patient's head to keep the drapes away from his mouth and nose and allow him to breathe comfortably.

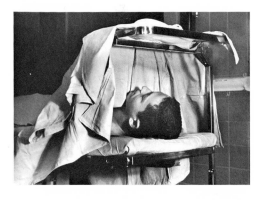

Always question the patient concerning the possibility of sensitivity to the local anesthetic agent. If there is a history of sensitivity to any one agent do not use it; there are plenty of different agents available. Make the initial local injection with your smallest needle (usually a 25-gauge). Begin subsequent injections through the area already anesthetized.

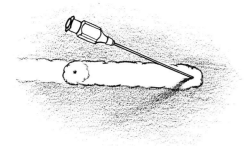

Always draw back on the syringe before you inject to make certain that you have not entered a vessel; keep the needle in motion while injecting. Detailed instructions on local anesthesia are found in Chapter 6.

Consider carefully the location of the incision. It should be placed so as not to damage an important nerve and so as to conform with the natural lines of the skin in the operative area. Never make an incision across a joint; if you do the scar will contract later and interfere with motion. The proper location for incision over a joint is the skin crease of the joint. Further exposure can be gained by extending the incision proximally and distally on either side of the extremity.

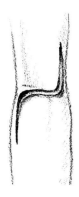

REGIONAL CONSIDERATIONS

SCALP

In most patients the scalp is covered with hair. To prepare the area, first cut the hair short with scissors. Shave an adequate operative area, but keep in mind the cosmetic effect. The field should extend approximately 1 cm. in all directions beyond the intended operative site. Local infiltration anesthesia is most satisfactory in this area. If it is conceivable that the lesion could involve the skull, investigate this possibility by an x-ray before operation. If the skull is involved the surgical problem is a major one and should be cared for by a neurosurgeon.

If the incision extends through all layers down to the bone, the galea aponeurotica must be closed separately.

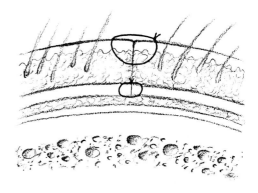

This will prevent a hematoma in the superficial layer from dissecting beneath the galea and raising the scalp from the bone.

FACE

Minor surgery about the face demands particular care. Scarring of the face or paralysis of any of the facial muscles can have tragic consequences. Before contemplating an incision of the face you must be thoroughly familiar with the anatomy of the facial nerve.

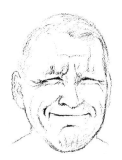

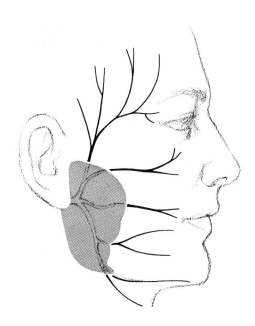

There is simply no excuse for damaging the facial nerve during minor surgery; procedures should be planned to avoid it. Obviously, major surgical procedures, particularly for malignancy, may necessitate damage to the nerve.

Incisions in the face should be made in the normal skin lines.

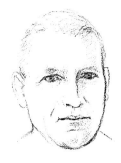

You can identify the less obvious skin lines by having the patient grimace immediately before you begin.

The location of the incision must be chosen before local infiltration with anesthetic solution is begun; the infiltration distorts the area and can mislead you as to the proper position of the incision. Keep the antiseptic solution out of the patient's eye. If working near the ear, pack it with cotton to keep out blood and antiseptic solution.

When operating about the face use fine instruments specifically developed for plastic surgery. Essentially these are smaller and more delicate than conventional instruments. Use a #15 blade on the scalpel. Use fine suture material, preferably silk (0000 to 000000). Approximate the deep tissues if necessary; this will minimize wide scarring. To close the skin use a small, round, cutting edge, plastic needle for suturing. Place the sutures just through the skin, no more than 2 mm. apart and only 2 mm. from the edge of the wound. Keep the wound covered for the first 24 hours. After that it can be left uncovered and the patient may wash directly over the area. Remove every other suture in three days and the remainder in six or seven days.

INTRAORAL. Any elective operation within the mouth should be done with an endotracheal tube in place, and no operation with a tube in place is a minor procedure. The novice must resist the temptation to operate on a minor intraoral lesion under local anesthesia; the danger of aspiration of blood is too great.

NECK

Lesions of the neck can be very deceptive; many which seem to be superficial may extend deep into the neck. Never undertake an apparently minor surgical procedure on the neck until the extent of the lesion has been appraised by someone with considerable surgical experience.

Incisions for superficial lesions in the neck should follow skin lines. These can be accentuated by having the patient flex his head. Decide on the position of the incision before you infiltrate the skin with local anesthetic solution. There will be some bleeding when you cut across vessels in the platysma. Once you have dissected below the platysma it is possible to develop a plane which allows more freedom to locate structures. The neck is crossed by many very important structures and a thorough knowledge of the anatomy of these structures is prerequisite to working in this area. For those without special training operations under local anesthesia should be restricted to the area superficial to the strap muscles.

Surgery on the deeper structures in the neck should be undertaken only when the patients have an endotracheal tube in place. Because of its abundant blood supply wounds in the neck heal rapidly. Every other skin suture should be removed in three days and the remainder in five days.

HAND

Incisions in the hand should be planned and made so as not to endanger nerves and to respect joint areas. Incisions should not be made over the pads of the fingers; when necessary in the distal portions of the phalanges they should be made over the medial or lateral aspects. When a joint is to be crossed the incision should be made down one side of the finger across the joint in the skin crease and then con-tinued down the other side of the finger.

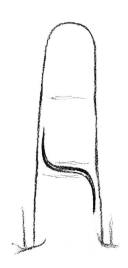

The nerve most likely to be injured is the digital nerve which lies on the medial and lateral aspect of the finger. If this is inadvertently divided, the ends should be sutured together.

Never immobilize a finger in extension because this will allow the lateral ligaments of the interphalangeal joints to shorten, causing permanent loss of joint motion. If it is necessary to immobilize the finger do so with the finger in flexion. In this position the lateral ligaments are extended. Furthermore, never immobilize more of the hand than is absolutely necessary. Sutures should be left in place for 10 days to two weeks if the wound is in position where motion puts tension on the suture line.

During operations on fingers hemostasis can be accomplished by placing a rubber band at the base of the finger. This will also enhance the effect of the anesthesia. A blood pressure tourniquet on the arm can be used for hemostasis, but it is not usually necessary for minor procedures.

FOOT

The skin on the sole of the foot heals very slowly. If you remove a minor lesion from the sole of the foot leave the sutures in place about twice as long as you would elsewhere in the body. Bed rest will usually allow an indolent lesion to heal. Slow-healing wounds of the foot frequently cause marked inguinal lymphadenopathy which can suggest the possibility of a malignancy. Resist the urge to take biopsies of the nodes; they will return to normal size when the sole wound heals.

SPECIFIC TECHNIQUES

The patient and the operative site are prepared as previously described. Factors related to specific anatomic sites are also applicable to these specific techniques.

Biopsy of Skin Lesions

This is indicated when precise histologic diagnosis of a skin lesion is required. If the lesion is small it can be removed in its entirety (excisional biopsy). If it is large, only a small portion is excised (incisional biopsy). For the latter remove a portion of the lesion including its junction with, and a portion of, apparently normal skin.

Either field block or local infiltration anesthesia may be used. Excise an ellipse of skin of the desired size. Begin by outlining the skin incision with a scalpel. Grasp one end with a thumb forceps or an Allis forceps and as you elevate it divide the deeper tissues with a scalpel. Compress the area of excision with a sponge for three to five minutes. During this period most of the tiny vessels will cease to ooze. Grasp the remaining bleeders with hemostats. Tie them with fine catgut or nonabsorable suture material. If the defect is wide, decrease the size with interrupted sutures in the subcutaneous tissues. Complete the closure with interrupted, fine, nonabsorb-

able sutures in the skin. Cover with a small, dry, gauze dressing.

Removal of Skin Papillomata

These are growths of skin on a small pedicle. Usually no anesthesia is required for their removal. Grasp the tip of the lesion with a forceps in your left hand and pull it up away from the skin. With a scissors in your right hand rapidly snip the lesion at the skin level.

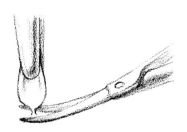

This is frequently accomplished without any bleeding. If the site does bleed, exert pressure for a few minutes and apply a dressing. This can be done so expeditiously that the patient has little or no discomfort.

Removal of Pyogenic Granulomata

These occur as a result of minor injuries to the skin which become infected. The resultant lesion is pulpy, friable, and bulbous, on a thin stalk. A granuloma can usually be excised without anesthesia. Lift the lesion with a forceps and excise it at the skin level with a scissors. It bleeds freely when it is first cut because the blood supply is made up of fairly large vessels in the stalk. Control the bleeding with compression and cauterize the bleeding point with a silver nitrate stick. This is usually all that is necessary. A small dry dressing completes the procedure.

REMOVAL OF NEVUS OR SIMILAR SKIN LESION

Infiltrate about the lesion in a field block anesthesia. If this is not practical, local infiltration directly into the area is satisfactory. Include the lesion in an ellipse of skin. The short diameter of the ellipse should be sufficient to extend beyond the edge of the lesion. The long diameter of the ellipse should be in the direction of the lines of force and approximately twice as long as the shorter diameter. This is a diagram of the lines of skin tension described by Langer.

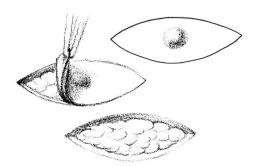

Usually one blood vessel supplies the nevus. After pressure has been applied for a few minutes and the oozing is controlled, grasp the vessel with a hemostat and ligate it; this will usually provide hemostasis. Approximate the subcutaneous tissues and close the wound with interrupted nonabsorable sutures. Cover with a small dry gauze dressing.

REMOVAL OF SEBACEOUS CYSTS

Sebaceous cysts are retention cysts caused by obstruction of a glandular duct. They consist of a thin wall encasing much sebaceous material. Occasionally they become infected; if treated in an infected state they should merely be incised and drained. This will control the infection but does not guarantee against recurrence; it is wise to tell the patient that there is reasonable possibility of recurrence after simple drainage. The proper treatment of a noninfected cyst is complete excision. Field block anesthesia is most satisfactory (p. 87). After waiting a few minutes to allow the anesthetic solution to take effect, make an elliptical incision in the skin over the cyst. The incision should extend beyond the edge of the cyst in each direction in its long length and cover about one-quarter of the diameter of the cyst in its short length. With a scalpel, carry the dissection through the skin down into the subcutaneous tissues, keeping the blade just lateral to the cyst. With a dissecting scissors, and a combination of sharp and blunt dissection, the cyst can be excised

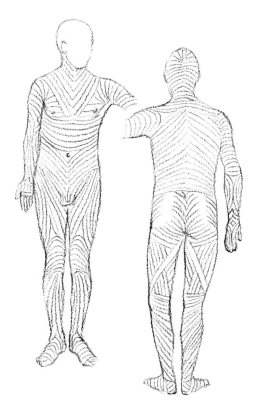

After the skin is divided lift one end with the forceps and divide the subcutaneous tissues.

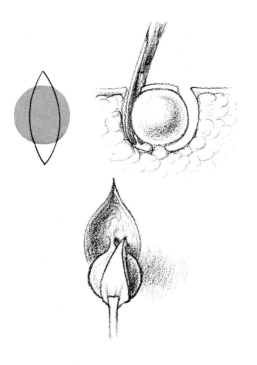

87), make a linear incision in a skin line directly over the area of the lipoma. Carry the incision down to the level of the tumor. Use a curved scissors to remove the mass. Insert the closed scissors alongside the lipoma and then open the scissors. Successive maneuvers of this sort will make it possible to "shell out" the lipoma. Usually there is very little bleeding. Maintain pressure for a few minutes; grasp residual bleeders with hemostats and tie with fine suture material. Close the dead space by approximating the deep tissues with interrupted sutures. Close the skin with interrupted sutures. Cover with a dry gauze dressing.

MUSCLE BIOPSY

The most common reason for muscle biopsy is to obtain a representative cross section of a small blood vessel for histologic examination. The procedure is sometimes used to rule out fungal infestation of a muscle. The muscles most commonly biopsied are the deltoid and the gastrocnemius. Infiltrate the skin, subcutaneous tissues, and muscles with 1 per cent procaine solution. Make a linear incision over the muscle to be biopsied. Carry this through the skin, subcutaneous tissues and the fascia overlying the muscle. Grasp a section of muscle with forceps or a hemostat and excise it. Control any bleeding. Close the rent in the fascia with interrupted sutures. Approximate the subcutaneous tissues and close the skin with interrupted sutures. Cover with dry gauze dressing.

without rupturing it. After the entire cyst has been removed, apply pressure to the area for three to five minutes. This will leave few vessels to tie. Should the cyst be ruptured during its removal, you need not worry that the sebaceous material will seed the area, but it is important to remove all the lining of the cyst. Grasp the lining of the cyst with a hemostat or forceps and, maintaining tension on it, remove every bit of it by sharp dissection. Again use compression for a few minutes to stop most of the bleeding. Control any residual bleeding with ligatures, approximate the deep tissues to remove dead space, and close the subcutaneous tissues and skin. Use interrupted sutures throughout. Cover with a dry gauze dressing.

REMOVAL OF LIPOMA

A lipoma is a fatty tumor that may appear in the subcutaneous tissues in almost any part of the body. It is not likely to become malignant but it may cause some disfigurement or discomfort. Under local field block anesthesia (p.

LYMPH NODE BIOPSY

This procedure is used in the diagnosis of malignancy or of certain granulomatous diseases which may involve lymph nodes. The nodes most frequently excised for biopsy lie in the cervical, axillary, and inguinal areas.

The most commonly removed cervical nodes are the supraclavicular. These nodes are rarely palpable under normal circumstances, and when they are they should be considered abnormal. An error in the identification and interpretation of a supraclavicular lymph node is frequently made on palpation of the area where the anterior belly of the omohyoid muscle crosses the scaleni. This is called the "junior resident's lymph node" and can be recognized by following the belly of the muscle beyond the one prominent point. In contrast to the supraclavicular region, nodes are commonly palpable in the axillary and inguinal areas. In these areas their significance is best interpreted by comparison with the opposite side.

Never attempt to remove a lymph node which you cannot feel before you begin the operation. Always palpate the node after the patient is positioned on the operating table. A node which is readily palpable when the patient is in one position may be very difficult to find when he is in another. If you cannot palpate the node return the patient to the position in which he was first examined and begin the excision with the patient in whatever position makes the node most accessible. A thorough knowledge of the anatomy of the area is prerequisite to successful operation. Infiltrate the area with 1 per cent procaine solution. Make a linear incision in the skin crease over the node. Carry the incision through the skin, subcutaneous tissue, and fascia. Before proceeding further, palpate within the wound to ascertain the position of the node. Set your retractors to position the node in the center of the incision. Using a forceps and dissecting scissors, remove the node by a combination of sharp and blunt scissors dissection, avoiding any important structures. It is sometimes helpful to grasp the node with an Allis or Babcock forceps and lift it as you cut it free. There is always a vessel which enters the hilum of the node and which will bleed freely when cut. If possible, grasp this vessel with a hemostat before cutting the node free. If you do not, you must pick up the vessel after the node is removed. Ligate the vessel; approximate the deep tissues with interrupted sutures; close the skin with interrupted sutures; and cover the wound with a dry gauze dressing.

Skin Grafting

Wounds that have insufficient tissue available to allow a primary closure may be left with a raw surface. Such defects granulate, but the process is time consuming and the resultant scar is usually unsightly, may be tender, and does not tolerate trauma. Such a result is undesirable on a weight-bearing area. The defect can be closed more rapidly and a more satisfactory scar effected by using skin grafts. Injuries or operations involving major skin grafting require the services of the accomplished surgeon. However, simple applications of the various types of skin grafts can immeasurably improve the results in minor surgery. The various grafts may be free or pedicled.

Free Grafts

Free grafts may be (1) small deep grafts, (2) split thickness grafts, or (3) full thickness grafts.

SMALL DEEP GRAFTS. Small deep grafts, better known as pinch grafts, are made up of small pieces of skin which include the full thickness of the skin. These grafts take hold in most wounds, even those that are not completely clean; many takes occur even in the presence of some infection. They are used mainly where it is doubtful that a more desirable type of graft would take. The result is unsightly and should not be used where the area is exposed or over weight-bearing surfaces. Contractures may form in the scar. The grafts are taken from the thigh, the abdomen, or the arm.

The area of injury is cleaned up with

saline compresses. The grafts can be taken from the forearm, the abdomen, or the thigh. After preparation of the skin, mark off the area with iodine or an indelible pencil. Anesthetize the area with field block anesthesia. With a needle pick up the skin to create a cone. Cut the skin at the base of the cone with a scalpel.

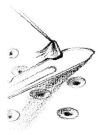

A properly cut graft is 2 to 4 mm. in diameter with a full thickness of skin at the center. Leave a space of 5 mm. between donor sites. Set the grafts on a piece of gauze soaked in saline until the desired number have been cut. Dress the donor site with a nonadherent dressing backed with dry gauze.

Place the grafts on the granulating area using two needles to position them.

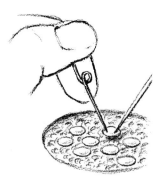

Set these 5 mm. apart and press firmly in the place with a cotton pledget. Apply a nonadherent dressing backed by absorbent gauze and held in place with a pressure dressing. If the dressing remains dry and there is no evidence of infection it can be left in place 10 days. If it is necessary to change the dressing

before that time do not disturb the grafts.

SPLIT THICKNESS GRAFT.   Split thickness skin grafts are the most widely used type of grafts because they are more easily cut and the percentage of takes is high. They may be obtained from the thigh, the abdominal wall, the chest wall, the back, or the arm. An effort should be made to match the skin of the recipient area. The cosmetic result is good, but they do not tolerate pressure well and contractures may occur. These grafts will take in areas that reject full thickness grafts and in the presence of mild infection. This type of graft can be used to cover large areas and for this purpose dermatomes are available.

After proper preparation of the skin, anesthetize the area with field block anesthesia. Have your assistant help you hold the skin taut with two sterile boards and, using a razor or a sharp scalpel, remove the graft.

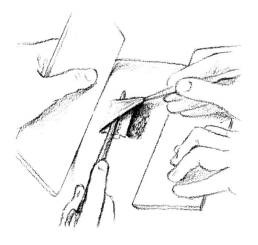

This is best done with a sawing motion. Small grafts can be cut with a razor blade held in a hemostat. A graft of proper thickness will uncover a white area with multiple punctate sites of bleeding. Place the graft over the recipient area. Perforate it so that fluid can drain through it and suture it in place. Leave the ends of the sutures long.

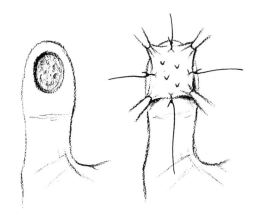

Put a piece of nonadherent dressing against the graft, back this with absorbent gauze, and hold these in place by tying the ends of the sutures in the edge of the graft over the top of the gauze.

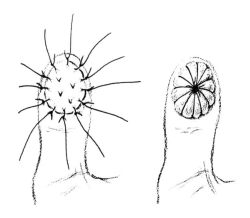

Cover the entire dressing with dry gauze. Leave in place for 10 days. If the dressing must be changed sooner because of drainage, change only the outer layers. Cover the donor site with a layer of nonadherent dressing backed with absorbent gauze.

A modification of split thickness skin grafting is the "postage stamp" technique. The graft is cut with a dermatone which has a special rubber backed adhesive sheet to which the graft is attached as it is cut. The firm sheet allows the graft to be cut into any size and shape with the backing in place. Commonly the graft is cut in squares approximately the size of a postage stamp. They are

then applied to the recipient area so that the best coverage is obtained. They are then managed as any other split thickness skin graft.

FULL THICKNESS GRAFT. A full thickness skin graft gives the best surface of all the free grafts, but has the disadvantage of being difficult to cut and less likely to take than other grafts. In general, the thicker a skin graft the more difficult it is to take hold. Full thickness grafts are used only on fresh wounds, particularly in areas where minimal contracture is tolerated, and on weight-bearing surfaces. After the proper preparation of both the donor site and the recipient area, anesthetize each with a field block anesthesia. The recipient area, which is usually where a scar has been excised, must be prepared with careful hemostasis. Attempt to outline the exact size graft you will need. Carry your incision directly through the skin along the entire outline of the graft. The graft contracts as soon as the edges are cut.

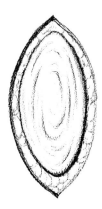

Lift the edge of the graft with a fine tooth forceps and using sharp dissection, cut the skin away from the underlying fat. Any fat adherent to the graft must be removed. Perforate the graft to allow drainage through it so that accumulation of fluid beneath the graft will not lift it from its base. Place the graft in the defect and initially suture all four quadrants.

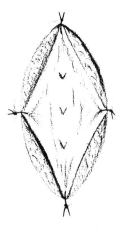

Follow with whatever sutures are necessary to complete the closure.

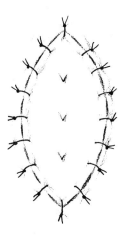

Cover the graft with a nonadherent dressing backed by a rubber sponge held in place by a pressure dressing. If the dressing remains dry do not disturb for 10 days. At this point remove the sutures but maintain the pressure dressing for 3 weeks.

Close the donor site with sutures; if this is not possible apply a split thickness graft.

Pedicle Grafts

Pedicle grafts are used in the repair of deep defects where skin grafts are inadequate and where more pliability and elasticity of the skin is required. Since both skin and subcutaneous tissues are transferred the result is more satisfactory but several operations are required. The original blood supply is left intact until the graft has taken hold; it is then cut free of its original site.

Pedicle grafts are used in all parts of the body and are best applied by a plastic surgeon. Simple pedicle grafts of the hand are demonstrated in Chapter 14, The Upper Extremity (p. 207).

Needle Biopsy

Needle biopsy has become an accepted method of obtaining representative tissue from deep within the body, areas which otherwise would have required a major operative procedure for exposure. Since the procedure is done under local anesthesia, the dangers of general anesthesia are avoided. There is no operative wound; therefore, the patient is relieved of the discomfort and the inconvenience of recovery from operation. Because the procedure is less formidable, the patient is more likely to accept it.

Indications

Needle biopsy is indicated when a representative sample of tissue is needed for diagnosis and when it seems possible to obtain this safely by the needle method. The technique may be employed to obtain a representative section of a tumor mass which is thought to be nonresectable to determine proper treatment, or to establish the nature of nonmalignant disease.

Contraindications

Needle biopsy is contraindicated: (1) when there is danger of seeding an operable tumor and making it inoperable (as in seeding cells of an operable tumor of the lung in the chest wall), (2) when the mass to be biopsied lies close to important structures which might be injured during the procedure and (3) when the patient has an abnormal bleeding tendency.

Limitations

It must be recognized that the probing needle is incapable of selecting the most representative portion of a mass. The pathologist can only diagnose the tissue presented him. There is no assurance that this tissue is typical of the entire mass. It is important to recognize that while positive diagnoses are reliable, a negative diagnosis may merely mean that a representative piece of tissue was not obtained.

Complications

Needle biopsy may be accompanied by any of the following complications:

HEMORRHAGE. The needle may strike a blood vessel in the area. The procedure should not be used in any area where there is danger of striking a major vessel. Bleeding from smaller vessels can usually be controlled with pressure.

INFECTION. This occurs as a result of lapses in proper surgical technique. If the area is properly prepared, one should not need to worry about infections.

SEEDING. When used in the diagnosis of suspected malignancy, needle biopsy carries the danger of seeding tumor cells in uninvolved areas. If the needle traverses only tissue which will be removed at subsequent operation there is no cause for worry. If this is not the case, the biopsy can spread the tumor, e.g., when the needle seeds cells from an operable tumor of the lung into the chest wall. These precautions are not necessary when the tumor is obviously inoperable and the tissue is needed to

determine the best type of palliative therapy.

Technique

The instruments needed consist of a local anesthesia set and a Vim-Silverman needle. The Vim-Silverman needle is the most important part of the equipment. It consists of a large bore, short bevel, carrier needle, an obturator the same length as the needle, and a forked inner needle for obtaining the biopsy.

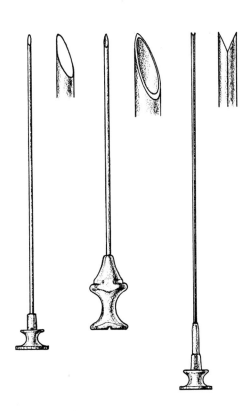

The forked needle is 2 cm. longer than the carrier needle. Shave the skin, prepare the area with alcohol and tincture of Zephiran, and infiltrate the point of puncture with procaine. Insert a longer needle through this area to infiltrate the deeper tissues. Make a small nick in the skin and fascia with a #15 scalpel blade to facilitate the passage of the needle. Pass the carrier needle, with the obturator in place, through the small incision and to the area of the mass. Remove the obturator and replace it with the forked needle. Insert this its full length, thereby putting it 2 cm. beyond the outer needle. Advance the outer needle over the forked needle; rotate both needles 180 degrees and withdraw them together. Remove the forked needle from the carrier needle. There will be a core of tissue 1 to 2 mm. in width and 2 cm. long within the groove of the forked needle. Slide this core from the groove in the carrier needle into a specimen bottle in which it is sent to the laboratory.

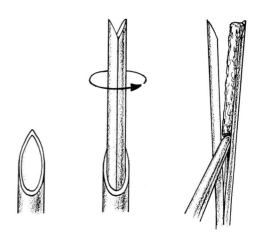

A small dressing over the needle hole is usually sufficient. The patient should be watched for any evidence of a complication related to the site of biopsy.

Chapter Eleven

Infants and Children

While the physiologic mechanisms of infants are similar to those of adults, differences in anatomic size and relationships demand that procedures in the infant be carried out differently than in the adult. This chapter describes only those techniques which are peculiar to infants and children.

VITAL SIGNS

PULSE

The pulse is counted by palpation of an artery. In the infant, few pulsating vessels are readily available for palpation. The most accessible is the femoral artery. Gently palpate the vessel immediately below the inguinal ligament. If this is not palpable count the heart rate by auscultation directly over the heart.

BLOOD PRESSURE

The blood pressure of infants and children should be measured in the same manner as in adults if possible. A mercury or aneroid type of manometer

can be used. The mercury manometer is more reliable, particularly if the surface level of the mercury is at zero. An aneroid manometer should be checked against a mercury manometer once a year. The size of the cuff is important. The cuff should cover approximately two-thirds of the upper arm or leg. Cuffs are available in widths varying from 2.5 cm. to 18 cm. The blood pressure should be measured with the child at rest. In older children a brief explanation will claim their cooperation; infants can be pacified with a bottle. If the child will not relax, sedation must be used. Measure pressures in the arm with the patient sitting or lying and pressures in the leg with the patient prone. Apply the completely deflated cuff snugly and evenly, with the bag over the artery, and the lower end of the cuff one cm. above the antecubital or popliteal fossa. The pressure may be measured by palpation or auscultation.

Palpation

The blood pressure should be determined first by palpation. Frequently,

159

palpation may be the only way in which the pressure can be measured. Palpate a pulse distal to the cuff and keep the finger over the artery. With the cuff in place gradually raise the pressure of the cuff until the distal pulse can no longer be palpated. Slowly lower the pressure in the bag and note the point of reappearance of the pulse. This is usually 5 to 10 mm. of mercury lower than the systolic pressure determined by auscultation.

Auscultation

Auscult directly over an artery distal to the blood pressure cuff. With the cuff in place raise the pressure to approximately 30 mm. of mercury higher than the systolic level measured by palpation and allow it to drop slowly. The level at which the first sound appears is read as the systolic pressure. (This is usually 3 to 4 mm. lower than that measured by a direct tap with an intra-arterial needle.) The level at which the sounds completely disappear is read as the diastolic pressure. When the sounds do not disappear the level at which the sounds become muffled is read as the diastolic pressure.

Flush Method

In many infants it may be impossible to measure the blood pressure by either palpation or auscultation. One must then depend upon the flush method which, while not as accurate, gives a good approximation of the blood pressure. Place a proper size cuff about the ankle or wrist and elevate the limb until it blanches. Mild pressure on the palm or soles assists blanching. With the extremity blanched in an elevated position raise the pressure in the cuff; lower the extremity to the level of the heart and gradually release the pressure. Lower the pressure 5 to 6 mm. of mercury and leave it at this level for 3 to 4 seconds while the extremity is inspected. Repeat this procedure until flushing is

observed in the blanched limb. A fine oscillation of the column of mercury may be noted 5 or 10 mm. above the flushing point, indicating the approaching end point. Flushing is manifest by a sudden pink coloration below the cuff edge that spreads distally. The manometer reading at this point is taken as the systolic blood pressure. Although deepening of the color will occur as the pressure is further reduced, the initial flush is the end point. This method yields measurements which average approximately 25 mm. of mercury below systolic pressure. Although the flush method measures only the systolic pressure and is not of the accuracy one would desire, it is presently the method of choice for the indirect measurement of arterial pressure in infants under one or two years of age.

Normal Range

In 24 newborn infants Woodbury, Robinow and Hamilton* obtained an average systolic blood pressure of 80 mm. of mercury with a standard deviation of 8.2 mm. by direct measurement. The systolic pressure rose 10 to 15 mm. of mercury during the first 10 days of life. Pressures in premature infants were lower: a 5-month fetus had a pressure of 39/21 mm. of mercury; a 6½-month fetus 55/25 mm.; a 7-month fetus 70/35 mm. and an 8-month fetus 75/45 mm. of mercury. They also found that crying raised the systolic pressure 10 to 45 mm. of mercury, with an average increase of 27 mm.

Using the point of complete cessation of heart sounds as the diastolic pressure and cuff widths that covered no more than two-thirds of the upper arm, Graham† made 25,000 determinations

---

* Woodbury, R. A., Robinow, M., and Hamilton, W. F.: Blood Pressure Studies on Infants. Amer. J. Physiol. *122*:472, 1938.

† Graham, A. W., Hines, E. A., Jr., and Sage, R. P.: Blood Pressure in Children Between the Ages of Five and Sixteen Years. Am. J. Dis. Child. *69*:203, 1945.

on 3580 school children in a long term study and found the normal blood pressure to be as follows:

Age	Systolic		Diastolic	
	Arithmetic Mean	Standard Deviation	Arithmetic Mean	Standard Deviation
5	93.9	7.04	54.9	4.33
6	100.0	7.47	55.5	4.05
7	102.2	7.49	55.8	4.00
8	104.7	7.86	56.5	4.74
9	106.5	7.97	57.0	4.73
10	108.6	8.20	57.7	4.76
11	110.9	8.57	58.5	4.99
12	112.7	8.84	59.0	4.94
13	115.2	9.27	59.6	4.87
14	117.9	9.32	60.5	5.19
15	120.8	9.35	60.8	5.13
16	121.4	9.68	61.1	5.19

GASTROINTESTINAL TRACT

GASTRIC LAVAGE

In Infants

Many pediatricians routinely intubate the stomach of the newborn to ascertain the patency of the esophagus. Furthermore, routine aspiration of the stomach of all newborns delivered by caesarean section has been shown to lower the incidence of pulmonary complications by preventing aspiration of amniotic fluid regurgitated from the stomach. Pass a #10 French soft rubber urethral catheter into the oropharynx, then slowly down through the pharynx and the esophagus into the stomach. A slow rotary motion of the catheter helps the descent. The catheter usually passes readily but if it kinks in the pharynx do not hesitate to use the fingers of your other hand to guide it. The catheter enters the stomach after a length of approximately 10 to 12 cm. has been passed. This length is equivalent to the distance from the bridge of the nose to the xiphoid process. Advance it a few more centimeters. Attach a 10-ml. syringe to the end of the catheter and exert mild suction. At the same time gently press over the infant's stomach which usually contains 14 to 20 ml. of fluid. Continue mild suction while the catheter is slowly and gently withdrawn. This procedure sometimes causes the infant to gag, cough and hold his breath. If he seems to have such difficulty give some oxygen until he settles down.

In Children

This technique is used in older children to wash out their stomachs. This may be done because of poisoning or to clean out the stomach in a toxic enteritis. Pass a #10 or #12 French catheter as recommended above. Ascertain that the tube is in the stomach by aspirating gastric contents. Aspirate all material which can be removed. Using a syringe, inject lavage fluid into the catheter and then aspirate the fluid. Repeat this maneuver with fresh lavage fluid until the return is clear. In cases of suspected poisoning save the aspirate for clinical analysis. Maintain suction on the tube while withdrawing it from the stomach.

GAVAGE

Premature infants and those who are very weak may be unable or unwilling to suck. If an infant cannot suck he probably cannot swallow. It is sometimes possible to maintain his nutrition by feeding directly into his stomach via a tube. Pass a small, smooth-tip polyethylene tube into the stomach via the nasopharynx. After aspirating gastric contents to make certain that the tube is in the stomach, you can begin feedings. Pushing air through the tube with a syringe and auscultating over the stomach helps you to locate the tip of the tube. Intermittent feeding is safer than a continuous drip. You can feed every one to two hours to every three to four hours depending on the patient. The amount fed will depend upon the number of feedings and the total caloric intake desired. The tube can be left in place. After each feeding push some water through the tube to prevent the feeding material from blocking the tube. When the infant begins to suck on the tube give him a few drops of water orally to determine whether he can swallow. When he begins to swallow satisfactorily he can be fed orally. If necessary the oral feedings can be supplemented by tube.

FARBER TEST

If one suspects atresia of the bowel in a newborn infant he can substantiate his diagnosis with the Farber test. Swallowed epithelial cells are present in meconium in the normal infant with a patent gastrointestinal tract. Demonstration of these cells in the meconium will rule out intestinal obstruction in the newborn. Prepare smears from the center of a representative specimen of meconium. Defat the smear by washing with ether for 3 minutes. Stain the slide with Sterling's gentian violet, wash with water, and decolorize with acid alcohol. Epithelial cells retain the stain. Such cells are not present with atresia.*

SWEAT TEST

Patients with fibrocystic disease of the pancreas excrete excessive amounts of sodium and chloride through sweat. Measurement of the sodium and chloride content of sweat is a worthwhile diagnostic test because a positive test is possible only with fibrocystic disease of the pancreas or adrenal cortical insufficiency.

After carefully washing the patient place him, nude, on a plastic sheet in a heating unit. Place infants under 6 months in an Isolette with a temperature of 35°C. and 100 per cent relative humidity. Place older children on a plastic sheet under a heat cradle containing a 100-watt bulb and cover with a blanket. Collect the sweat with a tuberculin syringe from the plastic sheet and the patient's back. If the patient urinates on the sheet it must be washed and the test begun again. Infants under 3 months rarely produce enough sweat to make the test worthwhile.

Whereas the sweat of a normal person contains 1 to 101 mEq./L. (average of 37) of sodium and 6 to 112 mEq./L. (average of 37) of chloride, patients with fibrocystic disease of the pancreas produce sweat containing 102 to 215 mEq./L. (average of 163) of sodium and 103 to 217 mEq./L. (average 162) of chloride.*

VASCULAR SYSTEM

It may be necessary to aspirate blood for diagnosis or to administer blood, fluids, or electrolytes for treatment.

ASPIRATION OF BLOOD

Antecubital Vein

Blood specimens can usually be obtained without difficulty in children over three years of age by antecubital vein puncture. Venipuncture of an antecubital vein in the adult is described on page 295. The technique is essentially the same in a child except that a smaller needle (#20 to #25) is used and the arm must be restrained in the younger children. Puncture of this vein can be used for therapeutic as well as diagnostic purposes.

---

* Farber, S.: Congenital Atresia of Alimentary Tract, Diagnosis by Microscopic Examination of Meconium. J.A.M.A. *100:*1733, 1933.

* Borbero et al.: Simplified Technique for Sweat Test in Diagnosis of Fibrocystic Disease of Pancreas. Pediatrics *18:*189, 1956.

Femoral Vein Puncture

This is the commonest site of blood-letting in the infant. Place the patient on his back and restrain both arms by wrapping him in a sheet or a blanket which encases his arms and trunk; abduct his legs and have an assistant hold him in that position. Palpate the pulsations of the femoral artery on the side where the vein is to be punctured just below the mid-point of the inguinal ligament. The femoral vein lies just medial to the femoral artery. After you identify the artery, sterilize the skin with alcohol; attach a 20-gauge needle to a 10-ml. syringe and pierce the skin 3 cm. below the inguinal ligament just medial to where the pulsation of the artery is felt.

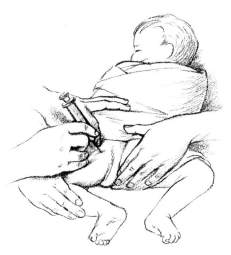

Maintain continuous back pressure on the plunger of the syringe as you advance the needle. As soon as the needle enters the vein blood will be drawn back into the syringe. After the desired amount of blood has been obtained, withdraw the needle and maintain pressure over the puncture point for several minutes with a cotton ball soaked with alcohol. If the femoral artery should be entered instead of the femoral vein, there need be no cause for alarm. Draw in the desired amount of blood and remove the needle and maintain pressure on the artery for 5 minutes *by the clock.*

External Jugular Vein

This is the next most common site for the withdrawal of blood from an infant. Restrain the infant in a sheet but do not extend this above the shoulder. Place the infant flat on his back with both shoulders touching the table; rotate his head sharply to one side and extend it over the edge of the table. He is supported in this position by an assistant who must hold the head still. The external jugular vein passes behind the angle of the jaw, crosses the sternocleidomastoid muscle toward the posterior border and enters the deep tissues just above the clavicle. Cleanse the area carefully with alcohol. If the child is made to cry the veins will become engorged and consequently stand out prominently. Using a 20-gauge needle attached to a 10-ml. syringe puncture the skin along the course of the vein directing the needle toward the chest.

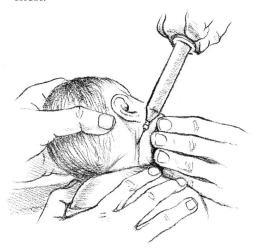

After the needle pierces the skin direct the needle into the vein, exerting constant back pressure on the plunger as the needle is thrust forward. Blood will enter the syringe as soon as the vein has been entered. After the desired quantity of blood has been withdrawn, remove the needle, exert pressure on the site with an alcohol sponge, and bring the child to an upright position. Maintain the pressure for several minutes.

Internal Jugular Vein

This vein is never used for the administration of fluids or medications and is used for aspiration of blood only when no other veins are available. Place the child in the position recommended for an external jugular vein puncture. Insert the needle lateral to the sternocleidomastoid muscle at the junction of its lower and middle thirds. Pass the needle beneath the muscle, aiming it at the sternal notch and advance it until it enters the vein. After completion of the procedure maintain firm pressure over the area for five minutes with the child in a sitting position.

Sagittal Sinus Puncture

This is used for the injection of fluid only in an emergency, such as shock, and for aspiration of blood only when no other vein is available. Restrain the infant in a supine position with the top of his head at the edge of the table. Shave the anterior fontanel and carefully sterilize the skin. Using a short bevel needle pass it into the sinus only deep enough to aspirate blood.

Arterial Puncture

It may be necessary to aspirate blood from an artery when laboratory studies demand arterial blood or when no vein is available. The femoral artery is most available. Position the patient as for a femoral vein tap. Palpate the artery below the inguinal ligament. Insert the needle attached to a syringe 1.5 cm. below the ligament, directly over the site of the pulsations, and advance it toward the pulsations while maintaining suction on the syringe. Arterial blood is evident by its color unless the infant has unsaturated blood. The blood will usually flow into the syringe without suction. After removal of the needle maintain pressure over the puncture site for 5 minutes *by the clock.*

BONE MARROW TAP

The most common site of bone marrow tap is the sternum. In infants less than one year old the tibia, just below the tubercle, is preferred. The iliac crest or the sternum may be used.

Sternal Puncture

If it is necessary to do a sternal tap in infants, insert the needle in the manubrium, just above the angle of Louis. In older children a point between the second and third costosternal junction, just lateral to the midline, is preferable. In infants use a 21 gauge spinal needle; in older children a 19 gauge spinal needle can be used.

Restrain the child by wrapping him in a sheet with his chest bared. In older children local anesthesia can be used. In younger, restless children preliminary sedation with Pentobarbital sodium followed by nitrous oxide-oxygen anesthesia is recommended. Insert the spinal needle containing an obturator through the outer plate of the sternum in a line perpendicular with the skin. When the needle goes through the outer plate it is apparent by the decrease in resistance. Decrease the angle of the needle and move it farther into the marrow cavity. Remove the needle and apply pressure to the puncture point for a few minutes with an alcohol sponge.

Tibial Marrow Puncture

Immobilize the leg of the infant on a padded long leg splint. Tape the leg to the splint at the ankle and above the knee. After proper preparation of the skin raise a wheal with local anesthetic solution over the proximal end of the tibia on the anteromedial aspect between the tibial tubercle and the medial condyle. Insert a trochar or a spinal needle through the skin and the outer plate of bone. You can recognize the "give" when the needle enters the marrow cavity. Attach a 10-ml. syringe and aspirate 0.5 ml. in infants or 1 to 2 ml. in older children. Make a smear immediately and send it to the laboratory. Pressure over the puncture site is usually adequate for hemostasis.

Administration of Fluid

When an infant is unable to take fluids orally they must be administered by one of the supplemental routes—subcutaneous or intravenous.

Hypodermoclysis

Fluids may be given subcutaneously when it is difficult to find a suitable vein. The loose subcutaneous tissues of the infant facilitate use of this route. Fluids which can be given by this route include physiologic saline, 2½ per cent dextrose in water cr physiologic saline, M/6 sodium lactate, or Ringer's solution. Blood or more concentrated solutions cannot be so administered. The fluids are usually given in either the scapular region or the thighs.

SCAPULAR REGION. This is the most common site for subcutaneous administration of fluids to infants. Place the infant on his stomach; prepare the skin over the scapula with alcohol. With your left hand pick up the skin over the scapula in a fold and insert the needle into the elevated skin at the lower tip of the scapula. Insert the needle, pointed cephalad, parallel to the chest wall in the subcutaneous level, and inject 25 to 30 ml. of fluid.

Repeat the process over the other scapula, injecting an equal amount. If you must give more fluid use the thigh area. The same areas can be used repeatedly after the injected fluid is absorbed. If the infant has respiratory difficulties, the thigh should be used rather than the scapular area.

THIGH. The thigh offers the advantage of allowing larger quantities of fluid to be administered and is a satisfactory site for a continuous or prolonged infusion. The fluid to be injected is contained in a sterile bottle connected by tubing to needles, which are inserted into each thigh so that fluid is simultaneously given bilaterally. Restrain the child so that he cannot remove the needles; both arms and legs must be restrained. Cleanse the skin of the thighs with alcohol, pick up a fold of skin between the thumb and forefinger on the lateral aspect of the thigh, and insert the needle subcutaneously in a cephalad direction.

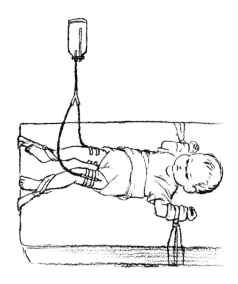

The needles can be taped in place until the desired amount of fluid has dripped in. The intravenous route is a more satisfactory means of replacing large volumes of fluid than either of these subcutaneous areas.

Intravenous Fluids

In older children the antecubital vein or the veins of the dorsum of the hand are quite satisfactory for the administration of fluid. If either of these are used the part should be properly supported and the other extremity should be restrained so that the child cannot pull out the needle. The technique of inserting the needle is similar to that described on page 295. If the antecubital and hand veins are not adequate, a scalp vein or a cutdown on an ankle vein should be used. The scalp vein is the method of choice in infants and the cutdown is preferable in older children.

SCALP VEIN. Restrain the infant with a sheet so that he cannot move his arms or legs and place him on his back. Turn his head to one side and examine the scalp for a prominent vein. The most accessible veins usually cross down in front of the ears. Shave the hair over the area of the vein to be used. Cleanse the skin with alcohol and make the infant cry, at the same time compressing the vein proximal to the point where the needle is to be inserted. This will cause the vein to become engorged and make it simpler to insert the needle. Use a 22-gauge short bevel needle attached to a short plastic tube running to a three-way stopcock. A 10-ml. syringe is attached to one end of the three-way stopcock and the other leads to a bottle containing the fluid to be injected. Insert the needle into the vein and check the position of the needle by drawing back slightly on the barrel of the syringe. When the needle is in proper position a small amount of blood will flow back into the tubing. After this has been accomplished, tape the needle in position. Stabilize the head by placing sandbags on each side.

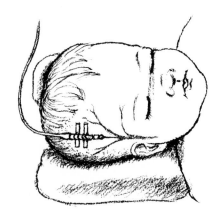

VENOUS CUT-DOWN. The older child rarely will hold his head still long enough to allow use of the scalp veins. Consequently, in older children, as well as in some infants, a venous cutdown must be employed. The greater saphenous vein, just anterior to and above the medial malleolus of the ankle, is one of the most uniformly located veins in the body and is the one most commonly used for cutdowns. Secure the foot firmly on a board as illustrated.

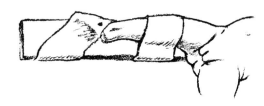

This procedure in an adult is described on page 298. Prepare the area with alcohol and infiltrate the area over the vein with procaine. Make a small incision parallel to the skin crease and perpendicular to the direction of the vein. Carry the incision through the skin. Using a small, pointed hemostat, bluntly dissect beneath the vein and lift it up into the wound. Place a piece of nonabsorbable suture material about each end of the vein. Tie the distal ligature; proximal to this ligature make a transverse incision in the vein wall sufficiently large to allow the insertion of the cannula or polyethylene tubing. Insert the cannula and tie the vein down over this with the ligature previously placed about the proximal end of the vein. If the polyethylene tube is used, it should be inserted about four inches. Place a sterile dressing over the wound and tape the needle or tubing in place. Attach it to tubing from a bottle containing fluids which are to be given. The leg should remain secured to the board and the board anchored to the lower end of the crib. Wrap the connection between the tubing and the cannula in the dressing of the leg so that pull on the tubing will be less likely to pull out the cannula. The intravenous drip must be continuous to keep the cannula patent. The rate must be set so that the total fluid requirements for the day will run for 24 hours.

EXCHANGE TRANSFUSION

Exchange transfusion has made it possible to save the lives of many infants afflicted with blood incompatibility, which ultimately would have resulted in the hemolysis of their circulating cells, irreversible brain damage, and death as a result of the elevation of the serum bilirubin. Breakdown of the cells does not begin until after birth. By removing most of the sensitized cells, the possibility of bilirubin elevation is eliminated.

Exchange transfusion also makes it possible to regulate the blood volume of the infant. Many of these children are born with an excessive blood volume and are in heart failure; this situation calls for an immediate exchange transfusion. Finally, most of these infants are markedly anemic and the exchange transfusion makes it possible to give the infant a larger amount of hemoglobin for gas transfer.

Exchange transfusions are indicated in erythroblastotic infants who are in cardiac failure or are so anemic that cardiac failure seems imminent, and also in Rh positive infants with a positive direct Coombs test who were born to Rh negative mothers with an Rh antibody titer in albumin of 1 to 8 or greater. If such infants are premature it would be wisest to perform an exchange transfusion even though the mother has an Rh antibody titer of less than 1 to 8 in albumin. Repeat exchange transfusions should be performed if the serum bilirubin approaches 20 mg. per cent or if the infant shows signs of central nervous system involvement.

One of the most serious complications of exchange transfusion is hypothermic shock. Often the procedure must be done as an emergency immediately after birth, and the blood bank has not been properly warned. Then the baby should be protected in some type of a heated bed. There are heated buntings manufactured specifically for this purpose which work quite satisfactorily. If it is anticipated at delivery that the baby will probably require an exchange transfusion, several technical points should be observed. The cord should be clamped at the earliest possible moment. This will deprive the baby of the 75 to 100 ml. of blood available from the placenta, but this blood is made up completely of sensitized cells which may break down and produce pigment and add to the problem of exchange. Furthermore, the additional load on the circulation may precipitate heart failure. The cord should be tied several inches from the abdominal wall to leave vessels available for cannulation. Two specimens of blood should be collected from the cord, one for the Coombs' test and a second for base line laboratory studies.

The team should be made up of at least three people. The transfusionist should have an assistant to help him with the cannulation and the transfusion. A third person should observe the infant and keep an accurate running record of the transfusion including the amount of blood injected and withdrawn, medications given and a careful check on the pulse, respirations and general condition of the patient. He should keep a close watch on the cardiac status to determine the need for intravenous calcium and the effect of the administration of this drug. The equipment consists of an exchange transfusion tray, a prep tray and a pack of drapes. A typical exchange tray consists of:

2 hemostats, straight, mosquito
2 hemostats, curved, mosquito
1 scissors, mosquito
1 forceps, tooth, mosquito
4 towel clips
1 probe
1 15 mm. stainless steel scale
1 knife handle, #3
1 knife blade, #11
1 umbilical cannula and 2 adaptors
1 pan, stainless steel, small
3 20 ml. Luer-Lok syringes
3 10 ml. Luer-Lok syringes
3 specimen tubes with corks
1 glass adaptor
1 piece of rubber tubing forty inches long
3 umbilical cord tapes

In addition to the trays, one should have available equipment for resuscitation. This includes an electrical aspirator, an infant laryngoscope and airways, an oxygen tank with a mask and a rebreathing bag, and the necessary drugs. The drugs should include:

1 1 ml. ampule of caffeine and sodium benzoate
1 1 ml. ampule of 1:1000 epinephrine
3 10 ml. ampules of 10 per cent calcium gluconate for intravenous use
1 500 ml. bottle of sterile physiologic saline solution for intravenous use
1 small sterile bottle of physiologic saline solution for intravenous use for mixing with the 1:1000 epinephrine
1 10 ml. bottle of heparin containing 10 mg. of heparin per ml.
1 6 oz. bottle of benzalkonium chloride 1:100
1 500 ml. bottle of O Rh negative blood less than five days old

There should be on hand several pieces of polyethylene tubing #190 and #200, cut in 30-cm. lengths. There are also commercial catheters available for this particular purpose.

Technique

The baby is placed in a supine position in the bunting or on the table with heat available and the abdomen exposed. The abdomen and the umbilicus are cleaned with the tincture of Zephiran. The umbilical cord is cut 1 cm. distal to the mucocutaneous junction. Bleeding usually does not occur unless the venous pressure is high. The two arteries are readily identifiable by the thickness of their muscular walls. The umbilical vein is the largest of the three vessels. If the vein is plugged with clots, these should be lifted out with forceps or sucked out with the polyethylene tube and syringe. Once the vein has been cleaned, one can then insert the polyethylene catheter. In inserting the catheter, there are two points of obstruction which are met within the umbilical vein. The first is 2.5 to 4 cm. proximal to the mucocutaneous junction of the umbilical cord at the point where the umbilical vein curves dorsally to assume an intraperitoneal position. The second obstruction is at the junction of the umbilical vein, the portal sinus and the ductus venosus at a depth of 8 cm. If you are able to get the catheter beyond the second obstruction, the transfusion goes very well. The insertion of the tubing 12 to 14 cm. will place the tip in the inferior vena cava in the average newborn.

The umbilical vein can sometimes be found in an infant who is as many as four or five days old by exerting traction on the dried cord and cutting across the base. If it is not possible to do this, you can cut down on the umbilical vein just cephalad to the umbilicus. This is made possible by the 2 to 4 cm. subcutaneous position of the cord. Make a small 1 to 2 cm. transverse cutaneous incision about 1 cm. cephalad to the upper margin of the umbilicus. This will expose the umbilical vein before it courses intraperitoneally. It is no problem to insert a catheter here. In the small number of instances where it is not possible to cannulate the umbilical vein the catheter can be inserted into the femoral vein through a transverse incision on the medial aspect of the upper leg midway between the inguinal ligament and the knee. The vein is cannulated at this level because tying it off here does not embarrass the collateral circulation and will not cause edema of the leg.

First measure the venous pressure. This is done by holding the cannula upright and, with a stainless steel ruler, measuring the height of the column above the abdomen. Those patients who are in heart failure show a remarkable improvement with removal of the excess fluid from the circulation. The normal range of venous pressure in the quiet infant by this procedure is 4 to 8 cm. If the pressure is in excess of 10 cm. the baby is probably in cardiac failure. Blood should be withdrawn in 10 to 20 ml. increments until the venous pressure has been reduced to 8 to 10 cm. Once this has occurred, the exchange transfusion can be started.

Oxygen should be administered continuously and the individual watching the baby should make certain that a satisfactory airway is present at all times. When there is time available the blood should be warmed to 37°C. in a water bath prior to its use. When possible, monitoring electrocardiography should be employed. Blood is exchanged by removing increments of 10 to 20 ml. of blood and replacing this with an equal volume of bank blood. The larger the increment the greater the number of red cells which might be removed. However, in those babies with cardiac failure it is probably safer to exchange in 10 ml. increments. The infant is receiving citrated blood which does not clot because the citrate has tied up the ionized calcium in a relatively non-ionizable union. Excess citrate in the donor blood ties up some of the calcium in the circulating blood of the infant. To offset this the patient is given 1.5 to 2 ml. of 10 per cent calcium gluconate for every 100 ml. of blood replacement. This dosage is adjusted as indicated by the cardiac action of the patient and the clinical picture (shivering movements, irritability, or retching). There is some difference of opinion as to the exact amount of blood which should be exchanged, but most agree that removal and replacement of approximately twice the blood volume will usually remove 85 to 95 per cent of the susceptible cells. Since this requirement is always met with a 500 ml. transfusion, this is the total used (in sick infants it is sometimes held to 400 ml.). Following the transfusion, the cannulas are withdrawn and the infant is placed in an Isolette under close observation. If his temperature is low it is gradually brought back to normal; he is given oxygen as needed. Antibiotics (penicillin and streptomycin intramuscularly) are given for three days. All feedings are withheld slightly longer than in normal babies. The serum bilirubin should be followed carefully and if the bilirubin shows evidence of reaching 20 mg. per 100 ml., the exchange transfusion should be repeated. The tendency to give the patient a little extra blood at the completion of the procedure or even to replace the excess blood which was withdrawn to lower the venous pressure should be avoided. This will only throw the patient into heart failure. Furthermore, the hemoglobin of the baby will usually be about 1 Gm. higher the day after the operation as a result of the excretion of the excess fluid of the citrate solution from the circulation.

URINARY TRACT

COLLECTION OF URINE

Collection of urine in infants is complicated by their small size and inability

to cooperate. Isolated specimens for analysis may be collected by:
1. Midstream sample
2. Containers attached to the infant
3. Catheterization

Midstream Sample

If the child is old enough to cooperate and sufficient nursing help is available, a midstream sample can be obtained. The genitals are carefully cleansed and the child is encouraged to void. After micturition begins the nurse collects a sample of the midportion of the stream by inserting a sterile specimen bottle into the stream. This method is adequate for routine analyses but if a truly sterile specimen is required it can only be obtained by catheterization.

Attached Containers

Samples for study other than bacteriologic can be collected by taping a test tube to the penis of a male infant and by taping a feeder from a bird cage over the perineum of a female. Cleanse the skin of the groin and perineum scrupulously, set the appliance in place and hold it in place with adhesive plaster. When urine has accumulated, the appliance can be removed; the urine is poured into a specimen bottle and sent to the laboratory.

Catheterization

Catheterization is the best means of obtaining a sterile specimen. The technique is the same as that used in an adult (p. 285) except that appropriate sized catheters are used and the fragility of the lower urinary tract must be appreciated. Catheterization of an infant should not be attempted by a person who has not had the opportunity to pass such a catheter under the direct guidance of an instructor.

CONTINUOUS COLLECTION OF THE URINE

Where continuous collection of all urine excreted is desired it is done as follows: In males tape a finger cot to the penis. Tie the distal end of the finger cot over a medicine dropper and attach this to the catheter leading to a collection bottle.

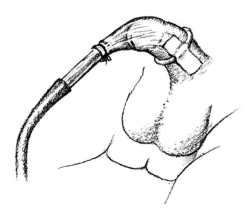

This is not possible in a female child. Continuous collection of urine from the infant female is best accomplished by using a metabolic bed: the infant is placed so that the perineum is over a hole in the mattress which holds a container to collect all urine and feces.

CEREBROSPINAL SYSTEM

Removal of spinal fluid is helpful in the diagnosis and treatment of many diseases, injuries, and tumors of the cerebrospinal system. This may be done via several routes.

LUMBAR PUNCTURE

This is the simplest and commonest method of obtaining spinal fluid in patients in whom there is no evidence of increase of intracranial pressure or of choked disks. The patient should be on his side with his knees drawn up and his head flexed so that his back is bowed toward the operator. Have your assistant or nurse hold the patient in this position by placing one hand behind the patient's knee, the other around the patient's shoulders and locking the hands together. Position the patient so that his back is at the edge of the table. Prepare the skin over the lower back by scrubbing with alcohol followed by tincture of Zephiran.

Depending upon the age of the infant, you may or may not wish to infiltrate the point of insertion of the needle with procaine. Introduce the spinal needle between the third and fourth lumbar vertebrae. (Review technique in adult, p. 79.) After the needle has entered the spinal canal as evidenced by clear fluid coming from the needle, allow about 8 drops of fluid to drop directly onto a chocolate agar slant for culture. Two other sterile tubes are used to collect an additional 5 ml. of spinal fluid. Send one sample for cell count and chemical analysis and the other for bacteriologic studies.

If indicated, measure the pressure of the spinal fluid by attaching a water manometer similar to that used for measuring venous pressure. Measurement of spinal fluid pressure is deceptive in children because of the lack of cooperation of the child and the amount of fluid needed to fill the manometer. To perform a Queckenstedt test gently compress the jugular veins. This causes an immediate rise in spinal fluid pressure which falls as the venous compression is released in the normal individual.

This response indicates that the spinal canal is open as evidenced by the direct relationship between venous pressure and intracranial pressure. This test should not be done if there is evidence of increased intracranial pressure. The experienced pediatrician can estimate the pressure by the bulging fontanel and the pressure with which the fluid is forced through the needle. Remove the needle and apply a small dry dressing when the test is completed.

CISTERNAL TAP

When spinal fluid cannot be obtained by lumbar puncture, or when there is evidence of increased intracranial pressure, a cisternal tap may be required. Shave the occiput and neck of the child. Prepare the skin with alcohol followed by Zephiran. With the head sharply flexed and the child in a sitting or lying position, introduce the needle through the skin in the midline at the base of the occiput. Direct the needle in a line from the base of the occiput through the external auditory meatus to the glabella.

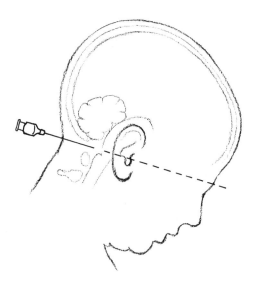

The cisterna lies at a depth of 1 to 2 cm. in infants. Do not penetrate too deeply. Introduce the needle, cautiously removing the stylet from time to time, until it enters the cisterna as evidenced by clear fluid in the needle; collect the fluid as recommended under spinal tap.

SUBDURAL TAP

Subdural tap is indicated when there is a suspicion of intracranial injury or infection. If a subdural effusion is found, subsequent therapeutic taps may be indicated.

The infant should be restrained in a sheet or a blanket so that he cannot move his arms or legs. The assistant holds the baby on the table in such a position that the entire top of the head is clear; the head is immobilized by a hand on either side. If the baby is given a nipple stuffed with cotton saturated with glucose solution he is usually pacified. Shave the scalp anterior to a line between the ears. Cleanse the skin with alcohol followed by Zephiran. Cover the posterior portion of the head with a sterile towel; excessive draping interferes with visualization of landmarks.

Using a 26-gauge hypodermic needle, raise a wheal with procaine at the point of entrance of the needle. This should be in the coronal suture just lateral to the fontanel. The point should be at least 3 cm. from the midline or at a point approximately in line with the pupil of the eye.

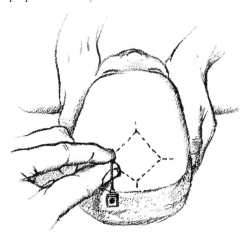

Introduce a short bevel, 20-gauge, 5 cm. lumbar puncture needle through the scalp at right angles to the skin surface. Rest the left hand on the head and steady the needle with the thumb and forefinger while you advance the needle with your right hand. In this way you can control lateral deviation of the point of the needle if the infant moves his head. Move the point of the needle along the bones until you find the suture line. Push the needle through the suture line slowly until the resistance is suddenly overcome. This is an indica-

tion that the subdural space has been entered. In older infants where union of the suture has begun it may be necessary to "screw" the needle until the dura is penetrated.

Since any excessive accumulation of fluid is always immediately beneath the dura there is no need to explore deeper. Remove the stylet and allow the fluid to drip from the needle. It may take a minute or two for flow to develop. It sometimes helps to rotate the needle to alter the position of the bevel. Do not move the point sideways and do not attempt to aspirate fluid through the needle. After 25 ml. of fluid has been removed withdraw the needle, apply pressure for a few minutes, and cover the puncture point with a sterile dressing.

When the tap is diagnostic it should be done bilaterally. If both taps are positive, remove 10 to 12 ml. Do not remove more than 25 ml. at a single tap. If one tap a day is not sufficient it should be done more frequently, but no more than 25 ml. should be removed each time.

Repeat taps should not be made through the same hole but the position should be varied slightly. Fluid collected for diagnosis is studied for appearance, pressure, cell count, sugar and chloride content, and bacteriology. Colloidal gold and cell blocks are done as indicated.

Normal fluid is clear and colorless. Normal pressure is 40 to 110 mm. of water in infants. It rises and falls promptly with gentle jugular compression. Normal cell count is 0 to 10 mononuclear cells. Depending upon the laboratory, normal protein values range between 15 and 45 mg. per 100 ml. The sugar values range between 40 and 80 mg. per 100 ml., depending upon the blood sugar, which is usually about 50 per cent higher. Normal chloride is 116 to 125 mg./L. There is an excellent table of the levels of these studies in various pathologic situations in an article by Frederic C. Moll on pages 234 and 235 of the February, 1955 number of Pediatric Clinics of North America.

Chapter Twelve

Gastrointestinal Intubation

The upper gastrointestinal tract may be intubated for any one of the following purposes:

1. Feeding
2. Aspiration
   a. For decompression
   b. For diagnosis
      Stomach—for determination of acidity and volume
      Duodenum—for assessment of biliary drainage
3. Compression

INTUBATION FOR FEEDING

INDICATIONS

Tube feeding is indicated when the patient is either unable or unwilling to swallow an adequate diet. This may be due to a local condition in the mouth or the esophagus which interferes with the ability to swallow, or to an intracranial lesion which interferes with the normal swallowing mechanism, or the swallowing mechanism may be normal but the patient unable to take food because he is unconscious. Some very ill patients cannot be persuaded to eat an adequate diet and the oral intake must be supplemented with tube feedings. Feedings may be instilled through a nasal feeding tube, a nasogastric tube, or through a gastrostomy or a jejunostomy tube.

NASAL INTUBATION

Nasal Feeding Tube

This is the simplest type and is used mainly for feeding. The commonly used nasal feeding tube is a standard 17 French rubber catheter passed through the nose into the upper esophagus.

173

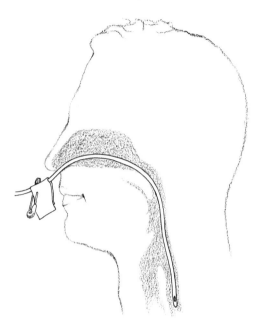

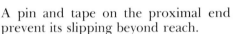

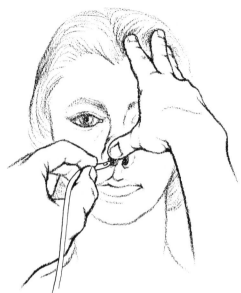

A pin and tape on the proximal end prevent its slipping beyond reach.

TECHNIQUE OF PASSAGE. Reassure the patient and explain the technique of passage as well as the purpose of the tube. Examine the nasal passages; one is usually larger than the other. If the mucosa appears swollen, or neither passage seems to provide adequate space for passage of the tube, dip a swab in ephedrine (2 per cent) and pontocaine (2 per cent) and apply topically to the mucosa of one nostril. After dipping the tip of the feeding tube in mineral oil gently introduce it into the nasal passage. Use the thumb and forefinger of your free hand to tilt backward the tip of the nose and then pass the tube along the floor of the nose beyond the turbinates.

Once the nasal passage has been cleared the next obstruction which may be encountered is the posterior wall of the nasopharynx. A stiff tube may run directly back against this. However, with a little gentle manipulation you can get past this point and into the oropharynx. Sometimes the nose-tilting maneuver already mentioned helps here also. After the tube has passed into the oro-

pharynx, encourage the patient to swallow the remainder of the tube himself.

It is anatomically possible for the tube to pass into either the esophagus or trachea; or the distal end may be regurgitated into the mouth. If the tip should be regurgitated into the mouth, pull back the distal portion of the tube until the tip is again in the oropharynx and repeat the procedure. If the tip should pass into the trachea, the patient will usually begin to cough. Tracheal intubation may also be recognized by a simple test: if the external end of the tube is placed in a glass of water bubbles will be produced during expiration. However, these signs may be misleading and the surest method is to insert a few drops of Dakin's solution into the tube. If this causes the patient to cough, the tube is in the trachea and must then be withdrawn and reinserted. Once you are satisfied that the tube is in the proper position, administer an ounce of water through the tube before you start the feeding and watch for reaction. These precautions are necessary for quite obvious reasons.

Important: Before attempting intubation review the possible complications (p. 188).

Nasogastric Tube

This is also a single lumen tube but it is longer than the nasal tube and is available in several diameters. While the nasal tube extends only into the upper esophagus the nasogastric tube passes through the cardiac sphincter into the stomach. In this position it can be used for aspiration as well as for feeding. The commonest nasogastric tube is a Levin tube, the diameter of which is 17 French.

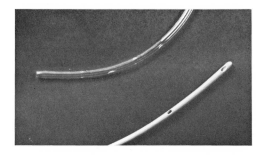

The original tubes were of hard rubber but a plastic variety is now available which, while having the same inside diameter, is softer and of a smaller external diameter. These features make the tube more comfortable for the patient. The small bore "Sustagen" tube has become popular as a feeding tube. Since the Sustagen feeding solution is thin, a considerably smaller tube may be used than is required for conventional nasogastric feeding.

The initial steps in the passage of a nasogastric tube are the same as outlined for the nasal feeding tube (p. 173). After the tube has been passed into the oropharynx give the patient a glass of water and have him sip it slowly. As he sips the water, slowly advance the tube until it enters the stomach. If it should slip into the trachea (as evidenced by coughing or bubbling from the end of the tube) or be regurgitated out through the mouth, pull it back until the tip is in the oropharynx and begin again to pass it through the esophagus. The *ability to withdraw gastric secretions from the tube* is proof that the tube is in the stomach. Pass the tube an additional four to six inches. This is usually to the second mark on the Levin tube. Once the tube is at a proper level secure it by taping it to the nose. Take the weight of the tube off the nose by attaching the tube to the forehead with a piece of tape.

Technique of Feeding

Clear the tube with a small amount of water and insert the feeding slowly by means of a syringe attached to the end of the tube. After the feeding flush with sufficient water to clear the tube. When feeding a patient who has not eaten for some time, start with a small amount and increase gradually. Begin with a 100 ml. feeding every waking hour and on succeeding days increase the amount and decrease the frequency until the patient is getting approximately 500 ml. four times a day. Some physicians allow a continuous drip of the feeding solution, but this should be done only while the patient is awake. Feeding patients while they are asleep or unconscious is hazardous because of the danger of aspiration. In many instances, patients may be taught to feed themselves.

The Feeding Solution

As mentioned earlier, there is a commercial product, called Sustagen, which can be mixed with either milk or water and which will provide satisfactory nutrition for the patient. It can be dripped in through the tiny feeding tube which has been developed by the same company. Artificial mixtures of basic dietary ingredients may also be used: every hospital has a basic formula for tube feeding. Finally, one can take an ordinary house diet, mix it in a blender and thin out the resultant paste as necessary with either milk or water. I prefer the last method because it allows an accurately composed, rounded type of diet for the patient. Its disadvantage is that it is too coarse a mixture to be passed through the tiny Sustagen feeding tube. On the other hand, it can be handled quite satisfactorily by the conventional types of feeding tube.

Important: Before attempting intubation review the possible complications (p. 188).

GASTROSTOMY

Technique of Intubating

A gastrostomy is a permanent or semipermanent opening through the abdominal wall directly into the stomach. It is used mainly for feeding purposes but under certain circumstances may be used for aspiration of gastric contents. There are two different types of gastrostomy. The more common type is serosa lined.

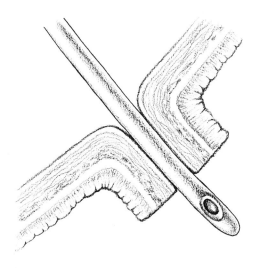

It is produced by invaginating the stomach wall and creating a tract with the serosa on the inner lining. This is a temporary type of gastrostomy and if the tube is removed and kept out for any period of time the serosa will seal to the serosa about the tract. This is an advantage when the gastrostomy is intended

to be temporary because the simple act of removal of the tube allows the tract to seal, and heal, thus avoiding a second operative procedure. On the other hand, the serosal type of tract is a source of potential difficulty while it is in use because if the tube should fall out and not be replaced without delay the tract might seal off and another gastrostomy would then have to be performed.

The second type is a mucosa lined gastrostomy.

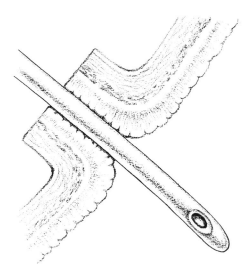

Since mucosa will not seal to mucosa, this is a permanent type of gastrostomy which is usually made when the stoma must be kept open indefinitely. One need not worry that such a gastrostomy will seal spontaneously and thus there is no need to keep a tube constantly in place to maintain patency. The tube need only be inserted for feeding and can be removed immediately thereafter. Closure of this type gastrostomy requires another operation.

Technique of Feeding

Depending upon the type of gastrostomy, a tube is either inserted into the tract or is already in place. *Before any material is instilled into the tube, stomach contents should always be aspirated.* Improper positioning of the tube, elsewhere than in the stomach, would be discovered at this point before any feeding was instilled. When proper positioning has been assured, wash out the tube with a small amount of water. Instill the feeding and follow this with enough additional water to wash the feeding through so that it will not clot in the tube. After the feeding the tube is clamped if the gastrostomy is a temporary type, or removed if it is a permanent type.

Type of Feeding

Hospitals usually have a routine gastrostomy feeding available. However, to ensure accurate control of the patient's diet, it is advisable to order an individualized gastrostomy feeding containing specific amounts of fat, carbohydrate, and protein as indicated by the patient's condition. You can also use a regular diet. To do this, have a regular diet portion sent to the floor. Blenderize it and thin it to the proper consistency with milk or water. Use as any other gastrostomy mixture. Start with small amounts. The first day give the patient 100 ml. every hour during his waking hours and on succeeding days increase the amount by 100 ml. and the interval between feedings by one hour until the patient is receiving 400 to 500 ml. four times a day. Note: If diarrhea develops first check the composition of the gastrostomy feeding. Routine hospital gastrostomy feedings commonly contain too much carbohydrate. This is a simple matter to correct. If this is not the case, decrease the volume and increase the number of feedings. If necessary give the patient ten drops of tincture of opium three times a day until the diarrhea is controlled. Dilute the medication with water and insert through the feeding tube.

JEJUNOSTOMY

A jejunostomy is a serosa lined tube. Occasionally it may be needed for aspiration, in which case the usual principles (p. 182) apply. Usually it is created for feeding purposes. Since a jejunostomy is serosa lined, a tube must be kept constantly in place. A moderate sized catheter, usually about a 17 French, is used. If the tube becomes displaced it should be replaced immediately. The ability to aspirate intestinal contents should be demonstrated before feeding is begun each time the tube is reinserted. Feeding via a jejunostomy requires considerably more care than feeding higher up in the gastrointestinal tract because the intestine at this point is quite sensitive to changes in the character of material entering it.

Technique of Feeding

There are many different methods of feeding including those used for some commercially available feeding solutions. The technique to be described utilizes homogenized milk and was described by Dr. Robert M. Zollinger. No food or fluid is given into the jejunostomy in the first 12 to 18 hours. During this period the tube may be clamped or connected to a drainage bottle at the side of the patient's bed. The day following operation give 50 ml. of 5 per cent glucose in water by asepto syringe every hour. The next day this can usually be increased to 100 ml. per hour. This should be continued until normal bowel activity has been restored.

Intestinal activity may be promoted by inserting 20 to 30 ml. of liquid petrolatum every 6 to 8 hours over a 24-hour period. Once normal peristaltic activity has been restored, milk feeding can be started. Begin with feedings of 50 ml. every hour gradually increasing this over the next three days to 200 ml. every two hours. Supplement this with intravenous fluids and electrolytes if needed.

If the jejunostomy feedings are planned for no more than two weeks the homogenized milk alone is adequate. An intake of 2000 ml. of homogenized milk provides approximately 1400 calories and 70 gm. of protein. In those cases where prolonged feeding is planned and more nutrition is desired, additional carbohydrate and protein may be added to the milk; however, such supplements should not be used until at least 7 to 10 days after construction of the jejunostomy. Add 30 gm. of starch hydrolysate and 50 gm. of protein hydrolysate to each 1000 ml. of homogenized milk. This provides 1000 calories and 70 gm. of protein per 1000 ml. of feeding. If the patient tolerates this, another 100 calories can be added by increasing the starch hydrolysate to 60 gm. This is usually as concentrated as can ordinarily be tolerated.

Individual variations affect the manner in which patients tolerate such a routine. If distention or cramps occur discontinue feedings and aspirate through the tube, if necessary, until the condition clears. Diarrhea most commonly occurs if milk is given too soon in too large amounts. Stop the milk and revert to glucose in water.

Advantages and Disadvantages of Intubation Feeding

The nasal feeding tube can be inserted by a specially trained nurse. Since it does not pass through the esophagogastric junction, the incidence of reflux esophagitis is lower. The nasogastric tube offers the advantage that the position of the tube can be ascertained before feeding is begun. Furthermore, certain conditions require aspiration of the stomach once a day. This could not be done with the shorter tube. An obvious advantage of both types is that neither requires an operative procedure for placement.

Gastrostomy is the route of choice when there is an obstruction proximal to the stomach. Jejunostomy should only be used when it is not possible to insert food into the gastrointestinal tract at a more proximal point.

INTUBATION FOR ASPIRATION

The purpose of decompression may be to place or keep the gastrointestinal tract at rest, or to remove the gastric and biliary secretions when the gastrointestinal tract is incapable of moving them along normally.

Nasogastric Tube

The nasogastric tube already described (p. 175) is probably the most commonly used tube in intestinal aspiration. Special circumstances may require that aspiration be carried out from low in the gastrointestinal tract, for which purpose longer intestinal tubes are required.

Long Intestinal Tube

To decompress the lower bowel the tube must be passed well down into the gastrointestinal tract, decompressing as it goes. In general, these long tubes may be divided into two groups: (1) double lumen tubes which depend on propulsion of an air-filled balloon to move the tube along and (2) a single lumen tube depending on the "free flow" of mercury in loose, balloon-tipped tubes. Both types depend on gravity and weighted tips to advance the tube into the duodenum.

Miller Abbott Tube

A typical example of a tube depending upon propulsion of an air-filled balloon is the Miller Abbott tube.

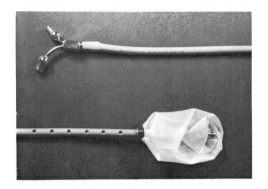

This is a double lumen tube with a metal tip. One lumen communicates with a balloon which is proximal to the metal tip and the other communicates with holes in the metal tip and in the tube proximal to the balloon. In this way decompressive suction is effected both ahead of and behind the balloon.

TECHNIQUE OF PASSAGE. Prepare the patient with a narcotic thirty minutes before the procedure. Reassure the patient and choose a nasal passage. Treat the nasal passage with a swab dipped in ephedrine (2 per cent) and pontocaine (2 per cent) prior to passing the long intestinal tube. Be sure that the tube is in good condition. The proximal end of the Miller Abbott tube is fitted with a metal connector containing two openings—one marked suction and the other marked air. Be certain that the connector is fixed to the tube properly. Next fill the balloon with air and test for leaks. Run some fluid through the suction lumen. Deflate the balloon. Lubricate the tip of the tube with mineral oil and gently pass it into the nose beyond the nasopharynx and into the oropharynx. Elevating the tip of the nose

and passing the tube along the floor of the nose aids passage. Give the patient a glass of water and have him sip it slowly. As the patient sips, advance the tube slowly and gently until it has entered the stomach, as evidenced by the ability to withdraw gastric contents. Apply suction to the tube until all of the contents of the stomach have been aspirated. If the gastric contents are thick, gavage the stomach with 50 to 100 ml. of normal saline between periods of suction to remove the particulate matter. After the stomach has been evacuated, withdraw the tube until the tip is at the cardia. If a fluoroscope is readily available time can be saved by fluoroscoping the patient at this time. Determine the level of the tube and position it so that the tip is at the pylorus. Turn the patient on his right side. After twenty minutes re-examine the patient fluoroscopically to see whether the tube has passed into the duodenum.

If a fluoroscope is not readily available a good approximation can be made by inflating the balloon and withdrawing the tube until the balloon meets resistance at the cardio-esophageal junction. Empty the balloon. Place the patient on his right side and slowly advance the tube about six inches. This should bring the tip to the region of the pylorus. Keep the patient on his right side for thirty minutes; this should allow the tube to pass into the duodenum. If it does, biliary drainage will be aspirated. If the tube has not passed into the duodenum one must use fluoroscopy. Reposition it under fluoroscopy so that the tip is at the pylorus. Keep the patient on his right side and return him to his bed for one hour. Check the position by fluoroscopy again after one hour. Further manipulation may be necessary.

Passing the tube into the duodenum is the most difficult part of using the Miller Abbott apparatus. Manipulation with fluoroscopy, inflation of the balloon to float the tip in, the use of stylets, magnets, and weighting of the tips have all been suggested. When we have difficulty passing the tube into the duodenum we insert 5 ml. of mercury into the bag to make use of gravity.

Once the tip has passed into the duodenum, advance the tube, with suction still on, an inch at a time until it reaches the third portion of the duodenum. At this point, insert 10 ml. of air into the bag. After the balloon has gone beyond the ligament of Treitz, add another 20 ml. of air to fill the balloon.

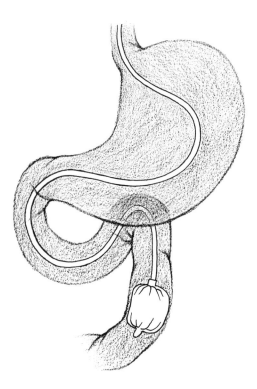

Do not anchor the proximal end of the tube to the nose or face. Advance the tube two inches every half hour. Intestinal activity should now take the tube down the intestinal tract.

Important: Before attempting intubation review the possible complications (p. 188).

Cantor Tube

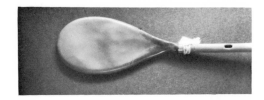

The Cantor tube is a single lumen tube with a bag loosely filled with mercury at its tip. Its lumen is considerably larger than that of the Miller Abbott tube. The end of the tube is not patent. A thin-walled rubber bag is fitted over the end of the tube. This bag is removable and can be replaced by another. First anchor the bag to the tube. Using heavy cord firmly tie the balloon over the tube. Put some mercury in a 10 ml. syringe with a 21 gauge needle. Insert the needle into the balloon and put in approximately 5 ml. of mercury.

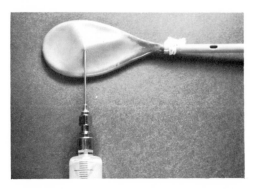

Draw off any air which might be in the balloon before withdrawing the needle.

Prepare the patient and the nasal passage as for insertion of the Miller Abbott tube (p. 179). Dip the tip of the tube in mineral oil. The patient may be either sitting up or lying flat so long as his head is hyper-extended and the nasal passage runs downward. Grasp the tip of the balloon and hold it up to allow the mercury to run to the neck of the balloon.

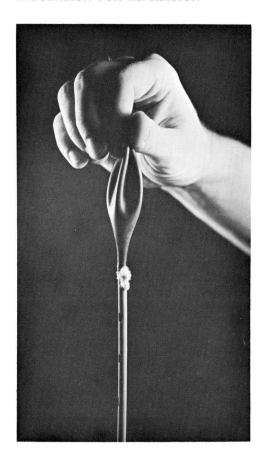

Trap it there with the thumb and index finger. This will allow you to fold the tip of the thin-walled balloon and insert it into the nasal passage.

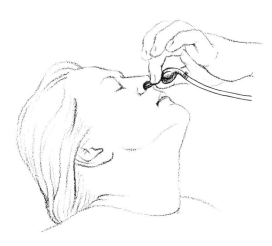

If you have difficulty you can push it along with a swab or a bayonet forceps. Once the tube has been passed back into the passage, release your finger and allow the mercury to run down into the tip of the bag. The weight of the mercury will assist in the insertion. After the tube has passed to the oropharynx, allow the patient to sit up and take a drink of water. The act of swallowing should carry the tube into the stomach. This will be evidenced by the ability to aspirate gastric contents. At this point, the S mark on the tube should be at the external nares. Pass along the tube to the mark P. This should put the balloon in the area of the pylorus.

Turn the patient on his right side, inclined face down, and raise the foot of the bed twelve inches. Keep him in this position for two hours which should allow the tube to pass into the duodenum as evidenced by drainage of bile. (If the tube does not pass have the patient ambulate; gravity should be effective.)

After the patient has been on his right side for two hours lower the foot of the bed and place him in the Fowler's position. Pass additional length of tube until the D mark is at the nose. The change of position should allow the tube to pass downhill to the ligament of Treitz. After two hours, turn the patient on his left side to pass the tube through the third portion of the duodenum and into the upper jejunum. This position is maintained for two hours and the patient is then encouraged to move about freely and sit in a chair if possible. The tube is not anchored to the patient and is allowed to move along at will.

Important: Before attempting intubation review the possible complications (p. 188).

After the tube has successfully accomplished its purpose it can be removed. Nasogastric tubes can be readily pulled out. Long intestinal tubes should be removed more slowly, withdrawing the tube 6 inches to a foot and waiting two or three minutes before withdrawing further. This will avoid drawing the intestine within itself, causing an obstruction.

Technique of Aspirating

Suction is applied to the appropriate orifice of the tube after it is in place. There are several different types of suction available:

1. Siphonage. This involves attaching the tube to a drainage bottle. The siphonage created by the fluid in the tube withdraws secretions. This is not so effective as methods utilizing external suction but is used where strong suction is contraindicated.

2. Suction created by a falling column of water.

3. Intermittent suction created by a pump.

4. Continuous suction created by a pump.

The suction apparatus is attached to the intestinal tube. Certain orders are necessary as an adjunct to intestinal suction:

1. Stop all oral feeding.

2. All intake and output should be carefully measured and charted. This includes urinary output.

3. The aspirating tube should be irrigated with an ounce of physiologic saline solution every hour.

4. Special attention to mouth care is necessary (p. 188).

5. Do not allow the patient to lie on one side for more than an hour.

6. Have the patient breathe deeply periodically to prevent atelectasis.

SELECTION OF ASPIRATING TUBE

Any of the tubes described can be used for decompression of the gastrointestinal tract. The results possible are related to the position of the distal end of the tube. The nasal feeding tube can aspirate only saliva and secretions from the pharynx. In most instances, aspiration is best accomplished by a nasogastric tube. This is easily and readily inserted to the optimal position. It can decompress the bowel if the obstruction lies at, or proximal to, the ileocecal valve.

The long intestinal tube is the tube of choice for use in the colon. It is the only tube which will be effective when there is an obstruction in the colon and the ileocecal valve is competent. Some prefer the use of the long tubes in obstructions in the lower small bowel. However, the disadvantage is the amount of time which must be spent in passing the long tube into the duodenum. On the other hand, the long tube is invaluable in getting past a fresh postoperative obstruction. In summary, the nasogastric tube is used in most cases of intestinal decompression, except where there is a fresh postoperative obstruction in the small bowel or any obstruction in the colon.

GASTRIC ANALYSIS

The stomach contents may be aspirated for diagnostic purposes. The Levin tube is most commonly used for this purpose. The contents are aspirated to determine acidity, the presence of tumor cells, and total volume.

A single lumen tube is passed into the stomach (pp. 173 and 174). The entire contents of the stomach are aspirated. The volume is noted as well as the presence of blood and the contents of free and total acid. The normal fasting stomach will hold 20 to 100 ml. yellowish or greenish fluid. Free HCl will range from 0 to 30 degrees and total acid from 10 to 50 degrees. The acid producing cells of the stomach are then stimulated by an injection of histamine subcutaneously (0.01 mg./Kg.) or by ingestion of a test meal. The stomach contents are withdrawn every 30 minutes for 2 hours and examined as before. Duodenal ulcer is associated with a high acidity which rises for approximately two hours. Gastric ulcer may be associated with a high, normal, or low acid pattern. A low acid curve in conjunction with a gastric ulcer suggests malignancy. The normal curve rises in about one hour to as high as 50 degrees free acid and 100 degrees total acid. It returns to approximately normal in two hours.

MEASURING AMOUNT OF PYLORIC OBSTRUCTION

In a patient with pyloric obstruction due to ulcer, part of the obstruction is a result of edema. The degree of obstruction which persists as the patient improves can be measured by passing a Levin tube and emptying the stomach. (The contents of the normal resting stomach should be no more than 100 ml.) The tube may be used also to feed the ulcer patient during the day and to empty his stomach at bedtime. The amount of residue at bedtime is a good index of the degree of obstruction present.

GASTRIC LAVAGE

Gastric lavage is indicated when the patient has swallowed a poisonous substance and in some instances when he has recently consumed an excessive amount of alcohol. It is possible to lavage the stomach with a Levin tube but it is more satisfactory to do so with a stomach tube which has a larger bore. Minimally a 24-gauge tube should be used in an adult and a 15-gauge tube in an infant. The stomach tube is stiffer and less likely than a Levin tube to coil as it is passed.

There is a great tendency for the patient to vomit and aspirate the vomitus during lavage. The only safe position for the patient is lying prone with his head projecting over the end of the table and facing the floor. Struggling children should be wrapped in a blanket before being placed in this position.

After the patient is placed prone on the table, any false teeth are removed and a gag is placed in the mouth to keep

it open. Before inserting the tube, mark with tapes or a pin the distance it is to be passed. Lubricate the tip of the tube with mineral oil and pass the tube through the mouth into the pharynx. Now pass the tube rapidly but not roughly through the esophagus into the stomach. This is necessary because many of these patients will be unconscious and others uncooperative, so that you cannot depend on their swallowing to help to pass the tube. Pass the tube to the predetermined level. It should now be possible to aspirate gastric contents.

Attach a funnel to the end of the tube and pour in 1 pint of tepid water ($\frac{1}{4}$ to $\frac{1}{2}$ pint in children). Then begin siphonage by dropping the end of the tube down into a pail at the head of the table. Set aside the first pint siphoned for later analysis. Continue the lavage a pint at a time until 16 pints have been used. Measure the volume returned at the completion of the procedure to be certain that most of the water is removed. If there has been any appreciable loss of fluid the possibility of a perforation of the stomach must be considered.

DUODENAL DRAINAGE

Technique of Passage

Duodenal intubation is now reserved for diagnostic work and these patients are all fasting. A small, single lumen, soft rubber tube with a weighted metal tip is used.

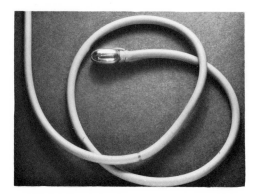

The many different types available are all variations of the same principle. Place the tube in a pan of ice water for approximately 15 minutes. Explain the procedure to the patient and attempt to put him at ease. With the patient sitting up insert the metal tip of the tube through his mouth far back into his pharynx and encourage him to swallow. As the patient swallows, advance the tube into his mouth until the tip reaches the stomach, where gastric contents can be aspirated.

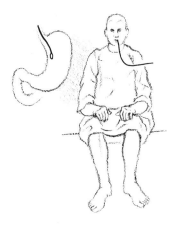

The tube will then be at approximately the 45 cm. mark. Now have the patient lie on his left side on a bed with the head elevated and advance the tube an additional 15 cm.

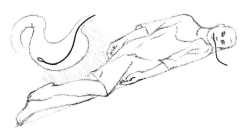

This maneuver will move the tube along the greater curvature of the stomach.

After about 5 minutes have the patient sit up, bend forward and take several deep breaths.

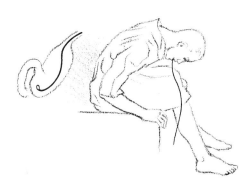

This maneuver helps the tip of the tube slip into the antrum as the anterior wall of the stomach falls forward. Next, position the patient on his right side in a head-down position for about five minutes.

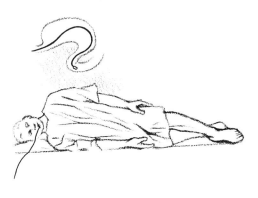

At the same time pass an additional 15 cm. of tubing. During this time the tip should pass through the pylorus into the duodenum. The aspirate should now contain bile. Have the patient turn over on his back for a few minutes, while still in the head-down position to pass the tube further into the duodenum.

He is now ready for the biliary drainage procedure.

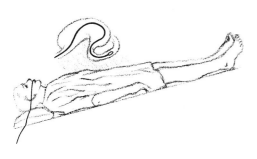

Technique of Biliary Drainage

With the tube in place in the duodenum, insert 50 to 100 ml. of sterile 25 per cent magnesium sulfate solution through the tube. This relaxes the sphincter of Oddi and induces drainage of the entire biliary tract. Aspirate the secretions into a series of sterile bottles. Golden yellow bile from the common duct appears very soon and is designated "A." After a few minutes this rather suddenly gives way to a darker, more viscid bile which comes from the gallbladder and is designated "B." This portion usually amounts to 30 to 75 ml. and is succeeded by a clear, light, yellow bile of low specific gravity which is assumed to be freshly secreted bile from the liver, and designated "C." The various portions are collected separately, and their color, viscosity, turbidity and general appearance noted, as well as the presence or absence of mucus. They are also examined microscopically for abnormal sediments and tumor cells and cultured for bacteria.

INTUBATION FOR ESOPHAGEAL COMPRESSION

Compression by tube is used to control diffuse bleeding in the lower esophagus or upper stomach. A typical example of the esophageal compression tube is the Sengstaken-Blakemore tube.

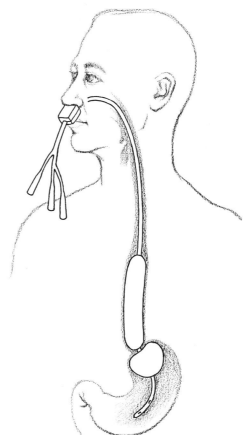

It consists of a triple lumen tube with two ballons attached. A large lumen, which extends beyond the balloons into the stomach, is used for aspiration and for feeding. Two smaller lumina communicate with the balloons. The distal balloon is just proximal to the perforated tip of the suction tube. This balloon lies in the stomach and compresses the gastroesophageal junction when traction is exerted on the proximal end of the tube. The proximal balloon is sausage-shaped. It lies in the esophagus and compresses the esophageal varices. The lower half of this balloon is doubly reinforced to prevent its expanding into the stomach.

Traction on the gastric balloon can be controlled by means of a headgear unit with a spring type strain gauge attached. The direction of pull on the tube is such that excess pressure on the nares is avoided.

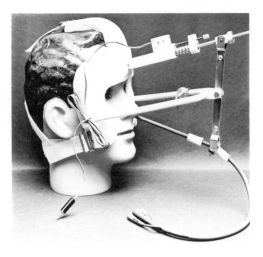

A cylinder reservoir unit is available that may be used to control the pressure in the esophageal balloon. It incorporates an alarm system which is set off by a decrease in either gastric traction or esophageal balloon pressure.

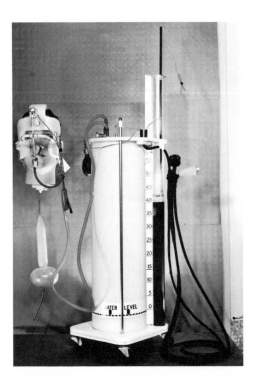

TECHNIQUE OF INTUBATING

Reassure the patient and spray the nostril and posterior pharynx with 2 percent pontocaine. Check each balloon to make certain that there are no leaks. Flush some fluid through the aspirating lumen. Deflate the balloons. Coat the lower half of the tube with mineral oil, or a thin layer of lubricating jelly. Gently pass the tube through the nasal passage into the oropharynx, manipulating it past the posterior wall of the nasopharynx. Tilting the tip of the nose and passing the tube along the floor of the nose will help. After the tube is in the nasopharynx, have the patient sip a glass of water while you pass the tube to the 50 cm. mark. This should put the tube well into the stomach as evidenced by ability to aspirate bloody gastric contents. Inflate the lower balloon with 200 ml. of air and withdraw the tube until you feel the resistance of the esophagogastric junction against the balloon. Put the plastic headgear in place and attach the tube to the strain gauges.

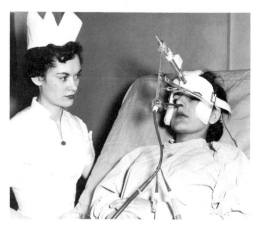

USE OF THE ESOPHAGEAL COMPRESSION TUBE

Aspirate the stomach so that all blood as well as air and swallowed water are removed. Interspace the aspiration with irrigations of the tube with 50 ml. of water to remove all clots. Adjust the pressure in the upper balloon until bleeding ceases, as determined by aspiration. The pressure usually required is 35 to 45 cm. of water. When the balloon is in proper position, the recorded pressure varies with cardiac and respiratory pulsations and with contractions of the esophagus which may raise the pressure to 70 mm. of mercury. The pressure should not be allowed to fall below 20 to 25 mm. Maintenance at this level usually requires about 50 ml. of air in the balloon; if considerably more air is required the balloon has slipped into the stomach. If this occurs, lower the esophageal balloon and reposition it. After sufficient air has been placed in the balloon the system can be sealed by means of a shut off valve. If the balloon deflates, the alarm system will be activated. Check the position of the tube by a portable x-ray. Connect the stomach aspiration tube to constant suction and irrigate the tube with 40 ml. of warm saline every half hour. The color of the aspirate should be recorded each time. This is an excellent means of detecting fresh bleeding in the stomach and also lessens the possibility of the tube's being obstructed by a blood clot.

It is important that the tube be kept in proper position and not regurgitated by the patient. The two most common causes of regurgitation are overdistention of the stomach with a liquid, and nervousness on the part of the patient. Keep the head of the bed elevated and keep the stomach empty. These measures decrease nausea and the gag reflex. The patient must be kept relaxed— not unconscious but rather in a slightly stuporous state. You can do this with the use of intravenous Amytal and small amounts of Demerol if necessary.

The inflated balloon should be kept at the minimal pressure required to control bleeding, for at least 48 hours and then slowly deflated. If no new bleeding occurs after 12 to 14 hours the tube may be slowly withdrawn, with very little danger of starting new bleeding. During the time the tube is in place, the patient must be kept hydrated and given nutrition intravenously. If things are going well, small feedings can be given through the stomach part of the tube, 100 to 150 ml. per hour, with the head of the bed elevated and the patient on his right side. The stomach should be aspirated just before feedings. Thick feedings must be avoided as they will clog the tube and remain in the stomach too long. Too much food in the stomach will increase the chance of vomiting the tube and, therefore, endanger the entire program of treatment.

Emphasize to the patient that he is to swallow nothing, not even saliva, once the tube is in place. When there is excessive accumulation of saliva the balloon may be deflated for a few minutes several times a day.

If, after the esophageal balloon is inflated to as much as 60 cm. of water, repeated aspirations from the stomach reveal bright red blood, this is evidence that the source of the bleeding is a coronary vein on the stomach wall. In this event give the patient additional sedation and increase the pull on the traction mechanism. Finally, inflate the stomach balloon gradually with more air. It may require a total of 300 to 400 ml. of air to arrest bleeding.

After the tube has been withdrawn, the patient may be given clear liquids and his diet slowly advanced to soft foods.

COMPLICATIONS

The use of an intestinal tube for feeding or for aspiration can be accompanied by complications. Complications resulting from intubation are:
1. Atelectasis
2. Stomatitis and parotitis
3. Ulceration of the nose and/or soft palate
4. Acute otitis media
5. Reflux esophagitis

Complications which may develop in association with feeding tubes are:

1. Regurgitation and aspiration of feeding
2. Diarrhea

These complications due mainly to aspiration include:

1. Dehydration
2. Electrolyte imbalance
3. Coiling of the tube
4. Intestinal obstruction

COMPLICATIONS OF INTUBATION

Atelectasis

The presence of any tube in the pharynx interferes with proper ventilation and tends to increase the incidence of atelectasis and retention of secretions. This should be constantly borne in mind. Keeping the patient properly hydrated and encouraging periodic deep breathing and coughing if necessary will help avoid these complications. Nasotracheal aspiration (p. 240) may be necessary. There is a definite hazard to intubation; the tube should be kept in place only as long as is necessary. Nasogastric tubes are best left in place for the duration of their use; nasal feeding tubes can be withdrawn and re-inserted as needed.

Stomatitis and Parotitis

With a tube through one of his nares (and almost invariably the more adequate of the two nasal passages), the patient usually becomes a mouth breather. As a result, there is increased drying of the mucous membranes. This is one of the reasons why the patient with an indwelling nasogastric tube complains so much of being thirsty. Drying of the mucous membranes tends to make them crack, then to become ulcerated, and finally to become infected. A high incidence of ulcers, stomatitis, pharyngitis and even parotitis is the result. The best

method of avoiding this complication is meticulous mouth care several times a day. The patient's mouth must be scrupulously cleaned at least four times a day. If the patient is able he should be encouraged to brush his teeth (and his tongue). He should follow this by irrigation with any conventional mouthwash and have the process completed by putting a drop of mineral oil on his tongue. If he is unable to do this himself it should be done by the nurse. If the tooth brush is too irritating, his mouth should be mechanically cleansed with moistened cotton swabs. If there is difficulty in cleaning the thick exudate from his tongue a solution of one part hydrogen peroxide and three parts water is helpful. After the mouth is cleaned rinse or swab with mouthwash. Finally coat the lining of the mouth with mineral oil. If the patient requires mouth care oftener than four times daily it should be given.

Ulceration of the Nose

If the tube is left in place too long, ulceration of the nose or of the palate may ensue. This is, however, not a very frequent occurrence, and I think its possibility has been considerably overemphasized. This complication can be avoided by withdrawing the tube two to three inches from the nose each day, coating it with an antibiotic ointment and allowing it to return to its former position. If ulceration should occur, the tube must, of course, be removed. If intubation is essential, the other side of the nose must be used or another orifice created.

Acute Otitis Media

Pressure of the indwelling tube over a prolonged period against the inner end of the eustachean tube can cause edema and obstruction with resultant otitis media. Some physicians believe that the patient with an indwelling tube should be kept on his back. I think it is sufficient to change his position regularly and not allow him to stay on one side for more than one hour.

Reflux Esophagitis

When a nasogastric tube is left in place lying through the cardioesophageal sphincter for a prolonged period of time, esophagitis may develop, probably because some of the gastric contents reflux about the tube. This condition is remarkably rare, but its possibility must not be overlooked; it is most likely to occur in the patient who has been desperately ill and whose general condition is poor. Naturally, in such patients the ability to tolerate the complication is also reduced. If there is anything about the patient's condition to suggest reflux esophagitis, a careful examination should be made immediately after the tube is removed. If inflammation is present a bland diet and antacids are prescribed. If constriction is a problem, bougienage will usually correct the situation.

COMPLICATIONS ASSOCIATED WITH FEEDING

Regurgitation or Aspiration

The feeding via the nasopharynx may enter the tracheobronchial tree directly via the feeding tube because of erroneous insertion, or indirectly by regurgitation and aspiration. A catheter in the trachea will cause most patients to cough and show some evidence of respiratory distress. But unfortunately, many patients who require feedings are quite ill and the cough reflex may be markedly diminished. Holding the tip of the tube below the surface of the glass of water and noting the presence or absence of bubbles is some help. Un-

questionably, however, correctness of positioning of a nasogastric tube is best determined by withdrawal of gastric contents from the tube. Such a demonstration is not possible with the nasal feeding tube which does not pass directly into the stomach. Instillation of a few drops of Dakin's solution through this type of feeding tube will cause no reaction if the tube is in the esophagus. If, on the other hand, the tube is in the trachea, the irritating solution will cause the patient to cough. One can confirm proper position by inserting an ounce of water prior to beginning the feeding.

There is also real danger of the feeding entering the tracheobronchial tree indirectly. In other words, the feeding may be instilled into the esophagus or stomach but the patient may regurgitate and aspirate the material into the tracheobronchial tree.

Probably the commonest prelude to this disaster is the habit of giving the patient a drip feeding while he is asleep or unconscious. It may also occur because the feeding is too large or given too rapidly. The unconscious patient who must be fed by tube should have a tracheostomy which will allow mechanical aspiration of any regurgitated material.

Diarrhea

A considerable proportion of patients who are fed by tube develop diarrhea. The commonest cause of this is excessive carbohydrate in the feeding. It is far better to order a specific diet according to the caloric requirements of the patient which is then blended and thinned. In the event that the patient develops diarrhea first consult with the dietetic department. If the composition of the diet is responsible, correcting the diet will solve the problem. Occasionally, the diarrhea will persist even though the makeup of the diet seems to be satisfactory. In this situation give paregoric (3 i q.i.d.) or tincture of opium (gtts. X t.i.d.).

COMPLICATIONS ASSOCIATED WITH ASPIRATION OF INTESTINAL TRACT

Dehydration

This results from removing more fluid than you replace. The patient's intake and output must be measured accurately. The amount of fluid necessary can then be calculated. (See Chapter 21.)

Electrolyte Imbalance

This is a consequence of improper replacement of the electrolytes removed. (See Chapter 21.)

Coiling of the Tubes

If the tube is advanced too rapidly, it may coil and develop knots. This complication is best prevented by slow careful passage of the tube. If knotting has occurred and the tube cannot be withdrawn, cut it off at the mouth and allow it to be passed by rectum. If it can be withdrawn up into the oropharynx, deliver the knot through the mouth and cut the tube. This difficulty is more likely to occur with the long tubes.

Intestinal Obstruction

The intestinal tract may be obstructed by the balloon of the Miller Abbott tube. This occurs if too much air or fluid accumulates in the balloon. As mentioned earlier, the proximal metal adapter may be in the wrong lumen. Even though the adapter is properly applied, the nurse may insert the irrigating solution into the wrong lumen. Finally, after a balloon has been in the gastrointestinal tract for more than five days a significant amount of gas may diffuse into the balloon. This can be evacuated through the proper ostium unless the tube has become knotted. In such a case treatment must be individualized. In the intact gastrointestinal tract, or if the balloon is proximal to the anastomosis, gentle traction on the balloon will gradually pull it back. Usually when it has been pulled back to the duodeno-jejunal flexure, it ruptures and removal is simple. If the distended balloon is beyond the anastomosis, do not pull it back because this maneuver may rupture the anastomosis. It is safer to cut the tube and let the balloon pass by rectum. If you elect to do this watch for signs of intestinal obstruction. If this occurs, try passing another tube proximal to the balloon. If this is not effective a laparotomy is required. It is not necessary to open the bowel. Manual compression of the gut will rupture the balloon and the tube can then be removed from above.

Chapter Thirteen

The Head and Neck

SCALP

Most of the blood supply to the scalp comes from the supraorbital, temporal, posterior auricular and occipital arteries. They anastomose profusely so that the healing properties of the scalp are excellent; large flaps readily heal and infection is rare. The blood supply comes up around the skull toward the top of the head. Consequently, a tight rubber band around the head just above the ears acts as a satisfactory tourniquet.

INJURIES

All injuries to this area should be considered as possibly involving intracranial injury. If, after study of the patient, it does seem that there may be damage, the patient must be managed as recommended on page 99.

Abrasions

Abrasions of the scalp are uncommon because of the protection afforded by the hair. Because of the resistance offered by the skull, blows to the head most commonly produce lacerations.

Lacerations

The free bleeding of scalp wounds can be controlled by pressing the bleeding area against the underlying skull. Cut the hair away and shave the skin immediately adjacent to the wound. An area of approximately one centimeter in all directions beyond the laceration should be cleared. Anesthetize the area by injecting 1 per cent procaine solution into the edge of the incision with a 25-gauge needle. Excise any devitalized skin. If the deep galea aponeuro-

191

tica is involved it must be sutured separately (p. 147). Close the wound with interrupted sutures. There is no need to drain the wound if it was properly cleansed. Apply one of the scalp dressings (p. 61) if the laceration is minor, or a recurrent head dressing (p. 62) if more extensive.

accidental tattoo

Hematomas

When they occur in the scalp they rarely become very large and rarely need aspiration. Most will resolve spontaneously. If aspiration is required, infiltrate the skin with procaine and insert an 18-gauge needle through the infiltrated area into the hematoma. Aspirate the hematoma, remove the needle, and apply a pressure dressing if there is reason to believe that the hematoma may recur.

INFECTIONS

Infections of this area are treated essentially as in other parts of the body (p. 113). Use compresses until the infection is localized and then employ surgical drainage.

SPECIFIC LESIONS

Any lesion of the skin which can occur elsewhere in the body may also be found in the scalp. The commonest lesion is the sebaceous cyst. Sebaceous cysts in the scalp have a special significance because they are more likely to become malignant and they must, therefore, be excised. The procedure is described on page 152.

FACE

The face also has a rich blood supply and, consequently, heals well. Sutures need not remain there as long as elsewhere in the body.

INJURIES

Abrasions

Abrasions of the face are common. They usually heal with very little treatment. Uncomplicated abrasions are treated by careful cleansing with surgical soap, gauze, and plenty of water. If dirt or other foreign bodies are imbedded in the wound each piece must be removed, with a pointed forceps if necessary; otherwise each will later represent a point of discoloration. No dressing is needed; the dried serum provides a satisfactory covering.

Contusions

The face is a common site for severe contusions, which are often accompanied by marked edema, ecchymosis, and sometimes fractures of the malar bone or the zygoma. Fracture should be suspected when there is a flatness of the injured side of the face and a lack of facial expression. If either bone is fractured, there is discoloration of the eyelid and gradually advancing subconjunctival ecchymosis 24 to 48 hours after the injury. If the ecchymosis becomes severe, double vision may occur as a result of secondary loss of function of the extraocular muscles. If there is considerable edema, the fracture may not be obvious and can be diagnosed only by x-rays. A fracture with no displacement requires no treatment, but if there is displacement the bone edges should be reapproximated as closely as possible to the normal position.

If no fractures are present, treat the contusion with cold compresses for the first 24 hours and with warm compresses thereafter. The area of ecchymosis will spread before it is absorbed. It is important to warn the patient of this; otherwise, he will mistakenly think that the injury is becoming more serious.

Lacerations

First anesthetize the area. This is most simply accomplished by injecting the skin edges at the raw surface with ½ or 1 per cent procaine solution using a fine hypodermic needle. If the wound is grossly contaminated, clean it first, but if the skin edges seem to be free of contamination, you can inject the procaine before you cleanse the wound. Hold a dry cotton sponge over the wound itself and carefully and vigorously clean the area about this. Débride the wound as necessary; usually debridement need not be extensive because the excellent blood supply to the face makes for good healing in most wounds. However, any obviously devitalized and/or dirt-impregnated tissue should be removed. Injury of deeper structures must be considered and ruled out. Lacerations of the cheek may damage branches of the seventh cranial nerve, the parotid gland, or Stensen's duct. Severed nerves should be repaired immediately. If the parotid gland is injured the capsule should be resutured and the wound drained. If Stensen's duct is damaged it should be repaired by passing a probe into the duct from within the mouth. The duct is repaired over the probe leaving the probe in place for 10 days.

The wound should be drained externally. If the depth of the wound can be completely cleaned, the defect can be closed with a careful plastic approximation. Close the deep tissues with interrupted silk sutures to take pressure off the suture line. Close the skin with fine plastic sutures (5-0 to 7-0) using interrupted over-and-over sutures 1 to 2 mm. apart. Small wounds of the face need no dressing and can be covered with a plastic spray or a small collodion dressing. On the other hand, if you are not certain that the wound is sterile, bring the wound edges together loosely to allow drainage between edges of the skin.

THROUGH-AND-THROUGH LACERATIONS. In treating through-and-through wounds into the mouth, after proper hemostasis and debridement, completely close the subcutaneous tissues and skin surface; leave the mucous membrane open or loosely approximate the tissues to allow drainage into the mouth. Irrigations with 3 per cent hydrogen peroxide solution, alternated at hourly intervals with the use of oral Varidase troches, will keep the intraoral wound clean and prevent the accumulation of eschar which usually occurs with incisions in the mouth.

LACERATION OF THE LIPS. The rich blood supply about the face allows rapid healing of the lips so that good approximation of the edges is important to the ultimate result. After cleaning the wound infiltrate the area with ½ per cent procaine. If the laceration has divided the orbicularis oris muscle, the cut ends must be approximated in a separate procedure. The vermilion borders must be carefully approximated to get a good result. Align these prior to closing either the skin or the mucous membrane. Close the skin with plastic, closely approximated sutures; close the mucous membrane portion of the wound by loose approximation only.

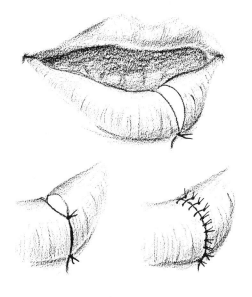

All sutures should be very loose because of the well known tendency of lips to swell. Puncture wounds of the lips, most of which are made by teeth, rarely require sutures. Proper cleansing is usually adequate.

LACERATIONS WITHIN THE MOUTH. General care of seriously injured patients with lacerations in and about the mouth is detailed in Chapter 7, Trauma. Bleeding is usually profuse, but in a remarkable number of these wounds there is spontaneous cessation of bleeding and local cleansing alone is required. If there is a significant defect it should be loosely closed with fine (5-0) nylon sutures. Irrigations with 3 per cent hydrogen peroxide should be alternated hourly with Varidase troches during the convalescent period.

Bleeding around a tooth will stop without treatment. If the tooth is loose, do not disturb it unless there is danger that it will fall out and be aspirated by the patient.

Lacerations of the tongue are usually self-inflicted as a result of falling and biting the tongue. Bleeding may be copious for a few minutes and then, surprisingly, often may stop. Consequently, lacerations of the tongue rarely need to be repaired to control hemorrhage. If the laceration is on either surface of the tongue, it is probably just as well to leave it alone. On the other hand, if it involves the margin of the tongue and creates a flap, it should be sutured. Suturing should be done anteriorly and posteriorly with fine nonabsorbable suture material after the tongue has been anesthetized with infiltration anesthesia. No dressing is possible. Have the patient irrigate his mouth with 3 per cent hydrogen peroxide solution interspersed at hourly intervals with Varidase troches to remove the eschar.

TONGUE FLAP SHOULD BE SUTURED.

Dislocation of the Mandible

Dislocation of the mandible is commoner in males than females, and the most frequent cause is a blow on the tip of the jaw when the mouth is open. The condyles are dislocated anteriorly and

superiorly. When this occurs, the lower jaw is more prominent and lies forward, and the mouth cannot be closed. It is often possible to palpate the abnormal position of the condyle.

TREATMENT. To reduce the dislocation wrap both your thumbs with protecting gauze. Insert one thumb over the lower molars on each side and steady the mandible with the external fingers. Press down firmly on the molar teeth and at the same time lift the tip of the jaw.

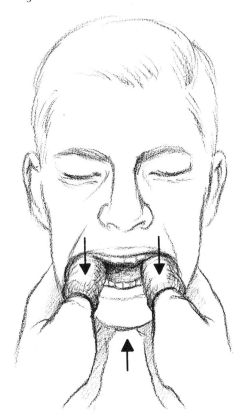

Continue to press down and back until the joint slips into place. In the majority of instances this will occur readily. In the occasional case it may be necessary to use general anesthesia. This problem may become chronic and the patient should be warned against opening his mouth widely and particularly against yawning. If necessary the jaw can be stabilized for a period with a Barton type dressing.

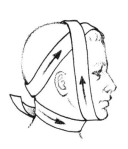 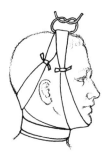

INFECTIONS

Superficial infections of the face are common. The face is exposed to trauma and has multiple orifices through which bacteria can enter. The area has an excellent blood supply, but since a portion of the deep venous return is by way of intracranial vessels, infection of the upper part of the face can rapidly threaten the brain. On the other hand, the lymphatics drain down into the neck away from the face.

One is hesitant to recommend surgery for infections of the face because of (1) the resulting scar and (2) the possibility of infection spreading within the cranium if the infection is incised too soon. For this reason, antibiotics, rest, and local compresses are used first. If there is no satisfactory response to antibiotics and nonoperative treatment within 48 hours one must resort to surgical intervention. Make the incision on one of the lines or creases of the face. These can be accentuated by having the patient grimace.

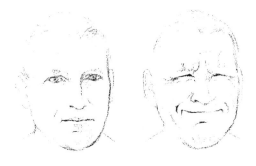

There is no need for through-and-through drainage. Culture the organism for antibiotic sensitivity and adjust the treatment as indicated. A thorough knowledge of the anatomy of the face, and particularly of the facial nerve, is a prerequisite to operating on the face (p. 148).

SPECIFIC LESIONS

Face

The lesions which may appear on the skin elsewhere also can be found on the face. Description of the surgical treatment of these lesions is contained in Chapter 10, Minor Surgery. Dissection must be based on understanding of facial anatomy and incisions should follow the natural lines of the face, so that a careful plastic approximation of the tissues can be done.

Lip

The commonest lesion of the lip is an ulcer. These are most frequently seen in persons exposed to excessive sunshine and in those who smoke pipes excessively. It is difficult to differentiate a malignant from a benign ulcer. Initial treatment consists of avoidance of trauma and of excessive exposure to the sun, plus local application of a bland ointment, such as lanolin, to the lips. If the ulcer does not clear with this treatment, a biopsy should be taken. If malignant, the lesion should be treated by complete surgical excision or radiotherapy.

Mouth

Several lesions may be found in the mouth which do not occur elsewhere. Retention cysts may develop as a result of blockage of a gland duct. These are characterized by a small nontender cystic swelling under the mucous membrane of the cheek, lips or tongue. They are treated by unroofing the cyst and removing the upper half.

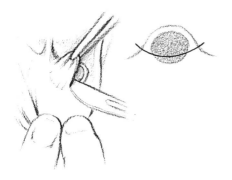

The inner, lower half of the cyst wall remains as lining of the mouth. The procedure is done under local anesthesia. If bleeding persists from the edge of the cyst wall, it can be sutured to the oral mucosa.

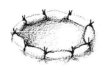

Ulcer

Trauma may produce in the mucous membrane of the cheek inflammatory lesions which ulcerate. These are of little consequence and heal without specific treatment. However, an ulcer may occasionally have a serious cause; it can be the result of tuberculosis, syphilis or cancer. If the lesion persists longer than 10 days a biopsy should be done.

Fibroma

A patient who repeatedly bites the mucous membrane of his cheek may produce a fibrous tumor or fibroma. Because of its bulk it is then more likely to be traumatized. Such a lesion should be excised at its base under local anesthesia. The base is usually sufficiently small that it can be closed primarily.

Leukoplakia

This is a white, plaque-like lesion which involves the oral mucosa and is thought to be due to irritation. It is particularly important because in some cases it is considered to be premalignant. Bernier* describes a benign lesion called pachyderma oralis and dyskeratosis. The latter is true leukoplakia but can be differentiated only by microscopic examination. Consequently, such a lesion must be biopsied for diagnosis. Treatment of pachyderma oralis consists of avoiding irritants (tobacco, condiments, and astringents). The treatment of dyskeratosis is excision.

EYE

INJURIES

Contusions

Because of the eye's loose tissues and abundant blood supply, blunt trauma to it may cause considerable swelling and ecchymosis of the lids, the periorbital tissues, and even of the eye itself. These swellings are usually absorbed without specific treatment. One must rule out the possibility of serious damage to the eye or to the bones of the face, either of which may be concealed by the local swelling.

Lacerations

Lacerations about the eye must be carefully and promptly closed to avoid interference with sight and to prevent disfiguring scars.

Superficial lacerations involving only the skin surfaces of the lids can be closed by simple suture. Linear lacerations can be closed by a subcuticular suture and irregular wounds can be closed with 6-0 black silk. Careful, accurate approximation of the tissues is necessary. No dressing is required. Remove the sutures in 3 to 4 days.

---

*Bernier, J. L.: The Management of Oral Diseases. St. Louis, C. V. Mosby Co. 1955.

Lacerations of the full thickness of the lids must be carefully examined to rule out the possibility of damage to the eye itself. If the laceration extends through the full thickness of the lid but does not involve the lid margin, only the two surfaces require suturing. Evert the lid and carefully approximate the conjunctiva with interrupted 6-0 black silk sutures. Close the skin wound with similar sutures. Close the lid and dress the repair with a layer of nonadherent dressing covered by a pressure dressing. Remove the pressure dressing in two days. The conjunctival sutures will slough out in a few days. Remove the skin sutures in 3 to 4 days.

Lacerations extending through the lid and involving the margin are more difficult to handle effectively. In such an injury, accurate approximation of the tarsus is essential to a good result. One can accomplish this by carefully suturing the divided edge of the tarsus. One is more likely to get a good result by a plastic repair. Split the lids into two layers for about 6 mm. on each side of the wound. Make the incision just anterior to the tarsus.

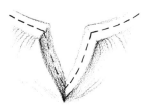

The anterior layer is composed of skin, subcutaneous tissue and orbicularis muscle and the posterior layer is composed of tarsus and conjunctiva. Remove a triangular wedge 3 mm. at its base from the anterior layer on one side and the posterior layer on the other side.

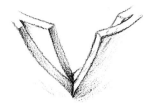

Approximate the layers with a mattress suture of which both ends are on the outside. Tie the suture over a button and carefully approximate the edges of the layers with interrupted 6-0 black silk sutures.

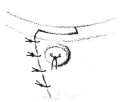

Close the lids and cover the repair with a nonadherent dressing covered by a pressure dressing. Remove the pressure dressing after 48 hours, Remove the skin sutures in 3 days and the mattress suture in a week. If the laceration involves the inner canthus or the duct, the patient should be referred to an ophthalmic surgeon.

Foreign Body

The commonest eye problem is a foreign body. The foreign body may have drifted into the eye from a dusty atmosphere, or it may have been imbedded in the eye as a result of some force as with flying particles from a grinding wheel. It may have gone directly into the eyeball, or it may have come through the lid and into the eyeball.

In many instances the patient is uncertain as to whether he has something in his eye, but he does complain of pain. Conjunctivitis may have developed and if sufficient time has elapsed before the patient consults you there may be a purulent reaction. The first problem is to determine the site of the foreign body. Have the patient either in a supine position or reclining in a chair with a head rest which makes him comfortable. A good source of light must be available and some type of magnification is necessary. Ask the patient to open his eye and inspect it thoroughly. One should attempt to see as much as possible before touching the eye. The conjunctiva of the lower lid, the lower fornix, and the lower part of the globe can be properly inspected by pulling down on the lower eyelid while asking the patient to look upward.

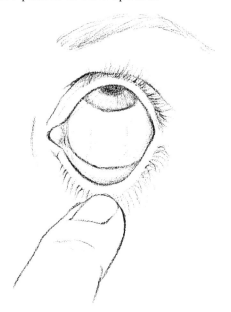

The most satisfactory method of examining the under surface of the upper lid is to evert the upper lid. Have the patient look down, grasp the eyelashes, and gently pull the upper lid down and out. Place the wooden portion of an applicator stick against the middle portion of the lid.

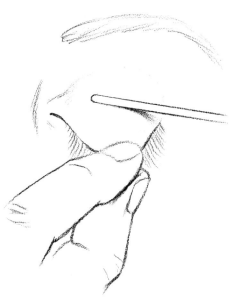

Push backward with the applicator stick and gently raise the lid upward with the eyelashes. This should evert the upper lid, exposing its conjunctival surface to your view.

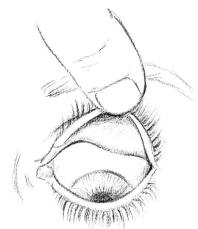

If you do not see any foreign body at this time and you believe that one is present it is probably imbedded in the eye. Place one drop of 1 per cent aqueous solution of fluoroscein into the eye and wash out the excess. This will stain areas of damage and make it easier to find sites of abrasion and foreign bodies.

If the foreign body is sitting loosely in the eye it can be readily removed by touching it with a cotton-tipped applicator soaked with either boric acid solution or normal saline. The foreign body usually adheres to the applicator. Frequently, more than one foreign body is present; after you have removed one you should search to ascertain that another has not been overlooked.

Imbedded Foreign Body

If there is any possibility that the foreign body has gone completely through the cornea, a dry dressing should be applied and the patient immediately put in the hands of an ophthalmic surgeon. On the other hand, if it seems that the foreign body has not penetrated, the cornea is anesthetized with one drop of an ophthalmic local anesthetic solution every one to two minutes until this has been done five times. Have the patient keep his eyes closed between instillations.

It is very important that the patient hold his eye steady. Ask him to stare steadily at a fixed point on the ceiling. With children this is not possible and they must be anesthetized. With the eye held steady, it is usually not difficult to lift out the foreign body gently with a sharp, pointed knife. In an emergency, the point of a hypodermic needle works well. Do not use a forceps because this will damage more tissue than the point of a knife. If the foreign body has been imbedded long enough to cause some rust spots to appear, these must also be removed in the same manner or they will stain the eye permanently.

After the foreign body has been removed, place 1 drop of 5 per cent homatropine into the eye to control the irritation of the iris. Cover the eye with a patch until the lesion has healed. Pain should not be treated with a local anesthetic; the patient should be given a systemic analgesia like codeine.

Laceration of the Eye

If there is any possibility that a laceration of the eye has extended through the cornea into the globe, many precautions must be taken to minimize loss of fluid from the globe. The patient should be placed in a supine position and kept in that position until a decision has been made as to the extent of the damage. The patient should be warned that touching his eye or putting pressure on his eyeballs in any way will cause further loss of fluid. In the course of the examination one should not exert any pressure on the eyeball, either with the examining finger or with a probing instrument. As soon as it has been determined that the eyeball is perforated no further examination is necessary. The eye should be covered and left undisturbed and arrangements made to transport the patient as soon as possible to an ophthalmic surgeon. He should be sent in either a supine or semi-recumbent position and warned against straining, stooping, or leaning over. No medication should be given into the eye; if he is having pain, he should be given systemic medication. Since vomiting increases intraocular pressure, codeine is generally used in place of morphine.

Vomiting increases intraocular pressure.

THE NOSE

INJURIES

Fracture of the Nose

Injuries to the nose are common; in an injury in which there is evidence of subcutaneous hemorrhage in the tissues of the lower eyelid, one must consider the possibility of fracture of the nose. Treatment of a fractured nose has two aims: one is relief of the obstruction and the second is correction of the deformity. Treatment must be carried out early because the excellent blood supply of the nose allows these bones to unite rapidly; if the position in which they unite is not satisfactory, a deformed nose will be the result. When the lesion is seen early and there is deformity, anesthesia is rarely necessary for correction because the nose is still numb. The simplest technique is to insert a hemostat or a similar slightly curved instrument into the nose and, using this as a splint, mold the fragments back into the proper position. In many instances, this is sufficient. If the position is not maintained a firm pack in the nose for a day or so will hold the fragments in proper position until they unite. Cold compresses sometimes hasten the disappearance of the associated ecchymosis.

Nose Bleed

Bleeding from the nose is very common and in the majority of instances is self limited; frequently no treatment is needed. In the majority of instances, when the bleeding is in the anterior portion of the nose, rolling a piece of paper

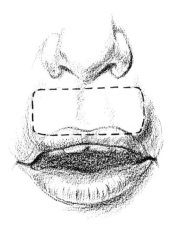

cardboard into a wad and inserting this under the upper lip will cause compression of the blood vessels which supply the anterior portion of the nose. This is a very simple and satisfactory method of controlling much of the bleeding in that area. If the bleeding persists and the lesion is within view, it may be stopped by inserting a cotton swab dipped in epinephrine solution. If this does not work it may be necessary to pack the nose with gauze.

Using a long bayonet tip forceps, pack the nose with a roll of narrow gauze. First pack the posterior superior area, folding the gauze on itself as you set it in place; next pack the anterior superior area, then the posterior inferior area, and, finally, the anterior inferior area. Hold the pack in place with a strip of adhesive plaster which covers both nostrils and is attached to the sides of the nose.

If the site of bleeding is located at the back of the nose, the pack described may not control bleeding. One must first place a pack in the posterior nasopharynx and then pack the remainder of the nose. Construct the pack by rolling a four-by-four gauze pad into a roll 2 inches long and approximately ¾ inch thick; fold the gauze on itself once

and roll in the long direction. Tie this roll in the middle with a heavy silk suture leaving one end long. Tie on three such sutures. Anesthetize the posterior pharynx with a spray of 2 per cent pontocaine. Pass a small rubber urethral catheter through the nose until it is visible in the oropharynx. Grasp the end of the catheter and pull it out through the mouth. Tie the end of one of the sutures to the catheter and pull it out through the nose. Repeat the maneuver through the other nostril so that there will be one suture coming out through each nostril and one through the mouth.

Test the pharyngeal wall to be certain that it is anesthetized. While gently pulling on the strings through the nares with one hand, use a finger of the other hand to pass the pack back through the mouth and into position in the posterior nasopharynx.

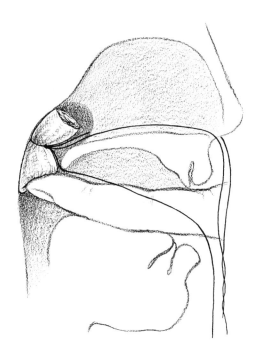

Tie the sutures through the nose loosely without pressure. Tape the suture coming out through the mouth to the tie side of the cheek. If bleeding through the nose persists an anterior pack can also be inserted as described above.

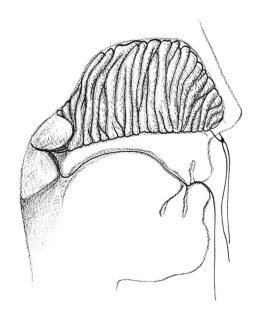

The posterior pack should be left in place not more than 24 hours.

Instead of using the posterior pack described above one can pass a Foley type urethral catheter into the posterior nasopharynx. Inflating the balloon on the catheter will provide satisfactory compression of the posterior naso-pharynx. If necessary this can be sup-plemented with an anterior pack.

Foreign Bodies

Children often insert foreign bodies into the nose. These produce symptoms of obstruction and may cause a sinus in-fection. To remove them, general anes-thesia is frequently required because children are uncooperative. The child is anesthetized and either a small slender probe with a hook on it or a fine forceps is used to lift out the foreign body. Ob-viously, the particular method depends on the type of foreign body and its posi-tion in the nose.

THE EAR

Injuries to the Ear

Lacerations

These should be immediately cleaned, any devitalized skin or cartilage excised to give good approximation, and the wound closed. A laceration of the cartilage can be repaired with fine nonabsorbable sutures. The skin closure should be sufficiently loose to allow drainage of serum. A pressure dressing should then be applied. Mold wet cotton into proper shape and apply both in front of and behind the ear so that the pressure will not cause deformity. Hold this in place with a circular bandage about the head.

Mold wet cotton

Hematomas

These commonly occur about the ears of boxers. When the hematoma is al-lowed to remain, it undergoes fibrosis and the resulting deformity is the well known cauliflower ear. Treatment, which should be undertaken early, in-cludes removal of the fluid by aspira-tion. With a small hypodermic needle make a wheal with 1 per cent procaine solution and then insert an 18-gauge needle and drain the hematoma. Apply a pressure dressing by putting a cotton mold about the ear and maintaining pressure with a circular dressing about the head.

Aspirate ear hema-toma c̄ 18 gauge needle

Foreign Bodies

The simplest and almost universally successful method of removing foreign bodies from the ear is by irrigation. A regular ear irrigation syringe is inserted into the external auditory canal. It should be inserted in such a way that the syringe tip never completely occludes the canal; otherwise, there would not be an exit for the pressure created by the syringe and the fluid would be blown into the middle ear. By leaving some space between the tip of the syringe and the canal wall you allow free escape of pressure and fluid. The fluid, reflected from the tympanic membrane, will usually remove the foreign body with it as it flows out of the ear.

INFECTION

Myringotomy

Although sulfonamides and newer antibiotics have materially reduced the complications of acute otitis media, there are still many instances of infection in this area which must be drained. This is done by an incision in the ear drum (myringotomy).

This can be done in children with local anesthesia (a few drops of warmed, 20 per cent cocaine instilled into the ear), but it is far more satisfactory to use a brief general anesthesia. Clean out the ear with alcohol on cotton-tipped applicators. Insert the largest possible otoscope speculum into the external meatus and examine the drum. The drum requiring incision will be bulging. Using a special ear knife, insert the blade into the drum at its most inferior point; carry the incision posteriorly and superiorly along the posterior edge of the drum slightly more than halfway.

The field will become obscured with blood and pus. Wipe this out and suck out the pus with a rubber bulb. After-care consists of keeping the drainage swabbed out of the ear.

NECK

INJURIES

Injury to the neck may damage the trachea or the major blood vessels to the head.

Injury to the Trachea

If severe blunt violence to the neck has smashed the tracheal rings, the patient may be able to exhale without difficulty, but the lack of support allows the tracheal walls to collapse on inhaling. Obviously, this patient needs immediate relief which is provided by tracheostomy. Tracheostomy should always be performed in any case in which there is the possibility of obstruction of the airway, and in any situation in which one seriously considers it advisable.

TECHNIQUE OF TRACHEOSTOMY. Tracheostomy can be done with the patient in his own bed. Place a folded pillow or sheet under the patient's shoulder to hyperextend the neck, and keep the chin in the midline. Infiltrate the midline of the neck with 1 per cent procaine. This is not necessary if the patient is comatose. If the patient's condition is rapidly deteriorating do not hesitate to proceed without anesthesia because the procedure may well be lifesaving. Hold the trachea in the midline. Make a vertical midline incision from immediately below the cricoid cartilage down to the suprasternal notch. These structures can be identified by palpation. Carry the incision in the midline directly down onto the trachea.

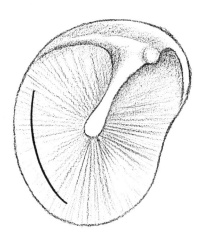

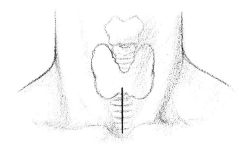

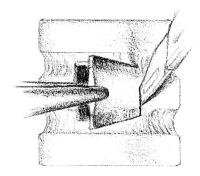

There will be very little bleeding if you keep the knife in the midline. The isthmus of the thyroid will obscure the trachea in the upper portion of the wound. In patients with a short neck the amount of trachea exposed between the isthmus and the sternum may be inadequate. A helpful maneuver in such cases is to apply an Allis clamp *around* the isthmus. Properly applied the apposing jaws meet behind the gland so that the gland is not damaged. One can lift the isthmus superiorly and anteriorly. In addition to exposing more trachea it also lifts the trachea forward and stabilizes it.

Using a pointed or small scalpel, make a vertical incision in the anterolateral aspect of the tracheal cartilage that you plan to remove. This should be the second or third cartilage below the cricoid. Grasp the anterior portion of the cartilage with a hemostat.

This frees the portion of the trachea held in the hemostat.

The tracheostomy tube consists of an outer and an inner tube and a stylet used while inserting the outer tube.

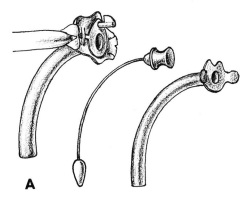

A

Insert the tracheostomy tube with the stylet in place.

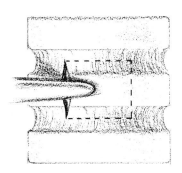

Remove the cartilage by making an incision in the membranous area above and below the cartilage and by dividing the ring on the opposite anterolateral surface.

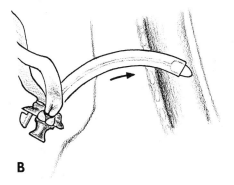

B

Remove the stylet, then check the position of the tube by determining the free flow of air through the tube. Insert the inner tracheostomy tube and turn down the clip which holds it in place.

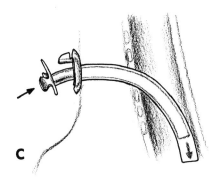

After checking hemostasis, close the wound loosely. Apply a dry dressing and tie the tracheostomy tape snugly with a tape about the neck.

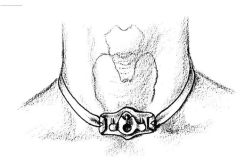

CARE OF TRACHEOSTOMY. A tracheostomy requires special care. Secretions must be periodically sucked out with a catheter. Aspiration through the catheter is maintained for only a few seconds at a time, but can be repeated until the tracheobronchial tree is clear. A few milliliters of saline can be inserted directly into the tracheostomy or through the tube as indicated to loosen secretions. Strict asepsis is essential. Furthermore, at the completion of the aspiration a few drops of saline should be instilled into the tracheostomy. This is because air going directly into the trachea is not humidified as is air going through the nasopharynx. Consequently, the air will tend to dry the trachea; a few drops of saline periodically will prevent this. The tracheostomy should be sucked out at least four times a day and perhaps as often as every ten minutes depending upon the condition of the patient. The nurse should remove the inner tube of the tracheos-

tomy at least four times a day, clean it well and reinsert it. There should always be a second complete tracheostomy tube in a sterile container at the side of the bed. The original outer tracheostomy tube should remain in place for 48 hours, after which a resident physician should change the outer tracheostomy tube every other day. When it is removed, the second tube should be immediately inserted in its place. The tube which was removed is then cleaned, sterilized, and left available at the bedside. The patient should be taught that he will have no difficulty talking if he places his finger over the end of the tracheostomy tube.

REMOVAL OF TRACHEOSTOMY TUBE. The tracheostomy tube should not be removed permanently until you are certain that the patient can get along without it. This ability is tested by placing a cork into the tracheostomy tube. If he accumulates secretions and has difficulty in breathing, remove the cork and aspirate the tube. Once you are satisfied that he does not need the artificial help, simply remove the tube and apply a dry firm dressing over the wound. This will leak for a few days but will ultimately close.

EMERGENCY TRACHEOSTOMY. In emergency situations the patient may need an adequate airway established immediately. The safest, quickest and most satisfactory way to provide an adequate airway is to insert an endotracheal tube. The tracheostomy, if it is still indicated, can then be done leisurely under optimal conditions.

If adequate help and *light* are available, the conventional type of tracheostomy can be undertaken immediately as described on page 202.

In the event of a *dire* emergency or if difficulty is experienced in finding the trachea quickly, an opening may be made through the cricothyroid membrane as a life-saving procedure. This portion of the airway is easier to enter than the trachea because it is much more superficial and is easily palpated immediately under the skin. A tracheostomy tube is not tolerated for long in this position, however, and has to be moved to the conventional position in the trachea as soon as feasible. I have always found that a conventional tracheostomy can be done expeditiously enough.

PERCUTANEOUS TRACHEAL CATHETER. Many thoracic surgeons have found a percutaneous tracheal catheter an effective means of cleaning tracheal secretions. The catheter does not aspirate the secretions; it provides a simple means of introducing a solution into the trachea which will thin the secretions and stimulate coughing.

Position the patient with his neck extended. Ask him not to swallow while the catheter is being inserted. Locate the peaked superior margin of the thyroid cartilage and palpate inferiorly until the lower edge of the cartilage is just passed. At this point the catheter will pass through the center of the cricothyroid membrane.

After proper skin sterilization, raise a small wheal of local anesthesia over the cricothyroid membrane. Introduce an 18-gauge thin-walled needle through the skin and into the trachea in a single motion. Check the position of the needle by attaching an empty syringe which should withdraw air freely. Angle the needle caudally and insert a 4-inch piece of polyvinyl tubing halfway into the trachea and remove the needle, leaving the remaining 2 inches outside the skin. Attach a blunt needle and every four hours insert enough saline or pulmonary detergent to initiate coughing.

Occasionally, a patient will sustain a laceration of the trachea and when this occurs there will be marked subcutaneous emphysema of the neck. Exploration of the wound and suture of the laceration is required. Tracheostomy is usually necessary prior to repair.

Injury to the Vessels

Any one of the major vessels of the neck may be damaged. These injuries are always associated with severe bleeding; the patient must be taken to the hospital very quickly or he will exsanguinate. These patients usually require replacement of 2000 to 4000 ml. of blood. The best treatment is pressure on the wound and the earliest possible operation. In the operating room, the vessels proximal and distal to the site of injury should be uncovered, the bleeding controlled, and the repair carried out as indicated.

INFECTION

The neck has many important structures encased in fibrous compartments. These fibrous compartments dictate the direction of spread of infections within them.

Acute Infections

Acute infections of the neck usually originate either in the tonsils or in the teeth. If superficial areas are involved, one follows the general principle of intervention when there is localization as evidenced by fluctuation. Incisions should be generous and should follow the direction of the elastic fibers of the skin. Deeper infections should also be drained, but the occasional or inexperienced surgeon should not undertake this procedure. This operation should be performed under general endotracheal anesthesia by an experienced surgeon. If there is any indication of closure of the glottis or difficulty in swallowing, drainage should be undertaken immediately even though no fluctuation can be appreciated.

Tuberculous Adenitis

The incidence of tuberculosis of the lymph glands of the neck with necrotic breakdown is decreasing but still occurs sufficiently often to be of clinical significance. Tuberculous glands can be differentiated from acute infections in that they appear as fluctuant, non-tender swellings without associated inflammation. An exception would be a fluctuant non-tender mass in the midline which would most likely be a thyroglossal duct cyst. If tuberculous adenitis is suspected, the patient should be put on a course of antimicrobial therapy (Para-aminosalicylic acid, 3 gm. q.i.d., and Isoniazid, 100 mg. t.i.d.) for two weeks, after which the area should be completely excised and the wound primarily closed. The antimicrobial treatment should be continued for 6 months. Remarkably few of these patients have pulmonary tuberculosis.

Supraclavicular Lymph Node Biopsy

The cervical region is a common area of metastasis of malignant disease from the head, neck, chest, and occasionally the abdomen. Consequently, in many instances a definitive tissue diagnosis can be made on the basis of a node removed from the neck. Before operation is undertaken one should be satisfied that one can feel the node. The simplest way of examining the supraclavicular area is to stand behind the patient and use the flat of the pads of one's fingers in palpating the area. It is common to mistake for a node the mass felt at the point where the anterior belly of the omohyoid muscle crosses the scaleni. Palpation further out in the line of the muscle will differentiate the muscle from a node. If a nodule can be felt, it should be excised. At the time of the excision, be sure again that you can feel the node, because a different position of the patient sometimes moves such nodes from accessible to seemingly inaccessible positions. Always begin the operation with the patient in a position in which the node can be felt. Infiltrate the skin in the line of the incision which should be in one of the normal skin folds of the neck. Carry the incision through the skin, subcutaneous tissues, and platysma. After this level has been reached it is possible to separate the tissues with a combination of blunt and sharp scissors dissection until the node is uncovered. The node is usually supplied by a blood vessel which runs into the hilum; if possible, clamp this before you divide it. Lift up the node with a Babcock forceps, clamp the vessel going into the hilum, divide it, and remove the node. Hemostasis is established and the wound can be closed without drainage, using interrupted, nonabsorbable sutures.

Commonly mistake anterior belly of omo-hyoid for node.

Chapter Fourteen

The Upper Extremity

DISLOCATION OF HUMERUS AT SHOULDER JOINT

The shoulder is one of the joints more commonly dislocated. Its wide range of motion, its exposed position, and the fact that the head of the humerus is larger than the glenoid fossa all make the shoulder joint vulnerable. Several types of dislocation are possible, but, since the acromium and the coracoacromial ligament prevent upward displacement of the head, most dislocations are subcoracoid.

The different types of dislocation have some common characteristics: The patient complains of pain and supports the elbow of his injured arm away from his body. Examination shows flattening of the shoulder and reveals that the head of the humerus is dislocated from the glenoid fossa and is in an obviously abnormal position. The patient is unable to touch the chest wall with his elbow when the hand of that arm is on the opposite shoulder.

Types of Dislocation

The various types of dislocation can be differentiated as follows:

Subcoracoid

The head of the humerus lies below the coracoid process upon the neck of the scapula. There is very little change in the length of the arm. This is the most common type of dislocation.

Subclavicular

The head is felt below the middle of the clavicle. This is usually an exaggeration of the subcoracoid variety.

Subglenoid

The head is felt in the axilla. It lies over the scapula below the glenoid cavity. There is marked lengthening of the arm and flexion of the elbow. This is the second most frequent type of dislocation.

Subspinous

The head of the humerus is felt behind and below the acromium. The elbow is displaced forward and the arm is rotated inwardly. This is a backward dislocation and is rare.

Dislocation of the shoulder is frequently associated with damage to the nearby ligaments and muscles as well as to the brachial plexus. The extent of damage should be determined. While not absolutely necessary, it is advisable to take an x-ray of the shoulder to rule out the possibility of a fracture.

TREATMENT

The dislocation should be reduced as soon as possible. If treated immediately or if the dislocation is of the recurrent type, little or no anesthetic is necessary. Often a narcotic is adequate. But if the dislocation cannot be readily reduced, the procedure should be done under general anesthesia. There are two widely accepted methods of reduction:

Kocher's Method of Reduction

This is aimed at disengaging the dislocated head of the humerus and rolling it back into position. In using this method you must appreciate that you have a great deal of leverage and can harm the patient if you perform the maneuver incorrectly. The patient may be sitting or in a supine position. If the right

shoulder is dislocated grasp the patient's elbow with your right hand and his wrist with your left. Slowly but firmly pull the humerus away from the shoulder with your right hand.

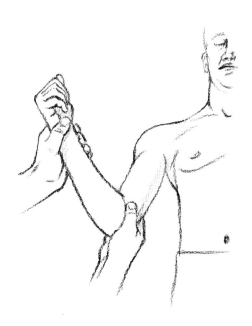

While maintaining the downward pull on the humerus, slowly rotate the arm externally by moving the wrist out until full external rotation of 90° is reached.

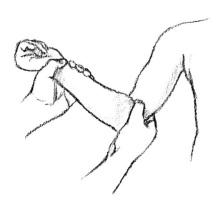

Keeping the arm in full external rotation, bring the elbow in across the chest to the midline of the body.

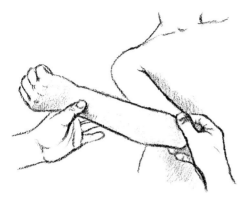

Holding the elbow in this position rotate the arm internally, bringing the hand over to the opposite shoulder.

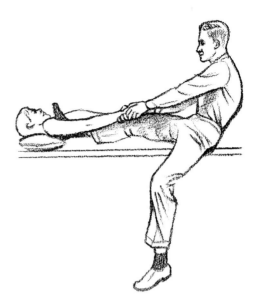

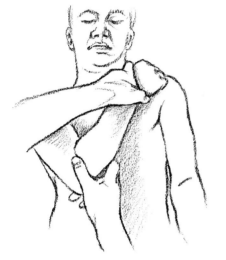

This should allow the head of the humerus to glide smoothly back into position in the glenoid fossa.

Hippocratic Method

The Hippocratic method utilizes manual traction and leverage over a heel placed in the axilla. The patient lies supine on a table. Sit facing the patient on the edge of the table on the side of the dislocation. Grasp the patient's wrist with both hands and place your stockinged foot (right foot for right shoulder) in the patient's axilla. Exert continuous, gradually increasing, traction on the arm, at the same time bringing it in toward the body.

This maneuver forces the head of the humerus outward. If the head does not readily slip into position external rotation of the arm may be helpful.

The reduction of the dislocation should be checked both clinically and radiographically. This injury often recurs unless the shoulder is immobilized. The shoulder should be immobilized by strapping the arm to the side and holding the forearm in a sling. No external rotation should be allowed for three weeks. Activity may be gradually increased after that time.

INJURIES TO FOREARM AND HAND

GENERAL CONSIDERATIONS FOR OPERATION ON HAND

Testing

The extent of injury to an extremity and particularly to the hand can often be accurately determined by examination of the part. Sensation should be tested over the forearm and on both the volar and the dorsal surfaces. The motor function of the hand and wrist should be tested. Applying counterpressure while a particular muscle is used is helpful in determining the motor function of that muscle. A careful record of these preoperative findings should be kept.

Anesthesia

Superficial minor injuries requiring only surface soft tissue repair without deep wound exploration can be operated under local infiltration anesthesia. Operating on the finger requiring more time (up to one hour) and deeper dissection can be done under digital nerve block (p. 94) anesthesia. Trauma to the deeper areas of the hand and most injuries which involve a tendon or a nerve should be treated under general anesthesia. When treating infections of the hand it is unwise to inject local anesthetic solution near the area of infection. Consequently, proximal nerve blocks or general anesthesia must be used.

The operation should be carried out in a bloodless field. This is best done with a special arm pneumatic tourniquet calibrated and stabilized to maintain pressures of approximately 250 mm. mercury. If none is available a blood pressure cuff may be used. The tourniquet is applied smoothly to the upper arm over a cotton gauze bandage. Prior to inflation the limb is compressed to render it bloodless by means of a rubber roller bandage applied from the tip of the fingers to the tourniquet. (The compression bandage is omitted in the presence of infection.) Once the tourniquet has been inflated, the rubber bandage is removed exposing the arm for operation. Two hours of tourniquet time under conditions of proper tourniquet application and function is usually safe. Longer periods have been tolerated. If, however, surgery in excess of three hours is contemplated, two periods,

each of 90 minutes with a 15 minute interval of tourniquet removal and limb perfusion between is recommended. Regardless of the stage of the operation a soft gauze dressing can be applied and held by the operator with the limb elevated during the period of restored circulation. With this light wound compression and elevation bleeding is rarely a problem during tourniquet release. The tourniquet is then reapplied.

The tourniquet is generally released at the completion of the operation. If overall wound hemostasis is considered inadequate, the tourniquet may be released prior to wound closure. Regardless of when the tourniquet is released a marked reactive hyperemia follows. The limb should be elevated for at least 5 minutes and the patient undisturbed. When tourniquet control is used brachial block on general anesthesia must be used.

Cleansing the Area

Accidents involving the upper extremity often occur in persons who are working with their hands. Consequently, the hands of the victim are often impregnated with grease and dirt and this must be removed before an operation is undertaken. Accordingly, at the operating table, after anesthesia has been induced, the area should be scrubbed with a brush and surgical scrub soap as long and as vigorously as necessary. A brush should not be used on open raw areas; these should be cleansed with soap and gauze. Do not hesitate to take as long as an hour, if necessary, for proper cleaning. After the area has been well scrubbed, it should be irrigated with copious amounts of sterile saline and finally treated with Zephiran. After the area has been properly prepared, the tourniquet should not be used until you are ready to begin the operation, unless it is necessary to control troublesome bleeding.

First débride all devitalized tissue. Injuries of this sort frequently have dirt ground into the skin edges and the subcutaneous tissues. After the loose material has been washed from the wound, sharp dissection may be necessary to remove the dirt-impregnated tissue. This will allow good clean skin edges for reapproximation.

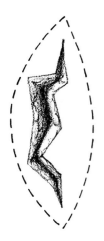 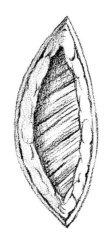

Any devitalized muscle must be removed. Viability in muscle is determined by (1) its color, (2) its ability to bleed when cut, and (3) its ability to contract when stimulated. After débridement is complete, the wound drapes should be changed before proceeding with the repair.

Incision

The wound will usually require further opening. In general, the incision should be made parallel to skin creases. If it is necessary to cross a joint, cut down one side parallel with the long axis, cut across the joint perpendicular to the length of the finger, and continue down the other side.

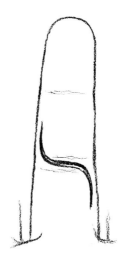

An incision directly over the joint and perpendicular to the crease results in a scar which restricts joint function when the scar contracts. Identify the separate nerves, tendons, and blood vessels. A simple method of determining the identity of the distal portion of the tendons is to grasp them with a small hemostat and pull on them. The finger action that results will identify the tendon. If the tendon is not evident, pass a hemostat into the canal and grasp it.

INJURY TO SKIN AND SUBCUTANEOUS TISSUE

Skin Defect

Direct primary repair is the most desirable closure of a skin defect. In such cases the skin can be approximated with interrupted silk sutures.

Wringer Injury

Often the hand of a child is hurt by being caught in the wringer of a washing machine. The damage may be greater than is at first evident. If the skin is intact, one may be tempted to regard the injury lightly; this could be disastrous. When next seen the patient may have marked swelling which could progress to necrosis of the skin.

Cleanse the extremity with surgical soap. Cover any raw area with a gauze dressing. Finally, cover the arm from the fingertips to the elbow with a pressure dressing. Wrap the area loosely with absorbent cotton building up to a thickness of three to four inches. Apply compression with a firm, cotton elastic bandage. Test for proper circulation in the extremity, evidenced by pink fingernails which blanch on pressure, and sensation in the fingertips. Keep the extremity elevated. As the edema subsides the pressure dressing will loosen and must be reapplied. In the first few days the dressing may require reapplication several times a day.

If the injury extends to the elbow causing hemorrhage of the area, Volkmann's ischemia becomes a possibility. This is characterized by edema of the elbow, loss of pulses, and congestion which changes to pallor, and is accompanied by loss of sensation in the hand. Under such circumstances the sub-fascial tension at the elbow joint must be relieved.

Avulsion of Skin of Forearm

A wringer accident or a simple "belt and pulley" accident may pull off the skin of the forearm in a manner similar to the removal of a sleeve.

If the skin is destroyed the area should be covered with a split thickness skin graft immediately after proper cleansing. The skin may be attached distally. There is a great temptation to cleanse the area and suture the skin back in position, a maneuver which will certainly meet with defeat. The entire sleeve of skin will slough. The proper technique is to convert this piece of skin into a full thickness skin graft. Detach the skin completely. Excise any devitalized skin or any portion impregnated with dirt. Remove all fatty tissue and fascia from the underside of the skin. Cleanse the forearm, establish hemostasis, and suture the skin back in place. If the entire piece of avulsed skin is available this is more than necessary and the excess should be cut off. If insufficient skin is salvaged for coverage the resultant defect should be covered with a split thickness skin graft. Cover the graft with a nonadherent dressing and a pressure dressing.

If the avulsed skin is attached proximally, do not overconfidently feel that you can sew this in place. Only the proximal hand's breadth will survive suturing. Leave approximately that amount (after checking viability), excise the remainder, convert it to a full thickness skin graft, and replace.

Note: See pages 121 and 123 for discussions of antibiotic treatment and tetanus prophylaxis.

Injury to Tendons

General Considerations

Divided tendons should be repaired at once if the patient is seen very soon after the injury and if the wound is clean. Ideally they should be repaired within 6 hours. They should never be sutured if (1) the wound is already infected, (2) the injury occurred more than 24 hours earlier, (3) there is crushed or devitalized tissue, or (4) the wound is badly contaminated. If any one of these problems exists it must be attended to and the tendon repaired later under good conditions. If both flexor tendons to the finger are severed between the distal crease in the palm and the middle joint in the finger, the sublimus tendon should be removed. If both are allowed to remain they will become adherent to each other. If only the sublimus is divided, remove it.

Identify the two ends of the tendon. First attempt to grasp the end of the tendon by passing a small, pointed hemostat into the canal of the tendon. The distal stump of the tendon can usually be grasped by this means. If unsuccessful, flexing the fingers in the case of flexor tendons, or extending them in the case of extensor tendons, will frequently force the distal end of the tendon back within reach of the hemostat. Similarly, an effort should be made to grasp the proximal end of the tendon by means of a small pointed hemostat passed into the canal. Flexion or extension of the wrist and milking of the forearm should assist in working down the proximal end of the tendon. When this maneuver is not successful you may have to follow the tendon high into the forearm to reach the proximal end. Do not make a longitudinal incision along the arm; this will destroy the gliding surfaces and pulley mechanisms of the tendon. Furthermore, the incision will go directly across joints causing late scar contractures. Make a small transverse incision higher in the arm and locate the tendon.

Suture materials in order of preference are #34 or #35 stainless steel wire, fine silk, or fine cotton. Catgut should not be used for the repair of tendons because the reaction which it produces may cause the tendons to adhere to adjacent structures.

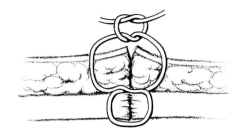

Use #34 stainless steel wire. This suture has very little strength because very little is needed. A good result can be obtained simply by approximating the ends. Immobilize the wrist in hyperextension with a volar plaster splint for three weeks, leaving the suture in place during that time. Removal of the suture at the skin level will also free it from the tendon.

Repair of Flexor Tendons

Two different methods of repair may be used: in one technique the suture is left permanently in place; in the other it is removed after three weeks.

SUTURE TECHNIQUE. Grasp each end of the tendon with a straight hemostat. Thread each end of a 12-inch silk suture through a fine, spear-point 2½-inch needle. Pass one needle through the tendon, perpendicular to it and ⅝ inch from the end.

Repair of Extensor Tendons

Extensor tendons are more accessible, more readily repaired, and heal more easily than flexor tendons. The two ends of the tendon are identified. This is usually accomplished simply by hyperextending the wrist and fingers. Cut the frayed ends of the tendon so as to have a clean right angle division at each end. Unite the tendon ends with a single figure-of-eight suture which connects the tendon ends with the deeper loop and the skin with the superficial loop.

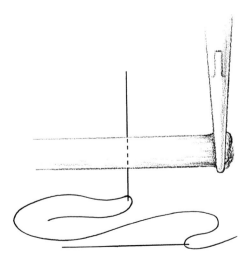

Pull the suture half way through. Simultaneously insert both needles, one from each side to cross the tendon in an "X."

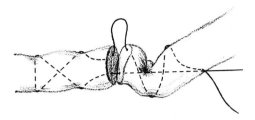

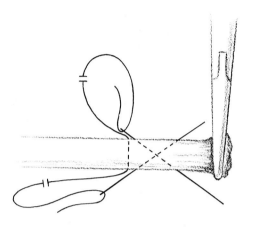

(Simultaneous insertion of the needles prevents either needle from penetrating the other limb of the suture.) Excise the jagged end of the tendon; reinsert each needle so that it emerges from the cut end of the tendon.

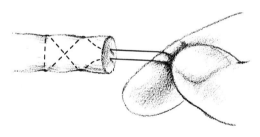

Partially divide the jagged end of the other portion of the tendon. Insert each needle in the end of the tendon and pass it diagonally through the tendon with one needle emerging on each side of the tendon. Simultaneously insert the two needles, crossing the tendon diagonally. Finally come directly across the tendon with one suture so as to have both ends together. To bring the severed ends of the tendon together, grasp one end of the suture and pull it taut and straight. If it is held straight the tendon can be easily slid forward.

Pull the second suture taut and tie the ends.

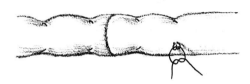

The tie will usually sink into the tendon substance. The aftercare is described on page 215.

PULL-OUT WIRE TECHNIQUE.   This suture may be used on any tendon anywhere but is most popular for suturing flexor tendons in the palm of the hand. The major advantage is that the suture may be removed after the tendon is healed. Thread spearpoint 2½-inch straight needles to each end of a strand of #34 stainless steel wire 12 inches long. Pass the first needle through the proximal segment of the tendon approximately ⅝ of an inch from the end. Pull the suture through to the halfway point. Pass the first needle diagonally across to the other side, advancing toward the end of the tendon. Again make a diagonal pass with the same needle but this time bring the needle out through the end of the tendon. Now pass the second needle diagonally across the tendon and then diagonally out through the end of the tendon in a similar position to the first needle. Before beginning the second needle, pass the pull-out wire beneath the wire suture. This wire is of similar size and approximately half as long as the suture and is placed beneath the proximal end of the suture. At this point use the pull-out wire and the distal end of the suture to move the suture back and forth in the tendon to loosen it and simplify removal three weeks hence. Twist the two ends of the pull-out wire together to prevent tissue growth between; thread the twisted wire on a curved skin needle and bring the pull-out suture out through the tendon sheath and the skin. Before threading the suture through the distal tendon grasp the end of the tendon with a hemostat. Partially divide this frayed portion before inserting the suture and complete the division after the suture is placed. Each end of the suture used in the repair is threaded longitudinally down the distal portion of the tendon for an inch or more. It is then brought out of the tendon and out through the skin, each end is brought out through a separate opening. Tie the distal suture outside the skin over a button. The pull of the proximal tendon puts tension on this suture. The button prevents the suture from cutting into the skin.

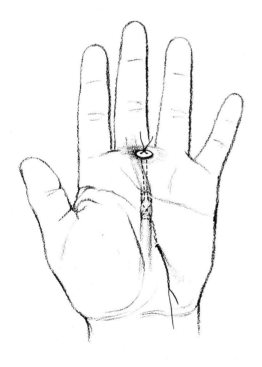

The suture acts mainly on the proximal fragment drawing it distally. As a matter of fact, when the tendon is divided in the narrow flexor tunnels, the repair su-

ture is placed proximal to the division and only very fine arterial silk sutures are used to approximate the ends. The chief purpose of the silk is to approximate; the tension is borne by the steel suture.

The suture is left in place for three weeks. No effort should be made to move the tendon during that period; this would only increase reaction about the tendon. To remove the suture cut it beneath the button. It should then be possible to pull out the suture by putting mild tension on the pull-out wire. If this is not possible, hook a rubber band to the pull-out wire and tape it to a point higher on the arm. The sustained tension will usually remove the suture overnight.

AFTERCARE. After the tendon has been repaired it should be covered by suturing the tendon sheath or by placing any nearby tissue loosely over the tendon. If sufficient skin is not available, a graft should be used because skin coverage is essential to a good repair. In flexor tendon repairs, immobilization is accomplished with the wrist flexed and the hand in a position of function. Extensor tendon repairs should be immobilized with the wrist somewhat extended. The simplest method of immobilizing the hand and wrist is to use a molded plaster splint (p. 73). The tendon should be completely immobilized for 3 weeks. Every day of the fourth week have the patient remove the splint, practice limited active motion without resistance, and then reapply the splint. Remove the splint entirely the following week and have the patient gradually increase activity. Exercises should be used many times every day. Since this becomes monotonous, it is far better to have the patient practice occupational therapy.

INJURY TO NERVES

General Considerations

Injuries to the upper extremity and hand frequently include damage to some of the nerves. No matter which nerve is injured an effort should be made to repair it because repairs to nerves in the hand and fingers yield better results than in any other part of the body.

Nerves cut in the distal part of the palm require slightly less than four months for full return of function, while nerves sutured in the proximal part of the palm require an average of seven months and nerves injured above the wrist require 13 months. After suture of a digital nerve, sensation returns at the rate of the length of one finger segment per month. The nutritional state of the hand is an important factor which influences nerve regeneration.

Regeneration occurs progressively down the extremity. The first sensation to return is coarse touch, followed by deep sensation and finally by light sensation. Paresthesias or tingling appear as sensation returns, but these ultimately vanish. As sensation returns the trophic changes in the area also disappear.

Sudomotor (sweat) fibers travel with sensory fibers. The absence of sweating in a denervated area complements the often more subjective finding of sensation to touch and pinpricks used in the diagnosis of nerve injury. Similarly, the return of sweating aids in the recognition of nerve regeneration following division and repair when the evaluation of the return of sensation may be more difficult.

Median Nerve

SENSORY LOSS. When the median nerve is injured sensation is lost over both the volar and dorsal surfaces of the distal and middle segments of the index and long fingers and the volar aspect of the thumb. The sensory loss may overflow these bounds or there may be very little sensory change.

MOTOR LOSS. Low divisions of the nerve paralyze the short thumb muscles, thus interfering with apposition of the thumb with the hand. The two outer lumbricales are also paralyzed. With the palm on the table, the index finger cannot scratch the table. With the two hands clasped the index and long fingers stand out without flexing. If the nerve is divided above the elbow there is loss of flexion of the thumb and the first two fingers; flexion and pronation of the wrist are weakened.

Radial Nerve

This is the most commonly injured of all spinal nerves.

SENSORY LOSS. When the injury is in the upper third of the arm, there is anesthesia over the back of the radial side of the hand and thumb. If the injury is lower, there is no sensory loss.

MOTOR LOSS. The most characteristic deformity caused by injury of the radial nerve is wrist drop. There is pronation and drooping of the wrist, thumb, and fingers. Flexion of the fingers is limited in this position, but if the patient passively supinates the arm, allowing the wrist to dorsiflex, he can make a fist. If the injury is below the elbow there may be no wrist drop, but only loss of extension in the thumb and fingers.

Ulnar Nerve

SENSORY LOSS. Sensation is lost on the palmar and dorsal surfaces over the ulnar border of the hand and on the little and ring fingers.

MOTOR LOSS. There is:

1. Paralysis of the inner two lumbricales and all the interossei, resulting in hyperextension of the metacarpophalangeal joints and flexion of the two interphalangeal joints.

2. Paralysis of the adductor muscles of the thumb and all the short muscles of the little finger.

3. Paralysis of the flexor carpi ulnaris and part of the flexor profundus, with weakened hand grasp and a tendency to radial abduction of the hand.

Ulnar and Median Nerves

SENSORY LOSS. The anesthesia covers the entire palm and the volar surface of all the digits as well as the dorsal surface of the last two segments of the long and index fingers, and the last segment of the thumb.

MOTOR LOSS. The wrist tends slightly backward and ulnarward and the hand inclines toward supination. The carpal and metacarpal arches straighten so that the hand is flat. The thumb is at the side of the hand, without power of apposition or adduction. There is clawing of the fingers, hyperextension of the proximal joints and sharp flexion of the distal two.

Repair of nerves is described on page 111. The repaired nerves should be properly covered. If no skin is available in situ use a graft.

The function of each muscle has an antagonistic function in another muscle. When a muscle is paralyzed it is unable to counteract the function of its antagonist, consequently the latter can overact. The hand must be protected from such overaction until the function of the paralyzed muscle returns. This is accomplished by applying a splint, maintaining the hand in a position of function.

Fractures should be immobilized in a position of function. Immobilization should be effected so that only the fractured bone is at rest; the patient is encouraged from the outset to use the remainder of the hand. In impacted fractures of the phalanges or metacarpals, immobilization in the position of function is adequate. If there is displacement, digital traction is necessary.

INJURY TO FINGERS

Contusion

Serious contusions of the fingers often result from having objects dropped on them or automobile doors closed on them. If the finger is intact, protection is all that is necessary. If the distal phalanx is fractured, cover the finger with gauze and a firm dressing which includes either a splint or plaster. Do not include the interphalangeal joint because immobilization of the joint, particularly in extension, may stiffen it. The fracture usually heals without difficulty.

Subungual Hematoma

Trauma to a fingernail may produce a hematoma under the nail. The most common cause is hitting the finger with a hammer. The hematoma is readily visible through the nail and there is exquisite tenderness at the site.

The best treatment is to decompress the hematoma. If the hematoma extends beyond the nail, elevation of the skin at the edge of the nail will relieve the pressure. However, in many cases the hematoma does not extend to the edge of the nail and it must be decompressed through the nail. This can be done by either of two methods: (1) Using a bayonet tip blade, bore a small hole in the nail directly into the hematoma. As soon as the blood escapes the symptoms will be relieved. (2) Straighten out an ordinary paper clip, heat the tip until it is red hot and burn a hole through the nail.

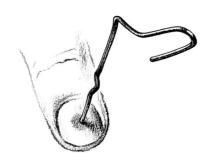

Surprisingly, this requires no anesthesia.

Amputation of Fleshy Tips

The tip of the finger may be cut off by a shearing accident. If the tip remains attached by any tissue whatever, it should be cleansed and sutured in place. After scrupulously removing all devitalized tissue and dirt, suture the tip using only interrupted nonabsorbable sutures in the skin. It will almost certainly "take" and provide an excellent result. In instances where the tip has been completely amputated, an effort should be made to cover the raw area with a graft. This is best accomplished by raising a flap on the hand. Clean the area properly, debride the injured finger, and establish hemostasis. Determine the position where the finger will meet the palm most comfortably. On the palm raise a skin flap of sufficient size to cover the defect in the end of the finger. Leave the flap attached on the proximal side. Suture the flap over the defect using interrupted silk sutures. The sutures are more easily placed if you do not pull up any suture until they are all in place.

After the desired number of sutures have been placed bring the open end of the finger in against the raw surface of the flap and tie down the sutures. This should satisfactorily cover the end of the finger.

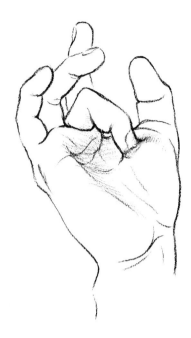

After five days, detach the flap from its base.

Another method is to apply a small, free, split thickness skin graft directly to the area. This is described on page 154. If this is not practical, the raw area can be treated with gentian violet, covered with a small piece of nonadherent gauze, and a dry dressing applied. The wound will heal without further treatment in about 10 days.

The pedicle graft will give a far better long-term functional result.

Traumatic Amputation of Finger

If the finger has been severed every effort should be made to save as much function as possible. The thumb should always be preserved, but any other digit that obviously will be functionless should be amputated. If a tendon is still inserted into a portion of a phalanx, an effort should be made to save the remainder of the phalanx. If the bone protrudes beyond the soft tissues, excise ¼ to ½ inch of this. Tailor the ends of the tissue so as to make an anterior and

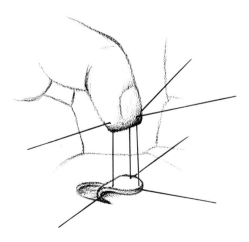

posterior flap, and suture these together with interrupted, nonabsorbable sutures.

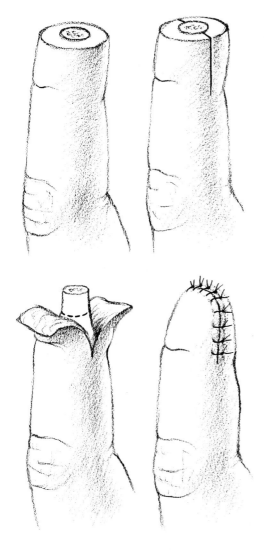

Excise the distal portion of the digital nerves to prevent a painful scar.

Baseball Finger

If force is applied sharply to the end of the finger the extensor tendon will frequently be avulsed from the distalphalanx. This produces a typical deformity characterized by partial flexion of the distal interphalangeal joint and inability to extend it actively. A faulty attempt to catch a baseball is the most common cause of this injury, known as a "baseball finger." Treatment consists of placing the joint in hyperextension and holding it that way for about 2 weeks by means of a splint. Run a tongue blade splint from the proximal interphalangeal joint to beyond the tip of the finger. Build up the splint under the distal phalanx so that when the splint is secured to the finger with annular strips of adhesive the distal joint will be in hyperextension. Another method is to make a tube of plaster of paris about the distal phalanges and hold the distal joint in a position of hyperextension and the proximal joint at 90 degrees until the plaster sets. Metal splints are available to hold the finger in such a position.

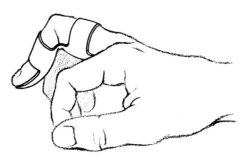

INFECTIONS OF FOREARM AND HAND

GENERAL CONSIDERATIONS

The fascial partitioning of the hand makes it possible for infection to spread rapidly along fascial planes and to permanently injure the functional capacity of the hand. An injury to a hand, with subsequent infection and permanent disability, can seriously interfere with a person's work.

Infections in the finger may occur: (1) in the pulp, (2) about the nail, and (3) in a joint. Infection in the hand may occur: (1) in the lymphatic system, (2) in the tendon sheaths, or (3) in the fascial spaces.

Fascial space infection or lymphangitis should always be treated with warm application, rest and antibiotics until there is evidence of localization. To open an inflamed area before localization is to invite spread of the infection. On the other hand, drainage is indicated after localization occurs. Fascial space infections should be drained, but this is not so urgent as in tenosynovitis where drainage must be immediate.

General anesthesia is most satisfactory. When local anesthesia is used, only the line of incision should be infiltrated. Ethyl chloride spray can be used when draining a superficial abscess where momentary anesthesia is adequate. A tourniquet can be used for hemostasis, but do not use an Esmarch bandage to compress the blood from the extremity. Merely raise the extremity until it has drained and rapidly raise the pressure in the cuff.

The area should be carefully cleaned and shaved. Any crusted material must be scrubbed free. Drainage should be carried out as recommended under the various sites of infection. Small catheters may be inserted in the wound for drainage and irrigation. The catheters should be covered with fine mesh gauze so placed that the catheters are not in contact either with tendons or with joint cavities. The catheters are led out through the dressings. A sterile medicine dropper is attached to the end of the catheter. Penicillin (250 U per ml.) or any other antibiotic solution can be injected into the bulb of the medicine dropper with a syringe and needle. Irrigations are made every three hours. The catheters should be left in place four days.

The hand should be immobilized in a position of function and kept elevated. Compresses applied should be intermittent, allowing an opportunity for the hand to dry in the interim period.

Infection of Finger

Felon

A felon is an abscess of the pulp space of the digit. This usually occurs as a result of a minor infection which burrows deeper. One or two days later, the distal portion of the finger is swollen, indurated, tense, and throbbing with pain. Pressure on the distal end of the digit will usually indicate *point tenderness.* This is usually the only indication of localization of an infection in this area. Treatment is immediate surgical drainage; if there is delay the pressure will destroy the underlying bone. In longstanding infections of this area, the possibility of existing bone destruction must be considered. This can be determined by x-raying the finger. If the bone has become necrotic it must be removed. When making the incision one considers the fact that the space is traversed by multiple septa which separate it into compartments. For satisfactory drainage, all of these must be incised. An incision can be made along either side of the nail, staying relatively close to the nail so as not to have a tender scar over the pad of the finger. The incision is carried the length of the phalanx and partially around the tip of the finger. The incision within the finger should extend across to the skin on the other side of the finger. In this way all the fibrous septa will be divided.

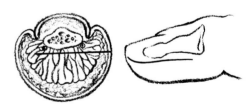

If there is a loose sequestrum it should be lifted up; if it is not loose, it need not be disturbed. Insert a thin strip of rubber drain into the wound; wrap with a loose recurrent dressing.

Paronychia

Infection of the area around the nail usually begins from a hangnail or a minor infection of the skin in that area. If the infection is treated when it first localizes, separation of the tissue from the nail, evacuation of the small amount of pus, and diligent application of warm compresses may suffice. The untreated infection spreads about the base of the nail and ultimately penetrates beneath the nail which must then be removed. Anesthesia may be accomplished by a nerve block at the base of the finger or at the wrist. Insert a scalpel blade between the nail and the tissue proximally and sweep out over the edge of the finger, raising the tissue from the base of the nail as you go. Repeat this on the other half of the finger.

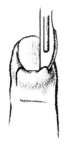

This will allow you to turn back the base of the tissue. If the infection did not extend below the nail, stop at this point; insert a thin rubber tissue drain beneath the tissue and wrap the finger with a recurrent dressing.

If the infection has invaded beneath the base of the nail, that portion of the nail must be excised to allow adequate drainage. Some surgeons remove the entire nail under such circumstances. This is not necessary, and the finger is less tender if the distal portion of the nail is left in place for protection. Remove the proximal one-third to one-half of the nail. This is done easily with a pointed scissors.

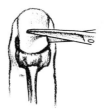

Insert a drain beneath the tissue. Cover the wound with a recurrent dressing.

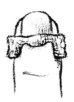

Infection from Human Bites

The human mouth is notorious for the wide range of bacteria which it harbors and infections of the hand resulting from human bites can be very serious. A frequent cause is a blow to the teeth with penetration of a tooth deep into the patient's hand and into a joint space. The injury is invariably infected. If the initial injury penetrated the joint space, a septic arthritis occurs. This is the most serious aspect of the infection, and if it is not properly treated immediately, the joint surfaces are destroyed and the function of the joint is lost. Treatment includes intensive antibiotic therapy, immediate complete débridement of the infected wound, including opening of the joint and providing adequate drainage. Obviously, the joint should be opened only if it has been involved. The hand must be immobilized in a position to maintain adequate drainage of the joint. Injury is usually sustained when the fingers are flexed and only in this position is the opening into the joint evident. For this reason, the hand should be fixed with the fingers in flexion and the joint left wide open.

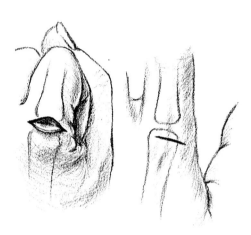

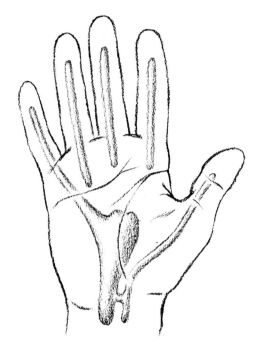

If need be, the joint may be irrigated with antibiotic solution. To do this, insert the smallest available urethral catheter into the wound, and incorporate it into the dressing.

INFECTION OF HAND

Tenosynovitis

This is an infection of the tendon sheath. It is far more serious and requires much more expeditious treatment than a fascial space infection. Pressure caused by infection within the sheath destroys the tendon very rapidly. If the tendon sheath of a digit is involved, the slightest motion, passive or voluntary, causes severe pain. The patient holds the finger semiflexed and rigid; there is tenderness over the affected sheath. The sheath of the middle three digits extends proximally to the knuckle joints. The sheaths of the thumb and little finger continue into the wrist as the radial and ulnar bursae. These two bursae frequently communicate.

Infection in the thumb and little finger rapidly spreads to the bursae and thence to the deep forearm. Infection from the tendons in the middle digits is more likely to spread to the fascial spaces in the hand. *Treatment is by immediate drainage* in which the tendon sheath or bursa is opened as well as the subcutaneous tissue. Make the incision in a midlateral position behind the nerve and blood vessels of the digit.

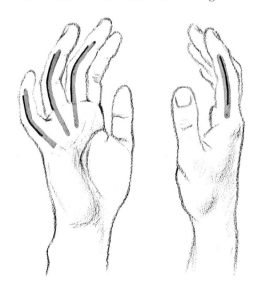

Expose the tendon and confirm the diagnosis by inspection. If the sheath is infected it bulges. Open an infected sheath along the entire length of the infection. Insert catheters into the wound but do not leave them in direct contact with the tendon. These will allow you to irrigate the wound after operation.

Fascial Space Infections

Fascial space infections are more common than synovial space infections but not nearly so crippling or severe. The fascial spaces which may become involved are the web spaces, the mid-palmar space, the thenar space, the hypothenar space, the dorsal subaponeurotic space, and the quadrilateral space in the forearm.

WEB SPACE. Although most of the pus in a web space infection is on the volar side, the abscess usually points dorsally. There is a tender red bulge in the distal part of the palm which soon extends dorsally in the web, earning it the name of a collar button abscess because of the appearance of a cross section. The base of one finger is swollen. There is no tenderness over the tendon sheath or pain on motion of the fingers unless the tendon sheath is involved. The condition is treated by surgical drainage, with a curved incision over the proximal portion of the swelling in the hand and a longitudinal incision dorsally over the web.

MID-PALMAR SPACE. The mid-palmar space is beneath the flexor tendons and superficial to the interossei muscles and is bounded on the radial side by a thin septum beginning at the third metacarpal and on the ulnar side by the fascia from the fifth metacarpal. This extends proximally to the carpal tunnel and distally to the tendon channel of the ring and little fingers. When it is infected palmar concavity is lost and there is tenderness over the entire area of the space. The palm is indurated and the distal crease is pale as a result of tension. The dorsum of the hand may be swollen. The middle and ring fingers are semiflexed; straightening the fingers causes pain. The space is drained through an incision in the palmar fascia. This parallels the distal crease in the palm and curves proximally down to the heel of the palm near the tendon of the little finger.

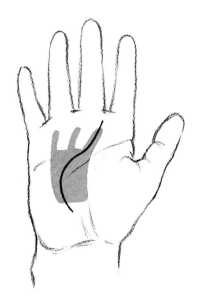

THENAR SPACE. The thenar space is on the radial side of the mid-palmar space. When it is infected there is a characteristic ballooning of the web of the thumb and a hard, red, tender swelling over the radial side of the index finger. There is abduction of the thumb and semiflexion of its distal joint. Move-

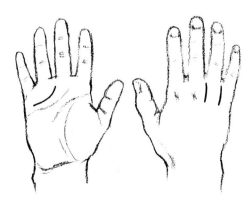

ment of the abductor pollicis against resistance causes pain. There is a semi-flexion of the index finger and pain on movement of the joint. Drainage is accomplished by an incision along the web of the thumb or curved along the radial border of the first interosseous muscle.

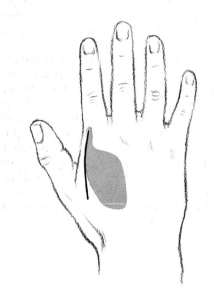

Some surgeons open the palmar surface of the thenar space, but this is dangerous because of the possibility of injuring the thenar motor nerve. Adequate opening of this space and proper drainage will cure the infection.

HYPOTHENAR SPACE. This is an infection of fascia overlying the hypothenar muscles. It usually points posteriorly and is drained by an incision directly over the inflamed area.

DORSAL SUBCUTANEOUS SPACE. This is an infection of the space between the skin and the aponeurotic layer over the extensor tendons on the back of the hand. There is swelling and tenderness over the dorsum of the hand. The infection may point anywhere in this area. Treatment is by incision and drainage at the area of pointing.

DORSAL SUBAPONEUROTIC SPACE. This is an infection between the aponeurosis of the extensor tendons and the skin. Pus which collects within the space

points at the webs of the fingers and at the periphery of the dorsum of the hand. It is drained at the area where it points.

INFECTION OF FOREARM

Radial Bursa

When the radial bursa is infected the patient holds the distal phalanx of the thumb in a semiflexed position. Even passive extension of this phalanx will cause pain. The hand is swollen and some of the concavity of the palm is lost. This is best drained through both proximal and distal incisions. The palmar incision skirts the ulnar border of the thenar eminence, extending from the region of the proximal flexion crease of the thumb to within a thumb's breadth of the transverse carpal ligament.

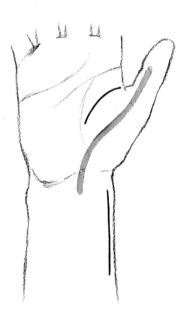

Carrying this incision higher would endanger the motor branches of the median nerve to the thenar muscle. The forearm incision is about three inches long just anterior to the radius.

Ulnar Bursa

The patient holds his fingers semi-flexed with the little finger most affected. There is pain on passive extension of the fingers. The little finger may have the classical signs of tenosynovitis. The hand is swollen, especially the dorsum, with some loss of concavity of the palm. There is fullness above the anterior annular ligament and point tenderness over that part of the ulnar bursa lying between the transverse palmar creases. If there is tenosynovitis, the tendon sheath should be opened as described on page 222. The ulnar bursa then must be opened in the palm and in the forearm. The palmar incision roughly parallels the hypothenar eminence and extends proximally to the transverse carpal ligament. The forearm incision is three inches long just anterior to the ulna on the medial side of the wrist.

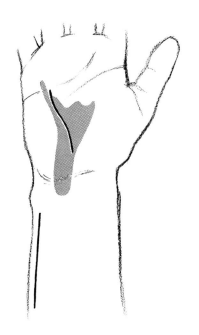

Infection of one bursa rapidly spreads to the other; both will be involved, in 80 per cent of the cases, within 48 hours. If both bursae are involved usually only one forearm incision is necessary and that should be the ulnar incision.

Quadrilateral Space of Forearm

Infection causes pain in the forearm which lessens when the nerve becomes numb. There is generalized, hard swelling on the volar aspect of the forearm beginning at the proximal edge of the transverse carpal ligament. The wrist is held flexed and extension is somewhat painful. Treatment is carried out in the lower part of the forearm. An incision is made just in front of the radius and just in front of the ulna. The radial nerve is displaced dorsally, and a dorsal branch of the ulnar nerve volarly. If the infection extends high into the forearm, an incision should be made between the flexor digitorum sublimis and the ulnaris muscles.

TUMORS OF FOREARM AND HAND

The skin of the upper extremity is subject to the lesions common to skin in any part of the body. Specific methods of treatment are described in Chapter 10, on Minor Surgery. The most common malignant lesion is carcinoma of the skin of the hand. This is treated by wide local excision with regional lymph node dissection if the nodes are involved.

GLOMUS TUMOR

A glomus tumor is an arteriovenous shunt surrounded by a network of nerves and occurs most commonly under the fingernail. It is truly a nerve tumor and is characterized by extreme pain. The nail is tender and pressure over it causes severe pain. An x-ray of the area will show erosion of the distal phalanx. The tumor can be excised under local anesthesia. Removal of the nail will cure the pain but not the tumor.

Xanthoma or Giant Cell Tumor

This is the most common tumor of tendons and tendon sheaths. It occurs as a firm, painless mass along the sheath. It does not become malignant. It can be removed under local anesthesia. Make a mid-lateral incision in the finger avoiding the digital nerve. Using blunt dissection free the tumor from the surrounding tissues and excise from the sheath.

Ganglion

A ganglion is a cystic swelling encased in a fibrous wall. It is usually found on the dorsal surface of the wrist, but may appear near any joint surface. Several types of treatment have been used: (1) rupture by external blunt force, (2) aspiration, (3) injection with sclerosing agents, and (4) surgical excision. The last has yielded the best results.

Infiltrate the area with a local anesthetic. Make a linear incision over the ganglion. With a forceps and scissors dissect out the ganglion down to its base. Excise the ganglion, its base and the surrounding tissue. Make no effort to prevent leakage of fluid from the joint capsule. Establish hemostasis. Close the dead space and approximate the skin with interrupted nonabsorbable sutures. Cover with a dry gauze dressing for a few days.

Chapter Fifteen

The Breast

TRAUMA

CONTUSION

The most common cause of contusion of the female breast is a kick by a child held by his mother. The patient consults you because of the intense pain and because of concern that the injury may produce a subsequent malignancy. On examination the breast is tender and edematous and there may be ecchymosis. Pressure and support by a tight binder or a snug brassiere will give some relief. Cold compresses during the first 8 hours after injury minimize edema formation, and warm compresses after that period promote absorption of the edema. The patient can be assured that there is no evidence that trauma to the breast causes malignancy.

Lacerations of the breast are treated as they would be in any other part of the body.

INFECTION

BREAST ABSCESS

The breast is a common site of abscess formation, particularly in the post-partum period. An abscess may occur in the superficial tissues, within the mammary tissue, or beneath it. If the abscess is in the superficial tissues, the area should be infiltrated with a line of procaine anesthesia radiating out from the nipple and an incision made directly into this. A small gauze or a rubber tissue drain should be inserted into the area and warm compresses applied. If the abscess is in the mammary tissue the incision should be radial from the nipple and carried directly down into the area of the infection. A finger should then be inserted to explore the depth of the abscess, breaking down any septa which loculate the suppuration. After the abscess space has been ex-

227

plored, an incision at a lower point may seem more practical. If this is so, do not hesitate to make the second incision and insert a rubber tissue drain to provide good dependent drainage.

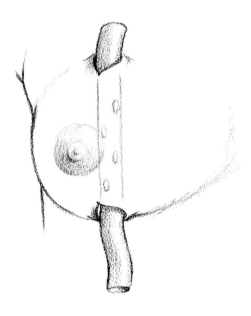

Warm compresses and specific antibiotic therapy are sometimes of value postoperatively. If the abscess should be in the retromammary area, it can usually be drained without cutting directly into the mammary tissue. Under general anesthesia make an incision in the line of the inframammary fold; with a finger locate and open the abscess, breaking down the septa compartmenting the suppuration. Insert a rubber tissue drain in position to accomplish good dependent drainage and use warm compresses in the postoperative period.

TUMOR

The breast is a common site of tumor. Both the public and the medical profession are well informed of the necessity of determining whether breast masses are benign or malignant. Consequently, masses in the breast are carried to a definitive diagnosis earlier than tumors elsewhere in the body. Even before the widespread practice of self-examination of the breast was adopted, most breast masses were found by the patient herself. She consults you for advice as to what to do about the mass. In order to form an opinion as to the nature of the mass you must examine the patient carefully. There are many good descriptions of a proper examination of the breast. The American Cancer Society publishes a good brochure on this subject* and Haagensen describes it in his book.† Comparison of any finding with the opposite apparently normal breast should not be overlooked. Any *isolated* mass or *isolated* area of involvement demands investigation.

Needle Aspiration

Many breast masses are merely cystic collections. Operation can be avoided if the lesion can be clearly identified as benign. Needle aspiration is of value in making this decision because a cystic mass may feel, to the touch, every bit as firm as a solid tumor. The possibility of the diagnosis of cystic disease is suggested by the occurrence of masses which enlarge and recede. On the other hand, it is possible for malignancy to develop in a breast where cystic mastitis already exists.

The technique of aspiration is as follows: Prepare the skin of the breast with alcohol and tincture of Zephiran. Raise a small wheal in the skin overlying the mass with 1 per cent procaine, using a 26-gauge needle. Through the wheal insert an 18-gauge needle directly into the mass and aspirate any fluid. If the aspiration results in the complete disappearance of the mass you may safely assume that it was a cyst. If any portion of

---

* Cancer of the Breast, American Cancer Society.

† Haagensen, C. D.: Diseases of the Breast. Philadelphia, W. B. Saunders Company, 1956.

the mass persists after aspiration, open biopsy is indicated.

Aspiration must not be confused with needle biopsy. Some surgeons perform needle biopsy of a lump in the breast, but this practice is not universally approved. The needle biopsy specimen reveals the histologic architecture of only the minute portion of the lesion removed. There is no assurance that another portion of the mass is not malignant. For that reason, all solid masses in the breast should be investigated with open biopsy.

BREAST BIOPSY

An open biopsy of the breast under local anesthesia is a simple technical procedure. Most surgeons prefer to perform this biopsy under general anesthesia, obtain an immediate frozen section and, if the lesion proves to be malignant, proceed immediately with a radical mastectomy. These possibilities are explained to the patient prior to the operation and, of course, are carried out only with her prior consent. While biopsy under local anesthesia is technically possible, it is felt that psychologically the patient is better off under general anesthesia during the period of anxiety while the report of the frozen section is awaited.

Some thought should be given to the position of the incision for a breast biopsy. The incision should be so placed that it will not be a problem to the patient later if the lesion proves to be benign.

INCISION

CIRCUMAREOLAR. Lesions beneath or near the areola can be reached by a circumareolar incision. The skin incision is made halfway around the areola at the junction of the areola with the breast.

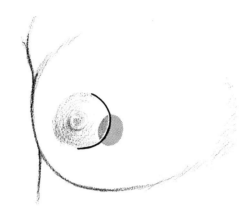

Do not carry the incision through the breast tissue because you will divide the ducts. After the skin has been divided you can separate the underlying breast tissue in a radial direction until you reach the tumor and excise it. After careful hemostasis the wound can be closed without drainage. The resultant scar is barely visible.

INFRAMAMMARY INCISION. If the lesion is very deep in the breast near its posterior surface the incision of choice is an inframammary incision. This incision is made in the fold where the skin of the breast reflects from the skin of the chest wall.

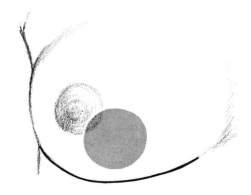

The incision is made as long as required; the breast is lifted up and the breast tissue is entered from the posterior surface to remove the nodule. With such an incision you can lift the breast from the chest wall and obtain access to any posterior area.

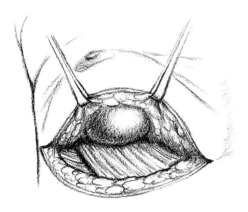

RADIAL INCISION. Other lesions in the breast are reached by a radial incision. This is made directly over the tumor and carried down to its level in a line which radiates out from the nipple.

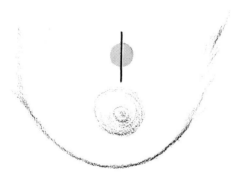

If the incision is not radial it will cut across ducts unnecessarily and possibly cause difficulty later in the lactating breast.

Closure of Biopsy Incision

After establishing hemostasis, the dead space in the wound should be closed by using over-and-over sutures to approximate the breast tissue. A thin rubber tissue drain is inserted to the deepest portion of the wound and brought out through the skin which is approximated with interrupted sutures.

A gauze dressing is used to cover the wound. Some surgeons use a compression dressing for hemostasis but not always successfully. Such a dressing sometimes prevents bleeding through the skin but the blood may dissect through the deeper tissues, causing a hematoma or extensive ecchymosis. With a drain in place and no compression, any drainage will be to the exterior. The drain is removed as soon as the drainage stops, usually on the second or third day. Most women are more comfortable if they are allowed to wear a brassiere immediately. A size larger than normally worn is more satisfactory. Never apply adhesive plaster to the breast and particularly not to the areola.

If the biopsied specimen proves to be malignant the wound should be properly closed, the entire wound reprepared, and all drapes and instruments discarded and replaced by a new set. This also includes the gowns and gloves of the operating teams. This is most simply accomplished by using only a Mayo tray with the necessary instruments for the biopsy. The bulk of the instruments are then still ready to use in the mastectomy.

EXCISION OF INTRADUCTAL PAPILLOMA

This lesion is manifested by bleeding from the nipple. One or several papillomata develop in one of the major ducts of the breast and cause the patient to bleed from the nipple. The tumor, if palpable, will be felt either as a small, elongated, thickening radiating out from beneath or near the areola, or as a round circumscribed mass near the areola. However, in many patients the tumor will not be palpable.

When you first see the patient, determine the quadrant from which the blood originates. Dry the nipple and selectively press on different areas of the breast until you find one which will cause blood to ooze from the nipple.

Once a satisfactory examination has been made it should not be repeated until the patient reaches the operating table. The operation is best done under general anesthesia. After preparation and draping of the operative area, press on the suspected area until blood exudes from one of the ducts.

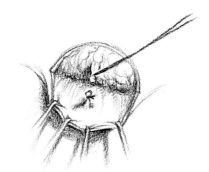

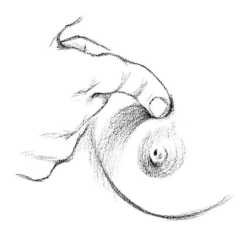

Lift the skin and subcutaneous tissue from the breast in the quadrant containing the duct and excise a wedge-shaped piece of breast tissue in continuity with the duct.

Insert the blunt end of a straight needle into this duct.

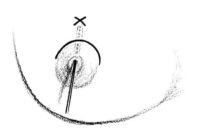

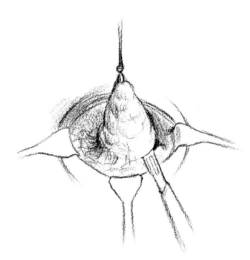

Using a circumareolar incision, cut down to the duct. Lift the areola and follow the duct to the base of the nipple where it can be divided.

Carefully examine the point of section to be sure that the papilloma does not extend beyond this point.

Chapter Sixteen

The Chest

TRAUMA

Many of the chest problems the young house officer has to face alone early in his career are caused by trauma to the chest. Some require immediate action by the first physician who sees the patient; others can be managed in a more deliberate fashion; all require some knowledge of cardiorespiratory physiology.

Rutherford and Gott* describe a rapid superficial estimate of ventilatory function made by simultaneously placing one's ear close to the patient's mouth and nose, watching the movements of the uncovered chest and palpating the pulse at the wrist. The force, duration and frequency with which the expired air strikes one's ear allow one to gauge the adequacy of ventilation. A strong blast of air eliminates the possi-

bility of significant interference with ventilation. If the exchange is feeble in spite of good effort, inspection of the chest may provide the answer.

An open pneumothorax is obvious, as is any paradoxical movement of the chest wall severe enough to cause respiratory embarrassment, since the flail segment usually involves the anterior or lateral thorax. On the other hand, if the exchange is poor in spite of symmetrical and vigorous respiratory efforts, airway obstruction probably exists.

If one hemithorax is prominent and does not move well with respiration, a large pneumo- or hemothorax probably exists. On the other hand, the involved hemithorax is diminished in volume when poor excursions are the result of splinting against painful rib fractures.

The neck should be examined to observe the relative position of the trachea, distended veins or subcutaneous emphysema. Tracheal shift to the opposite side as well as a prominent hemithorax with diminished breath sounds may be seen in both tension

---

* Rutherford, R. B. and Gott, V. L.: Thoracic Injuries. In Ballinger, W. R., Rutherford, R. B. and Zuidema, G. D.: *The Management of Trauma,* Philadelphia, W. B. Saunders Co., 1968, p. 285.

pneumothorax and massive hemothorax. Tension pneumothorax is more likely to be associated with subcutaneous emphysema and prominent neck veins, but a hyper-resonant percussion note is of even greater diagnostic significance. Massive hemothorax produces a flat percussion note and the neck veins are not full.

A diminished pulse in the face of adequate ventilation suggests cardiac tamponade or massive hemothorax. Cardiac tamponade should be suspected if there is a wound over or near the precordium. Central venous pressure is the best means of differentiating these two conditions.

CHEST WALL

INJURY

The chest may be injured by a crushing external force or by flying objects. Injury to the chest wall and injury to the intrathoracic structures present different problems; they will be discussed separately.

Contusion

A contusion of the chest wall may be the result of a blow, a fall, or a vehicular accident. If the contusion is complicated by fracture of the ribs, the ribs are of primary concern. If the patient has only a contusion, without any damage to the underlying ribs or intrathoracic structures, heat applied locally and salicylates for analgesia are usually all that is necessary.

Laceration

Most lacerations in this area do not interfere with any vital structures unless the wound extends into the pleural cavity. Treatment consists of débridement of the wound and primary closure after proper cleansing. This can usually be carried out under local infiltration anesthesia.

Rib Fracture

Trauma to the chest often causes fracture of one or more ribs. The pain accompanying a simple fracture of one, two, or three ribs may interfere with the normal excursion of the thorax and hence with normal ventilation. A fractured rib causes sharp, knife-like pain when there is motion of the chest. Consequently, the patient's respiratory excursions are markedly diminished, with splinting of the affected side. Physical examination reveals restriction of motion of the rib cage on the affected side. Physical examination reveals restriction of motion of the rib cage on the affected side. There is point tenderness over the area of fracture and external pressure elsewhere on the rib cage will cause pain at the point of fracture. Rib fractures may be associated with other less obvious injuries and the possibility of these must be considered. A sharp end of rib may lacerate the lung and produce a slow air leak which could ultimately result in a tension pneumothorax. An intercostal vessel might be lacerated, causing severe intrathoracic bleeding. A complete examination of the chest is in order to determine whether the lung is fully expanded or whether there is an accumulation of air or fluid within the hemithorax. The examination should be repeated some hours later to rule out slow accumulation of air from a small tear in the pleura.

It is common practice to treat fractured ribs by strapping the chest, thus restricting the excursion of the hemithorax. While this procedure usually reduces the pain, it may contribute to some of the complications of the fracture of the ribs. Only those patients should be strapped who have some flail character to their injury which can be stabilized by the external support. The pain of the fractured ribs is far better treated by an intercostal nerve block (p. 95). Inject not only the nerve of the rib involved, but also the two nerves above and the two nerves below the fracture. A patient may obtain relief for from 2 to 10 days with a single injection. The injections can be repeated if severe pain returns.

Fracture of the ribs may be complicated by:

PNEUMOTHORAX. The jagged end of the fractured rib will tear the lung if it touches it. There may be an extensive tear causing a large air leak; more commonly it is not so extensive. There may be a simple tear which readily seals and the resultant limited pneumothorax will be spontaneously absorbed. More dangerous is the small tear with a flap which operates as a ball valve. This could ultimately lead to a tension pneumothorax (p. 246).

If the pneumothorax is small (less than 20 per cent of the lung collapsed), is not causing respiratory distress, and is not accumulating (obvious only by repeated examinations), nothing need be done about it. If more than 20 per cent of the lung is collapsed the air should be evacuated by thoracentesis (p. 242). If the pneumothorax recurs or is found to be under tension, intercostal tube drainage (p. 244) is indicated.

HEMORRHAGE. If the rib tears an intercostal vessel, a hemothorax or a hemopneumothorax (if the lung is also torn) results. This should be treated as recommended on page 245.

RETAINED SECRETIONS AND ATELECTASIS. The pain associated with free movement of the chest makes the patient with a broken rib reluctant to breathe deeply. As a result respiratory motion is considerably restricted and some patients develop atelectasis. This is particularly true in the older age group. The treatment of the atelectasis should include relief of pain by intercostal nerve block, proper hydration of the patient, encouraging him to breathe deeply and, when necessary, nasotracheal intubation (p. 240). Rarely one must include bronchoscopy.

FLAIL CHEST. When there are multiple fractures of the ribs or the sternum and particularly when these are bilateral the patient may develop a flail chest. In the uninjured chest the motion of the lung is entirely a result of the expansion and contraction of the thoracic cage and diaphragm. When the thoracic cage loses its rigidity as a result of multiple fractures, it becomes susceptible to the negative pressure created within the chest and caves in during inspiration instead of expanding the lung by outward excursion. There is, of course, associated dyspnea. When you see a patient with a flail chest, auscultate the chest immediately. If the lungs are aerating you know that the dyspnea is due to a mechanical problem resulting from unsatisfactory expansion of the lungs, rather than to collapse of the lungs. As an emergency measure the situation can be controlled by inserting an endotracheal tube (p. 239), attaching the tube to an ordinary anesthetic machine and compressing the bag synchronously with the patient's inspiration. An intermittent positive or an intermittent positive and negative pressure machine which can follow or control the patient's respiration is even better. This aid to respiration can be continued until such time as it is possible to stabilize the chest. A satisfactory method of stabilization is external traction. Frequently a single point of traction is adequate, with fixation at the center of the greatest amount of laxity of the chest wall, but occasionally one may feel impelled to apply bilateral traction. The traction is applied by making a small incision under local infiltration anesthesia down to the rib. A sterile towel clip is clamped to the rib and is connected to continuous traction.

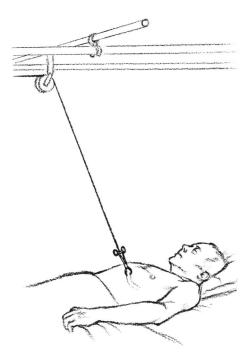

The pull should be from overhead and about 5 pounds of weight is usually sufficient. Traction is maintained until the ribs have healed sufficiently to give stability to the chest wall.

If there are multiple rib fractures, and particularly if there is more than one fracture of the same rib, it may not be possible to stabilize the chest by external traction. The cage must then be stabilized by intermittent pressure from within. As already mentioned this can be done by intermittent manual compression of the rebreathing bag of an anesthetic circuit, which is attached to an endotracheal or tracheostomy tube. However, it is far simpler to use a mechanical apparatus. There are many such machines available which deliver either intermittent positive pressure or intermittent positive and negative pressure. Some alternate at a definite time interval, others follow the patient's respiratory efforts, and still others can do both. The most desirable machine is an intermittent positive and negative pressure machine which can follow the patient's respirations but which will initiate respirations if the patient does not

breathe often enough. The pressures should be adjusted to effect adequate excursions of the patient's chest. At the same time the pressure pattern should exert a mean pressure approximating atmospheric. Respiration should be initiated approximately 15 times per minute if the patient does not breathe spontaneously that often. Continuous ventilatory support is discussed in greater detail on page 249.

Unfortunately, the automatic apparatus does not work well when attached to a tracheostomy tube because tracheostomy tubes are deliberately designed to occlude only part of the tracheal lumen (so that accidental occlusion of the tracheostomy tube does not occlude the airway). The mechanical breathing apparatus is activated by the negative pressure of inspiration. When the tube is not snug in the airway the negative pressure may not be transmitted. To accomplish a closer fit, remove the tracheostomy tube and insert a flexible endotracheal tube (McGill type) with a cuff. This must be smaller than usual to fit through the opening in the trachea. The cuff is then inflated and the tube attached to the machine.

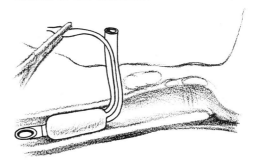

This arrangement may be used for weeks if necessary, until the chest wall is stabilized. Tracheostomy tubes with balloons attached are available commercially.

These patients require a great deal of care. They should be under continuous observation because if the tube becomes occluded the trachea will be blocked, and occlusion is likely because there is an excessive amount of blood and secretions in the tracheobronchial tree. The tube should be aspirated at least every hour and, if necessary, every 15 minutes. Later the interval can be extended. Three milliliters of sterile saline solution can be inserted to loosen secretions before aspiration. This can be repeated as often as necessary, but each increment of saline should be aspirated before more is inserted. The periods of suction should be only a few seconds. Wait until the patient recovers from one aspiration before you repeat it. At the completion of the aspiration, insert 3 to 5 drops of saline into the trachea. Whenever the patient seems to be having any respiratory distress, repeat the aspiration.

The patient with a tracheostomy has lost the humidifying effect of the nasopharynx. This is why you should insert a few drops of saline at the conclusion of the aspiration. Further humidification can be obtained by spraying a mist into the apparatus. Most machines have a small spray attached which is kept filled with sterile saline.

These patients are prone to develop pulmonary infections. In addition to the large doses of antibiotics recommended on page 123, they should be given an antibiotic to protect them against hospital bacteria. The sputum should be cultured every 4 or 5 days and the antibiotic treatment adjusted accordingly. In spite of all such measures these patients tend to accumulate material in the tracheobronchial tree. Consequently, early in their illness they require frequent bronchoscopic toilet to keep the tracheobronchial tree open. As the patient improves, the interval between bronchoscopic aspirations is lengthened.

Fracture of Sternochondral Junction

An injury which clinically simulates a fractured rib, but which cannot be visualized by x-ray, is most likely a fracture at the sternochondral junction. Physical findings are essentially the same as with a fractured rib. The patient has pain on deep inspiration.

There is point tenderness over the site of the fracture, and pressure elsewhere on the chest will cause pain at the sternochondral junction. Such a fracture is less likely than a fractured rib to produce the complications of bleeding or pneumothorax. It is treated in exactly the same way although healing is somewhat slower than with fracture of the ribs.

Avulsion of Muscle from Thoracic Cage

Occasionally a muscle will be pulled free from the thoracic cage at its point of attachment. This causes pain over the area and there is point tenderness. Use of the muscle causes pain at the point of injury. Local infiltrations to that area relieve the pain and the injury usually heals without further treatment.

Penetrating Wounds of Chest Wall

The damage produced within the thoracic cavity determines the significance of most penetrating injuries of the chest wall. The care of the patient depends more upon the extent of the deep injury than upon the superficial wound. A small penetrating wound, produced by a contaminated instrument, should be cleaned and debrided but not closed.

An unusual situation is that produced by a bullet which enters the subcutaneous tissue of the chest and richochets around the chest wall without ever penetrating deeply into the thorax itself. It is often possible to identify the site of entrance, determine the missile's course by following the ecchymotic area about the chest wall, and palpate the metallic object subcutaneously. If the bullet is causing the patient no difficulty it is probably wise to leave it alone for one week or so until some of the reaction subsides and then remove it. If there is evidence of infection it should be treated as any other infection in that area. Thoracotomy is indicated if the patient shows evidence of continued or uncontrolled serious bleeding or if an abdominal viscus or the mediastinum has been entered.

Sucking Wounds of Chest

If there is an open wound in the chest wall, air is sucked in through it rather than through the trachea during inspiration. This brings air into the pleural space and interferes with proper expansion of the lung on that side. The air which was in the collapsed lung moves over to the other lung. Expiration reverses the process. Consequently there is no movement of air through the trachea and little fresh air reaches the lungs.

If the opening in the chest wall is smaller than the diameter of the trachea the patient tolerates it fairly well. However, if the diameter of the opening in the chest wall is greater than that of the trachea the patient is in serious respiratory difficulty. The method of management is to immediately cover the defect with petrolatum gauze and a heavy gauze dressing to make it airtight. The air within the pleural space should be aspirated and the patient taken to the operating room.

BIOPSY OF LESIONS OF CHEST WALL

Tissue samples of a mass in the chest wall can be taken by open biopsy (p. 152) or by a Vim Silverman needle (p. 255). The open biopsy is more satisfactory because it yields a larger and more representative piece of tissue and, since the procedure can be done under local anesthesia, the major advantage of the needle biopsy no longer pertains.

STERNAL BONE MARROW BIOPSY

The bone marrow is frequently aspirated when there is a question of a blood dyscrasia and when anemia is being investigated. Marrow may be obtained from the sternum or from the crests of the ilium. The sternum is the more common site; the iliac crest is the primary site of biopsy when one is attempting to find malignant cells originating in a nearby tumor.

A special sternal puncture needle may be used, but this is not absolutely necessary. One can get satisfactory results with an 18-gauge spinal puncture needle. Have the patient lie flat in bed with his head extended. Prepare the skin over the body of the sternum with alcohol and tincture of zephiran and drape the area with sterile towels. Infiltrate the midline area immediately below the sterno-manubrial junction with one per cent procaine. Make a small nick in the skin with a bayonet tip blade to allow the spinal puncture needle to pass through the skin and fascia. Insert the needle, with its stylet in place, through the opening; push it obliquely into the sternum at an angle of 60 degrees to the surface of the chest until you feel the needle give. After the needle has passed through the anterior plate of the sternum, depress the needle so that it is at an angle of about 30 degrees. At this point, remove the stylet and aspirate the marrow. Usually a few milliliters are adequate for laboratory purposes. Direct smears can be made at the bedside and sent directly to the laboratory in oxalate solution. After the procedure has been completed, withdraw the needle and apply a small dry dressing.

RESPIRATORY SYSTEM

The major portion of the respiratory system lies within the chest. However, a discussion which did not include its components in the neck and head would be incomplete. Injuries to the head or neck can interfere with the airway to the lungs.

LARYNGOSCOPY

The larynx may be examined directly or indirectly. The indirect method is easier, but the direct method makes it possible to palpate structures with a probe and take biopsy specimens of any suspicious lesion.

Indirect Laryngoscopy

Indirect laryngoscopy is carried out by using a laryngeal mirror. The most common source of light for the examination is a standard lamp placed at the left side of the patient and reflected by a head mirror worn by the examiner. The examiner and patient sit facing each other in a darkened room with the patient leaning slightly forward. Ask the patient to grasp the anterior edge of his protruded tongue with a piece of gauze. Have him pull out his tongue as far as possible without causing pain and ask him to breathe quietly. Warm the laryngeal mirror in a medicine glass of warm water so that it will not fog from the patient's breath. Shake off the excess water; without touching the tongue pass the mirror back into the pharynx. If the patient gags remove the mirror and spray the pharynx with 2 per cent pontocaine. Reinsert the mirror and pass it back until it lies against the uvula.

Tilt the mirror forward, pushing the uvula and soft palate backward. This exposes successively the base of the tongue, the valleculae, the epiglottis, and finally the larynx. Various portions of the larynx may be seen as the mirror is moved about. Ask the patient to say "Eee." This should bring the cords into apposition. Remember that you are looking into a mirror and are seeing the structures in reversed position.

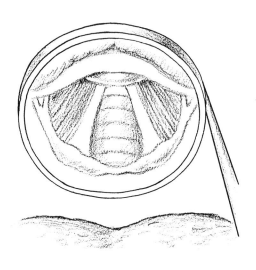

Direct Laryngoscopy

Direct laryngoscopy is used in young children and in adults in whom indirect laryngoscopy was unsuccessful; for biopsy; for removal of foreign bodies; and for insertion of an endotracheal tube for anesthesia. Except for children for whom general anesthesia is necessary, most direct laryngoscopy is done under local anesthesia. The pharynx is anesthetized with a spray of 2 per cent pontocaine. The patient should have received a barbiturate (100 mg. Nembutal) and a narcotic at least one hour prior to the examination.

The battery in the handle of the laryngoscope provides a source of light. The patient lies on the operating table in a supine position with his head and shoulders extending beyond the end of

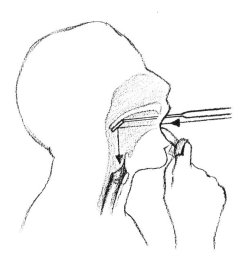

the table. An assistant sits on the right side and passes his right hand underneath the patient's neck so that the hand comes to rest on the left side of the patient's face. With his left hand he supports the patient's head. If there is no assistant, the operator must support the head with his own body. The head is extended, but the neck is brought forward to bring the mouth, the throat, and the trachea into a straight line. Insert the laryngoscope over the dorsum of the tongue; place your finger between the barrel of the laryngoscope and the patient's teeth to prevent damage to the teeth or lips. Pass the laryngoscope over the edge of the epiglottis and while lifting the entire scope forward (not tilting it on the teeth) advance it until the larynx is in view.

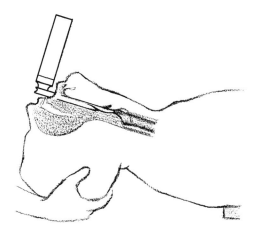

If the patient gags as the glottis comes into view a small swab soaked in pontocaine solution can be momentarily held against the area with a forceps. This is usually adequate to relieve the reflex of the glottis. You can then biopsy a lesion or insert an endotracheal tube if that was your purpose.

Insertion of Endotracheal Tube

An endotracheal tube is used for the administration of endotracheal anesthesia and to provide an adequate airway when the normal airway is obstructed. Its advantages during anesthesia are that the respiratory dead space is halved and that the patient's lungs can be ventilated with positive pressure without forcing gas into the stomach. Such a system allows one to anesthetize the patient without using excessive amounts of anesthetic gases and assures a patent airway into the lungs.

Endotracheal tubes are of varying diameters and are long enough to reach low in the trachea. The tubes are noncollapsible; some are made of plastic, some of heavy rubber, and some of thin rubber over a wire reinforcement. A cuff low on the tube can be inflated to provide a snug airtight fit. Since the tube is flexible, its insertion requires the use of a rigid stylet, which stiffens the tube during passage and is then removed.

TECHNIQUE. First make sure that all your equipment is functioning satisfactorily. Using a 10-ml. syringe, blow up the inflatable cuff to detect any leaks. If it is not working properly, replace it. Apply a thin coat of lubricating gel over the lower end of the tube. Perform direct laryngoscopy as described above. Once the larynx is in view, pass the tube through the cords when they separate and remove the stylet.

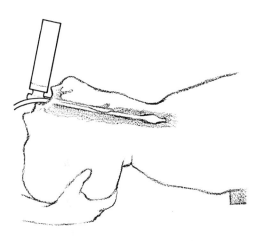

Ascertain that the tube is in the trachea by feeling air escaping from the tube when you press on the chest or by noticing that the chest expands when you blow into the endotracheal tube. If these signs are absent the tube is not properly placed; withdraw it *slowly* and reinsert it as directed above.

COMPLICATIONS.   Insertion of the endotracheal tube may be associated with the following complications:

1. Contusion or laceration of the lips or tongue. This occurs when the structure is caught between the laryngoscope and the teeth; careful insertion can prevent this.

2. Broken or knocked out teeth. This occurs as a result of using the teeth as a fulcrum while putting pressure on the laryngoscope. The scope should be held in such a way as to have the pressure on the end of the laryngoscope. If possible keep a finger or at least some gauze between the instrument and the teeth.

3. Contusion of the soft tissue of the pharynx. This is most commonly due to improper sedation and anesthetizing of the patient. The patient should be sedated with a barbiturate and a narcotic prior to the procedure. Adequate topical anesthetization should be carried out prior to insertion of the scope. Most contusions are due to gagging on the tube. If this occurs stop the laryngoscopy and apply more topical anesthetic solution.

4. Contusion of the larynx. This is due to efforts to ram the tube into the larynx without proper visualization. With sufficient time and patience, the larynx can always be brought into view and only then should the tube be inserted.

5. Laryngospasm.   Irritable vocal cords may go into spasm when disturbed. This complication is more likely to occur when Pentothal sodium anesthesia is used. It may be produced if the endotracheal tube is rapidly pulled out through the cords.

If the patient is receiving intravenous Pentothal sodium inject an additional amount; when the anesthesia deepens the cords frequently relax. Using the laryngoscope, expose the cords. Often the cords will then part enough to allow ventilation. If air is getting through between the cords do not disturb them, simply maintain this position until the spasm disappears. On the other hand, if the airway is occluded by the spasm and additional anesthesia does not relieve it, push the endotracheal tube between the cords. This can be done more easily than is generally appreciated.

INJURY TO EXTRATHORACIC STRUCTURES

With injury to the neck the patient may aspirate blood and mucus or the trachea may collapse on inspiration because of damage to its supporting wall. These problems are discussed in detail on page 202 and should be treated by tracheostomy.

Retained Secretions and Atelectasis

When the patient has in the tracheobronchial tree secretions that he is unable to raise, nasotracheal aspiration should be attempted. This is very useful in treating atelectasis caused by retained or aspirated secretions.

NASOTRACHEAL   INTUBATION. The patient should be in a sitting or in a semirecumbent position. The head should be thrown back but the neck brought forward. A sterile urethral catheter, about 14 F. with additional holes in it, is used. Wet the catheter; using sterile gloves insert it through one nostril and as it is passed back into the nasopharynx ask the patient to stick out his tongue. With your other hand, grasp the tongue, using a gauze square for traction. As the patient inhales, pass the catheter rapidly into the trachea. If the catheter slips into the trachea, it will encounter no resistance.

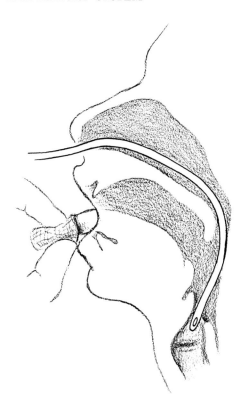

If the catheter does not slip into the trachea, the patient will gag and regurgitate the tip of the catheter through the mouth. If this happens, pull the catheter back until the tip is again in the oropharynx and proceed as before. When the catheter is in the trachea it moves along readily. The patient may have a violent paroxysm of coughing and insist that he cannot breathe. The fact is he cannot talk very well. Reassure him and point out that if he does not try to talk he can breathe adequately without difficulty. Next, apply suction to the end of the catheter for just a few seconds. The use of suction for any prolonged period deprives the patient of oxygen and can have lethal consequences. On the other hand, regardless of how ill the patient is, the catheter can be left in place for a long period and the offending secretions aspirated by applying suction for just a few seconds at a time. If the secretions are viscid or do not seem to be profuse, they can be thinned with saline. Inject 2

ml. of sterile saline together with some air into the catheter synchronously with an inspiration of the patient. This will cause a violent paroxysm of coughing and frequently the patient will cough up a fair amount of mucus around the catheter. After the patient ceases to cough and begins to breathe normally, aspirate any remaining saline and/or mucus. After an interval of a minute or two the insertion of saline can be repeated as often as necessary until the lung is completely clear.

In the event that you have difficulty in passing the catheter into the trachea, or if the patient requires such frequent nasotracheal aspiration that it seems to be wearing him out, bronchoscopy should be performed. If repeat bronchoscopy is necessary, it is far wiser to perform a tracheostomy (p. 202).

The technique of percutaneous endotracheal catheter is described on page 205.

INJURY TO INTRATHORACIC STRUCTURES

Any intrathoracic structure may be damaged. For our purposes we will discuss separately those injuries that cause hemothorax and those that cause pneumothorax. There are, of course, circumstances where a hemopneumothorax occurs.

HEMOTHORAX. Bleeding may be a result of damage to any of the major vessels, damage to the lung with bleeding of the pulmonary vessels, or damage to the vessels of the chest wall. When it occurs two problems are encountered: (1) The loss of blood from the cardiovascular system, and (2) the mechanical interference with lung expansion, cardiac action, and cardiac return by accumulation of blood within the chest. Frequently, the latter effect is more harmful than the loss of blood itself. In many instances the accumulation within the chest includes air as well as blood, thereby more seriously interfering with circulation. Often correction of the hemothorax relieves many of the symptoms.

THORACENTESIS. A thoracentesis should be done to determine the extent of bleeding and to remove the accumulated blood. When the intrapleural pressure is greater than atmospheric, it is probably better to insert an intercostal drainage tube (p. 244). Thoracentesis, or needle aspiration of the pleural space, is indicated:

1. To remove accumulated fluid and/or air so as to decompress the chest and expand the lung

2. To establish a diagnosis

3. In the treatment of empyema

The equipment tray for thoracentesis includes:

1. Sterile gloves for the operator

2. A metal container for antiseptic solution for preparation of the skin

3. Gauze squares for the preparation of the skin

4. Towels for draping the wound

5. Needles for the injection of the local anesthetic. These should include a 25- and 22-gauge 1½ inches long

6. 1 10-ml. syringe for the injection of the procaine

7. 1 medicine glass into which the procaine solution is poured

8. 1 short bevel 18-gauge needle at least 3 inches long

9. 1 50-ml. syringe

10. 1 three-way stopcock to fit the syringe

11. A rubber tube with a metal adapter to fit into the three-way stopcock

12. 1 hemostat

13. A container for the collection of the fluid

14. 2 sterile test tubes with corks for the collection of fluid to be sent to the laboratory

TECHNIQUE. Place the patient in a comfortable position. It is probably best to have him sit with his legs over the side of the bed and with his feet on a chair beside the bed. Roll up the movable support which he normally uses as a bed table and set this at such a height that he can comfortably lean upon a pillow placed on the top.

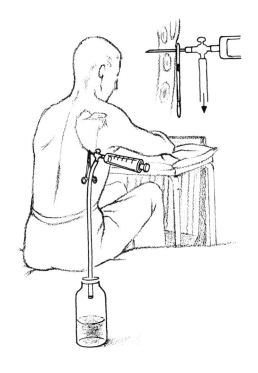

A thorough knowledge of the underlying anatomy is important. Obviously, one should not do a thoracentesis directly over the heart. If you are attempting to insert a needle in a localized area of collection, PA and lateral films of the chest are necessary. In addition, percussion is helpful in deciding where the needle should be introduced. In dealing with a free pleural space, insert a needle in the second interspace, anteriorly if you are only removing air, and directly under the tip of the scapula posteriorly in the midscapular line if you are removing fluid. After the skin has been prepared, infiltrate the skin at the point of insertion of the needle with a small wheal of procaine, using the 25-gauge needle. Attach a longer needle and infiltrate the tract with procaine, giving particular attention to the area just beneath the ribs. Since the thoracentesis needle is a short bevel needle, you may have difficulty passing it through the fascia. This difficulty can be obviated by making a small incision in the deep fascia by a stab with a bayonet tip scalpel blade. Before inserting the needle, make certain that the syringe and the three-way stopcock are functioning well. Attach the short bevel needle to the three-way stopcock which in turn is attached to the small syringe. Insert the needle through the anesthetized area and aim it at the lower portion of the interspace, barely passing over the top of the lower rib. The intercostal vessels are under the upper rib in the interspace; keeping the needle low in the interspace should avoid injury to these vessels. Puncture of the pleura is readily recognized by the sudden change in resistance as the needle goes through the pleura. Aspirate by withdrawing the plunger of the syringe. It may be necessary to reposition the needle to readily aspirate the fluid or air. Once you are satisfied with the depth of penetration of the needle, anchor the needle by grasping it with the hemostat at the point where it enters the skin. Turn the three-way stopcock so as to close the end of the needle and replace the small syringe with the 50-ml. syringe. You can withdraw whatever amount of fluid you desire. With the rubber tubing attached to the remaining side of the three-way stopcock, the fluid can be expressed from the syringe without detaching the needle. You can run fluid through the rubber tubing into the collecting bottle or basin. Fill each specimen tube with fluid; send one tube to the laboratory for study and tape the second to the head of the patient's bed to give all other interested physicians opportunity to see the gross characteristics of the fluid. It is also available for gross comparison with fluid from later taps if necessary. If the fluid is infected, you may only want to draw off a small amount to decide the nature of further treatment or you may want to empty the chest. The latter can best be done by attaching the rubber tubing to a needle and inserting the needle into a vacuum bottle used for the collection of blood. If this withdraws the fluid too rapidly, you can control it by partially occluding the rubber tube

between the vacuum bottle and the thoracentesis needle. When sufficient fluid or air has been removed to allow the lung to expand and come out against the needle, you can feel the lung bumping against the end of the needle. This can be corrected by withdrawing the needle slightly until all of the fluid or air has been removed. After this has been completed, insert 1,000,000 units of penicillin dissolved in a few milliliters of sterile saline into the pleural space. After the needle is removed, apply a small dressing to the area. In hemothorax, it is not always possible to remove all the fluid because of reaction in the patient. As more fluid is removed, the patient may experience thoracic discomfort, become dyspneic, or cough. This is relieved by stopping the aspiration at this point or by inserting air as the fluid is withdrawn. Usually inserting one syringe full of air for each two syringes of fluid withdrawn is adequate.

COMPLICATIONS. This procedure may have early or late complications. The early complications have to do with improper insertion of the needle. The needle may be inserted into a major vessel, into the heart, or into the liver. If this occurs and is recognized, it usually is not serious.

In many instances, the effusion in the chest may be sanguineous. It is often difficult to determine by inspection whether the fluid withdrawn is blood or a sanguineous effusion. Usually a hematocrit study is required to determine how much blood is contained in a sanguineous solution. The best means of determining whether one is withdrawing fluid directly from the circulatory system is to see whether it will clot. An easy way to do this is to ask your assistant to agitate the solution in a pan for a few moments. If it clots, it is not an effusion but blood. There are rarely any effects of simple penetration of a vessel.

Occasionally, moving the thoracentesis needle about a good bit tears the surface of the lung and results in an air leak. This may cause a pneumothorax; this usually is not serious because the lung rarely collapses more than 10 to 20 per cent. However, occasionally the tear in the lung may have a ball valve effect. This will ultimately result in a tension pneumothorax which must be treated with *immediate* intercostal tube drainage. The chest should be examined immediately after thoracentesis and several hours later. If the breath sounds have diminished, a chest x-ray or repeat thoracentesis should be performed. If the lung is more than 50 per cent collapsed, or if the intrapleural pressure is above atmospheric, intercostal tube drainage should be set up without delay.

INTERCOSTAL TUBE DRAINAGE. This can usually be set up in the patient's room under local anesthesia. The tube is inserted in a high interspace on the anterior surface of the chest wall sufficiently lateral to avoid the heart and the mediastinal structures. After the skin has been prepared with alcohol and tincture of Zephiran, infiltrate the area with one per cent procaine solution for a distance of 3 cm. directly over and parallel with the interspace. Using a scalpel, divide the skin and the pectoral fascia. Insert the scalpel parallel with the ribs and into the lower portion of the interspace.

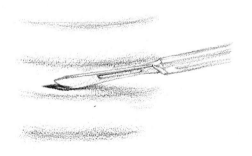

Grasp a urethral catheter (18 F. to 22 F. containing additional holes) with a hemostat so that the tip of the hemostat protrudes beyond the catheter. Force the hemostat and tube through the incision and into the pleural space.

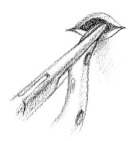

This must be done forcefully to get it through the chest wall. Entrance into the pleural space is easily recognized by the flow of air in and out of the catheter. Hold the catheter, unlock and pull out the hemostat, leaving the catheter in place. Anchor the catheter with a skin suture and reinforce this with adhesive plaster. Attach the catheter to a tube which leads to an underwater seal.

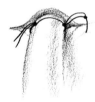

CHEST DRAINAGE (WATER SEAL). A functioning chest drainage setup merely requires that the drainage tube from the chest be inserted beneath the level of water in a container. The end of the tube should be only approximately one centimeter below the level of the fluid. If the pressure within the chest rises above one centimeter of water, fluid or air will be blown off. If the pressure within the chest drops below atmospheric, fluid will be drawn up in the tube by an equivalent amount. This allows for the exhaust of excess fluid or air but prevents the sucking of air from the atmosphere into the chest. It is common practice to attach an extra bottle to the system; this acts as a trap to collect the fluid which comes out of the chest.

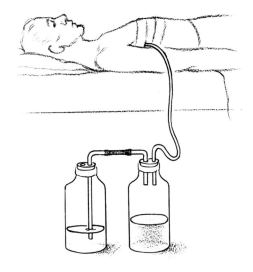

This additional bottle permits accurate measurement of the chest effusion and allows the differential between the level of fluid in the blow-off bottle and the tip of the tube to remain unchanged. When the pleural space is properly drained, bleeding will often cease. Evacuation of the pleural space allows the lung to come up against the chest wall, encouraging hemostasis. Blood lost should be replaced by an equal volume of blood. The replacement should be slow until the pleural fluid and/or air has been drawn off, to avoid overloading an already precariously balanced circulation. However, if one has difficulty sustaining the patient's blood pressure the replacement can be rapid. Once the blood pressure has been raised to approximately normal levels, give another 500 ml. rapidly and then continue to replace the estimated blood loss at a slower rate. In many instances, removal of the blood and air from the chest and blood replacement suffice to stabilize the patient and little further treatment is necessary. On the other hand, if the patient's blood pressure should again drop after the pleural space has been decompressed and 2000 ml. of blood has been given, or if these measures have failed to re-establish an adequate blood pressure, the patient should be operated upon immediately. If blood is needed immediately and is not available, the blood aspirated from the chest can be strained and used. It is rarely necessary to add anticoagulant to this blood.

CLOTTED HEMOTHORAX (TRAPPED LUNG). If, in a hemothorax, the blood is not removed, it may trap the lung in a collapsed position. This can sometimes be corrected by means of chemical debridement: if thorancentesis is unsuccessful in removing the blood or if after thoracentesis the lung is still collapsed by a layer of fibrin, attempt expansion with streptokinase and streptodornase.

TECHNIQUE. Perform a conventional thoracentesis. After all free fluid has been withdrawn, inject into the hemithorax the contents of one ampule of streptodornase and streptokinase dissolved in 50 ml. of saline. On each of the next two days, aspirate any liquid from the hemithorax. If necessary, you may repeat the insertion of enzymes on the second day.

Enzymatic therapy may produce a relatively severe pyrogenic reaction which is often misinterpreted as a spreading infection, but this is not an indication for discontinuing the treatment. The reaction usually disappears when the liquefied exudate is removed from the hemithorax. After the maximal benefit has been obtained by this method, the lung may not yet be fully expanded. If the hemithorax is not infected, there is no need for immediate surgical intervention. The remaining material may be absorbed over the next few weeks without further specific treatment. If the lung is not expanded in six weeks, operative decortication is indicated.

Pneumothorax

When the lung is torn, air leaks into the pleural space and a pneumothorax results. In the simple pneumothorax, excursion of the chest wall is limited on that side, the percussion note is hyperresonant, and no breath sounds are audible. The extent of the collapse should be checked by x-ray. If there is not more than 20 per cent collapse and the patient is comfortable, there is no need for any special treatment unless the condition progresses. The patient should be rechecked several hours later to rule out progression of the pneumothorax.

Complete pneumothorax and massive air leaks may occur as a result of extensive laceration of the trachea or bronchi. These patients are short of breath and have a considerable amount of subcutaneous emphysema. Thoracentesis and intercostal tube drainage should be set up as soon as possible. If the patient continues to have difficulty breathing, perform a tracheostomy. This has the added advantage of diminishing leaks from the trachea or main bronchi because the endotracheal pressure will no longer rise above atmospheric levels. A high volume suction pump is useful if the water seal does not seem to be adequate. Air leaks do not demand immediate operation. Many will seal once the lung is brought out against the chest wall. In injuries of the trachea and bronchi, the serious leak will persist and the laceration will have to be closed directly. In such cases, it is more important to stabilize the condition of the patient and have good anesthetic assistance available than to do an emergency procedure.

Subcutaneous Emphysema. Some of these patients develop a severe degree of subcutaneous emphysema. This is frequently very upsetting to the patient. These drawings of the same man indicate how much subcutaneous emphysema can distort an individual's appearance.

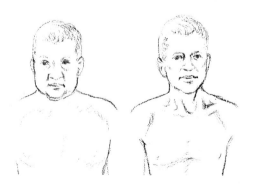

Air insufflates the subcutaneous tissues from hips to forehead. Palpation reveals crackling of the tissues. The emphysema may even cause the eyelids to puff and interfere with vision. If this occurs, the patient is particularly disturbed. Reassure him and demonstrate that he can open his eyes by milking the air out of the eyelids. Some of the air can be expelled by making small incisions in the skin of the neck and milking air out through these but this is only rarely necessary.

Subcutaneous emphysema is dangerous only when there is sufficient air in the mediastinal tissues to compress the trachea. Once a tracheostomy has been performed and chest drainage established, the situation is not hazardous. The air will ultimately be absorbed from the tissues. The subcutaneous emphysema will subside more rapidly if the patient breathes high oxygen mixtures.

Tension Pneumothorax

One of the most serious conditions and one which requires the most prompt care is tension pneumothorax. This occurs following extensive damage to the lung, but it may accompany minor lung damage where an air leak has a ball valve effect. The air can get into the pleural space during inspiration but cannot get out during expiration because the ball valve closes the exit. Air gradually accumulates in the pleural space, causing a shift of the mediastinum. Sudden death may result from kinking of the great vessels.

Tension pneumothorax is readily recognized if one considers the possibility. The patient is quite dyspneic. There is no movement of the affected side of the chest. The percussion note is hyperresonant and no breath sounds can be heard on that side. The trachea is shifted to the opposite side along with the other mediastinal structures. The situation requires immediate attention. Immediate thoracentesis is indicated without delay for permission or consultation. The needle should be left in place, attached to an underwater seal. The needle can be stabilized by putting a cork about the needle and taping the cork to the chest wall.

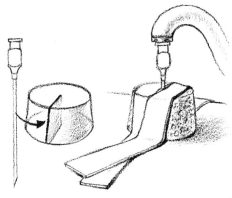

If necessary, an emergency water seal can be made by fitting a piece of rubber tubing over the end of the needle and running it beneath a fluid level in any available container. It must be emphasized that this is a temporary arrangement which should be continued only until replaced by intercostal tube drainage. The latter is frequently all that is necessary. If it is necessary to move the patient before a conventional water seal arrangement is available, set up a flutter valve on the end of the tube by attaching a condom or a piece of thin-walled drain.

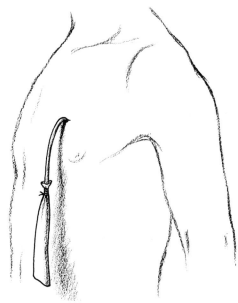

If the water seal drainage system does not have adequate capacity, attach a high volume suction pump. This will solve the problem unless there is a major tear in the trachea or in a main bronchus. These require thoracotomy and direct repair, but only after the condition of the patient is stabilized and good anesthetic support is available.

RESPIRATORY FAILURE

Respiratory failure is the inability of the lungs to maintain physiologic levels of oxygen and carbon dioxide in the blood. There are four basic causes of respiratory failure: (1) increased metabolic rate, (2) increased physiologic shunting of blood, (3) decreased oxygen transport in the blood and (4) increased pulmonary dead space.

Elevated metabolic rate is seen in the classic picture of the patient with airway obstruction and decreased compliance who must work so much harder to breathe. Agitation is often a major component of the increased work of breathing. There are numerous pathologic states which cause perfusion of non-ventilated areas of the lung and ventilation of non-perfused areas. Abnormalities in the relationship between ventilation and perfusion result in diminished oxygen transport in the blood, increased shunting and increased dead space. Increase in physiologic dead space is seen in patients with tachypnea owing to the uneven ventilation due to rapid respiratory rate. In caring for the patient with pulmonary failure it is important to delineate which of these states exists.

From the standpoint of therapy, it is often useful to divide the causes of respiratory failure into two broad categories: intrapulmonary and extrapulmonary. The most common type seen on the surgical service is the intrapulmonary type in which pathologic changes take place in the tracheobronchial tree and lung parenchyma. Common causes are pneumonia, atelectasis, chronic bronchitis, emphysema and pulmonary fibrosis. With the changes in the tracheobronchial tree and pulmonary parenchyma there is usually associated decrease in compliance with an increase in airway resistance. This is especially true in obstructive lung disease such as emphysema, bronchitis and bronchial asthma.

In restricted lung disease such as pulmonary fibrosis, edema and pneumonia there is also reduced compliance. Often, however, airway resistance is normal and presents no difficulty.

The extrapulmonary type of pulmonary failure is the less common of the two types and usually is easier to treat. This is seen in the patient with a muscular, neurologic or neuromuscular abnormality, but without any structural or functional pulmonary abnormality. Because compliance and airway resistance are usually normal in this group, it is easier to assist ventilation.

In the patient with compromised pulmonary reserve, a surgical procedure is often the precipitating factor that causes respiratory failure. Anesthesia and pain superimposed on pulmonary function may result in pulmonary failure. This is especially true in patients undergoing cardiac or pulmonary operations, but can be equally true in other types of surgery.

DIAGNOSIS

The diagnosis of pulmonary failure in the surgical patient is usually not difficult. The cardinal findings are dyspnea, hypertension, hypoxia and hypercapnia. Associated findings which may be present include pallor, sweating, tachypnea, cyanosis, tachycardia and clouded sensorium. The patient may have to work so hard to move enough air for adequate ventilation that if allowed to continue he will ultimately exhaust himself. The late manifestations include hypotension, tachycardia, anuria and finally generalized collapse. It

is often impossible to make an early diagnosis on clinical grounds alone. Arterial blood gas studies are the best method of diagnosis and of monitoring function in patients with suspected pulmonary failure. Analysis of the arterial blood usually shows the pH to be in the range of 7.30 or below, a pCO_2 of 50 mm. of mercury or greater and a pO_2 of 75 mm. of mercury or less. These values are highly variable and are related to pre-existing chronic lung disease, the type of care being given to the patient and the degree of compensation.

It must be established that the somnolent patient is not suffering from prolonged effects of anesthetic gases, narcotics or curare-like drugs. Narcotic-induced depression of ventilation is common in postoperative patients. Unless this is recognized, unnecessary radical therapy may be instituted. However, intensive therapy may be necessary in these patients to insure survival during the period of respiratory depression.

TREATMENT

Treatment consists of establishing an adequate airway and supplying an adequate volume of ventilation.

Establishment of An Adequate Airway

An airway is assured by either passing an endotracheal tube or establishing a tracheostomy.

PASSAGE OF AN ENDOTRACHEAL TUBE. The tube may be passed orally or through the nares. With some practice one can pass a large nasotracheal tube without undue difficulty. This tube is more convenient and better tolerated than one inserted through the mouth. The universal fitting on the proximal end of the tracheal tube allows the attachment of a respirator. The naso-tracheal tube insures adequate access to the tracheobronchial tree and permits one to begin immediate support of the ventilation. At the same time one can delay a decision as to whether pro-longed ventilatory support and a tra-cheostomy are necessary. With a naso-tracheal tube in place many patients can be carried through the initial period of difficulty. In an occasional patient the irritation of the nasobronchial tube is sufficient stimulation to adequate breathing. The standard catheter avail-able may be too short for adequate aspi-ration through such a tube. If an emergency situation arises, a sterile Levin nasogastric tube may be used.

An endotracheal tube provides a very adequate conduit for the passage of air in and out of the trachea. However, in the presence of pulmonary sepsis it is not the ideal means of pulmonary toilet. If one expects to remove particulate matter from the tracheobronchial tree, one should use a tracheostomy.

TRACHEOSTOMY. When it is antici-pated that a patient will require continu-ous ventilatory support, the advisability of doing a tracheostomy must be consid-ered. Generally we have been reluctant to leave a nasotracheal tube in place for more than 36 hours in an adult. If the patient needs continuous support beyond that period, we remove the tube and perform a tracheostomy. A large tracheostomy tube having a cuff of low elasticity and a large volume should be used. The balloon should be checked prior to the insertion of the tube. One must avoid tearing the larger volume cuff when inserting the tube through the opening in the trachea.

In patients who require immediate continuous ventilatory assistance, the support should be instituted wherever they are in the hospital. They can then be moved to a unit for specialized care. In transit they are ventilated and given additional oxygen, usually manually by an Ambu bag into which additional ox-ygen is flowing.

RESPIRATORY THERAPY

As soon as the patient arrives in the special unit he is attached to a ventilator, preferably a volume-controlled respira-tor. This must control the patient's res-piration to be effective. The initial phase of respiration therapy is usually the most difficult. The patient is often restless, synchronization with the respi-rator is poor and adequate ventilation may be difficult to establish. By venti-lating the patient at a rapid rate with adequate tidal volumes, pCO_2 will in most cases be lowered to apneic levels at which the ventilation can be controlled. Hyperventilation is accomplished using either an Ambu bag or the ventilator it-self. In those patients who cannot be hy-perventilated to apnea, careful drug ad-ministration is usually necessary. The drugs depress the respiratory drive so that the patient ceases to "buck" the res-pirator, allowing better ventilation with reduction of the pCO_2. Narcotics, alpha-prodine (Nisentil), hydromorphone (Di-laudid), morphine or meperidine (Dem-erol) have been used effectively. We usually begin with small doses (10 to 20 mg.) of Nisentil intravenously. This drug is a strong respiratory depressant, and in most instances this dose has been sufficient to suppress the respiratory drive for short periods. For a more prolonged effect twice the intravenous dose can be given intramuscularly. Once the patient has been controlled, drugs such as phenobarbital or hydroxyzine (Vistaril) are used to maintain sedation. Patients who are restless owing to postoperative wound pain usually respond to Demerol, Dilaudid or mor-phine. Hyperventilation has been cred-ited with reducing the need for narcot-ics for pain.

Resynchronization of the patient's respiration with the ventilator may be a problem after the patient has been dis-connected from it in order to be as-pirated. The nurses can usually hyper-ventilate the patient to apnea manually using an Ambu bag. If this is not possible, some suppression by drugs will be necessary.

Adjustment of Ventilator

Proper management of continuous ventilatory support requires monitoring by means of blood gas analysis. It is desirable to maintain the pCO_2 and the pO_2 of the arterial blood near normal. These values can be individually influenced by adjusting the composition and volume of the ventilatory gas. Increasing the volume of ventilation will wash out additional carbon dioxide and lower the pCO_2. The pO_2 of the blood varies directly with the concentration of oxygen in the inspired gas. In the Engstrom ventilator, which we use, the volumes of oxygen and of room air can be adjusted separately. This allows more complete control of the pO_2.

A blood sample is analyzed for pCO_2, pO_2 and pH as soon as the patient is stablized on the machine. If gas values are not optimal, the ventilation is adjusted and the blood analyzed again after a period of 30 minutes. This routine is repeated until satisfactory values are obtained. The minute volumes of oxygen and room air used to maintain optimal values are kept constant until there is evidence for change on the basis of later blood gas analysis.

Once the patient's ventilation has been stabilized at the desired level, the normal range of gas tensions can be continued by maintaining the ventilation unchanged. The blood studies should be repeated daily for the first two or three days. When the patient is kept on the machine longer and remains stable, it is possible to extend the interval to two or more days.

Considerable nursing care is required for any patient receiving continuous ventilatory support. A specially trained nurse should be in attendance at all times. A cuffed endotracheal tube is used routinely. It must be remembered that with such a device there is no airway about the tube such as exists when a regular tracheostomy tube is in the trachea. If the tube blocks, the patient cannot breathe, and the tube must be unblocked immediately or he will be asphyxiated. The trachea must be aspirated as often as necessary; this may be as often as every 15 minutes when first begun, but after stabilization and control of any infection a few times a day is sufficient.

To avoid serious pulmonary infections as a result of the tracheostomy special precautions must be taken:

1. A sterile catheter must be used each time the trachea is aspirated.

2. The nurse aspirating the trachea must wear a sterile rubber glove to handle the catheter.

3. The catheter is irrigated with sterile saline from a sterile cup, which is changed for each aspiration.

4. Tracheal aspiration must be limited to 3 to 5 seconds at a time to avoid precipitating cardiac arrest. On the other hand, the number of aspirations is not limited, provided the patient is allowed to recover between aspirations. The secretions may be thick or crusted. Two to 5 ml. of saline instilled just before aspiration will thin the secretions and facilitate removal. A special tracheostomy aspiration kit with sterile equipment is made up by the hospital. This consists of:

    A. a rubber glove

    B. an aspirating catheter

    C. a 5-cc. syringe

    D. a disposable cup

A large pack containing five or ten such kits can be kept at the patient's bedside.

Choice of Respirator

The ventilators available can be divided into three main categories, depending upon the principle controlling inspiration and expiration. In *pressure cycled respirators,* the inspiratory phase ends when a preset pressure has been reached. In *volume cycled respirators,* inspiration ends and expiration begins when a preset volume has been delivered. In *time cycled respirators,* inspiration and expiration are controlled by a preset rate and preset duration. Time cycled respirators are now less frequently used than pressure cycled and volume cycled respirators.

Proper use of any of the presently available ventilators will result in successful management of the great majority of patients in respiratory failure. Pressure regulated respirators, which are usually patient triggered, are used in most hospitals today. The patient must begin to inhale to trip a valve in the machine which initiates inspiration. Inspiration then proceeds until a predetermined pressure has been reached in the tracheobronchial tree, at which time the flow to the patient is terminated and a passive expiratory phase occurs. This works in most patients. However, in patients with bronchospasm, the increased intrabronchial pressure forces the machine to terminate the flow of gas prematurely, causing a decrease in tidal volume. As the tidal volume decreases, hypercapnea increases, and the patient attempts to take more breaths, thereby triggering the machine again and again, creating more bronchospasm and causing earlier termination of inspiration and faster breathing. In this way, a vicious cycle is formed.

In most patients the use of bronchodilators locally or systemically will help to avert bronchospasm and its associated effects. Persistent bronchospasm is most often seen in patients with chronic bronchitis and emphysema. On occasion we have seen several such patients who were unresponsive to bronchodilators and to ventilation with pressure cycled ventilators. We have found it possible to ventilate such patients with a volume cycled respirator.

This apparatus will maintain sustained pressure at a selected level until a preset volume of gas has been delivered. The pressure of gas delivered by this apparatus to a patient in bronchospasm rises rapidly also. However, when the selected pressure is reached, the gas that would raise the pressure higher is blown off through a safety valve, but the inspiratory phase continues until the present volume has been delivered. Additional portions of this gas insure that the alveoli behind the more stenosed bronchi get as large a share of the predetermined volume as possible. As the ventilation increases, hypercapnea is reduced and bronchospasm eases, thus facilitating better ventilation.

Controlled Versus Assisted Ventilation

The ventilation may be controlled. The patient makes no effort to breathe, and the ventilator initiates and carries out each breathing cycle. Or the ventilation may be assisted. In this, the inspiratory effort of the patient triggers the machine, which assists inspiration; expiration is passive. In most instances it is easier for the patient to adjust to assisted ventilation because the machine follows the patient's lead. However, when the patient is quite ill, the ventilation should be controlled because the patient is spared the energy required to breathe, an important consideration in a desperately ill patient.

Management of the Cuff

It is desirable to keep the pressure within the cuff in the range of 40 to 50 cm. of water. This is possible only if one uses a tube of adequate size and a large volume cuff of low elasticity. When the tracheostomy tube is inserted the cuff should be inflated until the trachea is just occluded. This is the point at which ventilated air ceases to come out through the mouth during the inspiratory phase. Adding an extra 2 or 3 cc. of air in the cuff may give a better seal but it will raise the pressure in the cuff to such a degree that it may cause serious damage to the trachea. The cuff should be left inflated until the tube is changed. This is usually every 48 hours.

Nutrition

On the first day of treatment the patient is fed intravenously. On the following day he is started on oral fluids if his gastrointestinal tract is functioning; the diet is then gradually increased. Patients on continuous ventilatory support can eat a regular diet after a few days. They can even get out of bed to eat while the ventilatory support continues. At such times the additional activities are less distracting to the patient whose ventilation is being assisted.

Stopping Ventilatory Support

Indications

A decision must be made as to when continuous ventilatory support should be discontinued. Continuous support not only provides more satisfactory gaseous exchange for the patient, but also markedly reduces the amount of effort the patient must expend to breathe. Consequently, an additional period of ventilatory assistance, beyond that required by the patient to adequately ventilate himself without support, may be utilized to diminish the work of breathing.

It is of interest that stabilization of the patient being artificially ventilated occurs at various CO_2 levels. The pCO_2 of a patient with chronic lung disease will often stabilize at a higher value than in one who has essentially normal lungs. Realization of this fact will often help avoid artificial ventilation for unnecessarily prolonged periods, since patients may be alert with relatively good pO_2 levels while the pCO_2 is elevated above 50 mm. of mercury.

After the patient has been stabilized on the basis of both clinical appearance and blood gas analysis he can then be given a trial off the ventilation. Ventilation is discontinued and blood gases are analyzed 30 minutes, two and four hours later. A drop in pO_2 does not necessarily signal the need for renewed ventilatory support. An oxygen collar can be put over the tracheostomy and oxygen administered at a rate sufficient to maintain a normal pO_2. On the other hand, if the pCO_2 rises or the patient must labor to keep it within normal limits, the ventilatory support is resumed. If the patient holds a normal pCO_2 without effort, the continuous support is permanently discontinued. An oxygen collar is put over the tracheostomy, and intermittent positive pressure breathing (IPPB) is used as often as necessary to maintain a normal pCO_2. The IPPB is best accomplished at intervals of two to four hours for periods of 20 minutes. It can be discontinued gradually as the patient progresses. The oxygen collar is usually necessary for a few days. The higher oxygen levels in the ventilating gases required during continuous support can be reduced after the ventilatory support is stopped. We use an oxygen collar at flows of 4 to 7 L. per minute of humidified oxygen. During the first few days of the weaning period we have returned some patients to continuous artificial ventilation during the night. This allows for better stabilization of the patient, reduces the work of breathing and enables the patient to sleep well with sedation. The tracheostomy may be plugged during periods of breathing ambient air. With improved ventilation, smaller tracheostomy tubes without balloons are used until the tracheostomy is no longer needed. At this time the patient is breathing well by the oronasal route and is able to expectorate tracheobronchial secretions.

Complications

INFECTION. Prophylaxis is the best approach to infection. The patient should be managed in an area where he is not exposed to serious infections. Good nursing care and aseptic management of the tracheostomy (page 202) are the best means of avoiding infection of the tracheobronchial tree. If the patient has an infection elsewhere, it should be cultured and appropriate antibiotic therapy begun. The tracheal secretions should be smeared and cultured twice weekly, and any bacteria found should be treated with appropriate antibiotics.

PULMONARY HEPATIZATION. Some patients requiring continuous ventilatory support have been found to develop a progressive coalescing atelectasis which makes the lungs look like liver when seen at autopsy. This is thought to be due to the high concentration of oxygen in the ventilating gas interfering with the surfactant, which normally allows the alveolar walls to maintain a proper surface tension. Once this process develops it is not reversible, and the patient develops hypoxia even in spite of the use of higher and higher concentrations of oxygen in the ventilating gas. The danger is in excessive oxygen in the ventilating gas and not an excessive pO_2 in the blood. One should make every attempt to limit the concentration of oxygen in the ventilating gas to 65 per cent even in the face of some hypoxia in the arterial blood, provided there are no adverse cardiovascular effects. If cardiac dysfunction or irregularity forces increases in the concentration of oxygen, it should be intermittent. Sometimes the problem can be solved without increasing the oxygen in the ventilating gas by increasing the resistance to expiration or by continuous positive pressure breathing.

BRONCHOSPASM. Many of these patients are in severe bronchospasm. This is usually due to retention of carbon dioxide, resulting in an elevated pCO_2. The bronchospasm interferes with efficient distribution of the gas, impairing good exchange. The bronchospasm can be relieved by merely increasing the ventilation and washing out the excessive pCO_2. Sometimes this is quite simple; at other times the spasm seriously interferes with the ventilation,

and one may have to use bronchodilators and suppress the respiratory drive with narcotics, making it easier to hyperventilate. In any event, the spasm can only be permanently cleared by bringing the pCO_2 back to normal.

EROSION OF THE TRACHEA. Serious erosion of the trachea and even death have occurred owing to the use of cuffed endotracheal tubes. Erosion was due to the pressures in the cuff pressing on the lateral tracheal wall. This can be prevented by following the routine detailed on page 239. If there is any question as to the level of the pressure, it can be measured at the tube connected to the cuff. If a high volume–low elasticity cuff is used, there should be little difference between the cuff pressure and the lateral tracheal pressure.

CARDIAC ARREST. Cardiac arrest may be caused by (A) Excessive tracheal suction (see page 250). (B) Obstruction to the trachea. If the tube plugs, the patient will asphyxiate, since the cuffed tube fills the trachea. The tube must be immediately unplugged. (C) Breakdown of the ventilator. If the ventilator stops, the desperately ill or paralyzed (medically or otherwise) patient cannot respire. If this happens the nurse must detach the ventilator and ventilate the patient manually.

Obviously, if either of the last two problems is to be properly handled, the patient requiring continuous ventilatory support must have an attendant present at all times.

THE HEART

INJURIES

Wounds of the Heart

The heart may be injured by nonpenetrating wounds, by penetrating wounds, or by perforating wounds. The majority of nonpenetrating wounds of the heart, or contusions, are probably never recognized. Penetrating wounds are those which enter the heart but do not break through into the pleural space. Perforating wounds, since they enter into the pleural space, cause massive bleeding.

The majority of perforating wounds produce a picture of hemothorax which cannot be controlled and which requires early operation. The only exception is the perforating wound in which blood is escaping from the ventricle more rapidly than it is escaping through the wound in the pericardium. In this situation, a picture of cardiac tamponade will exist.

Cardiac Tamponade

Cardiac tamponade is the major clinical feature in patients with penetrating wounds. Blood escapes from the wound in the heart into the pericardium, where it is trapped. As the pressure rises within the pericardial sac—a tough, nondistensible structure—there is corresponding interference with filling of the heart by blood from the cavae. The pressure within the cavae is relatively low, and thus the pressure within the pericardium need be elevated relatively little to ablate a flow of blood from the cavae into the right atrium. The patient with cardiac tamponade has low blood pressure, low pulse pressure and high venous pressure which is readily evident by distension of the neck veins. The heart sounds are distant and there may or may not be an increase in the area of cardiac dullness. On fluoroscopy the heart may not seem to be enlarged but there is an absence of pulsation. The main defect is the elevated intrapericardial pressure raising the intraventricular and intra-atrial pressures, and interfering with blood flow from the cavae. The patients show remarkable improvement when even a small amount of blood is removed from the pericardial sac because this lowers the intra-atrial pressure below the caval pressure, and allows blood flow to con-

tinue. Much of the blood enters the sac before there is any significant rise in pressure. It is the last small increment of blood which causes the significant rise in the pressure in the pericardial sac, and conversely its removal causes the most significant drop in pressure. A high percentage of these patients can be properly treated by pericardiocentesis.

PERICARDIOCENTESIS. This is most safely done via the left costoxiphoid route. A 10 cm. 18- or 19-gauge, short bevel needle is used. Infiltrate the skin about 2 cm. below the costal margin to the left of the xiphoid with 1 per cent procaine; puncture the skin and subcutaneous tissues with a bayonet tip knife blade, insert the needle at an angle of 45 degrees to the abdominal wall and pass this upward toward the pericardial cavity. When you feel that you have entered the pericardial cavity, withdraw the stylet from the needle. If no blood drips out, reinsert the stylet and carefully pass the needle somewhat further. Continue this until you obtain blood. If the needle comes in contact with the ventricle, you can feel the thrust of the ventricle against the needle and you can pull back the needle. Withdraw as much blood as you are able to obtain readily and withdraw the needle.

It is remarkable how much clinical improvement occurs following the removal of small amounts of fluid from the pericardial sac. In the event that the blood within the pericardial sac is clotted and you cannot draw a sufficient amount to improve the patient, immediate operation for evacuation of the clot and repair of the wound is indicated.

As soon as a patient with compression of the heart is admitted, the operating room should be prepared and the patient observed there. If the patient responds after pericardiocentesis, continue to observe him closely. If tamponade recurs, repeat the tap. If it recurs again, immediate thoracotomy is needed. Thoracotomy is also done if the tap fails to relieve the tamponade or if there is continued bleeding into the pleural space. Most patients with injuries to the heart who reach the hospital alive can be managed successfully without thoracotomy.

NEEDLE BIOPSY OF INTRATHORACIC TUMORS

Needle biopsy may be a means of avoiding a thoracotomy in a patient with an intrathoracic tumor. Initially, this was considered a reasonable means of diagnosis of all intrathoracic masses. However, after several reports of seeding of the chest wall, this procedure has been restricted to biopsy of tumors which are obviously inoperable or are discovered on thoracotomy to be deep in the lung. Percutaneous needle biopsy of a lung tumor should be reserved for patients whose tumors are inoperable by reason either of extension of tumor or of the general condition of the patient. In such patients the exact nature of the mass is of value in deciding further therapy. Such tumors should not be biopsied if they are close to the heart or the great vessels.

TECHNIQUE

Identify the exact position of the tumor. Posterior-anterior and lateral views of the chest are usually adequate for this purpose, particularly if the tumor is adherent to the chest wall in any area. Occasionally, fluoroscopy is necessary. In this instance, the procedure should be done in the fluoroscopic room.

Prepare the skin with alcohol and tincture of Zephiran. Make a skin wheal with procaine and infiltrate the deeper tissues. Make a small incision in the skin with a bayonet tip scalpel blade. Insert the carrier needle with the obturator through the incision and into the chest. Pass the needle low in the interspace to avoid the intercostal blood vessels. Insert the needle into the tumor. If fluoroscopic guidance is necessary it should be

used at this time. After the needle has been inserted into the tumor, remove the obturator and insert the forked needle to its full length, which brings it several centimeters beyond the carrier needle.

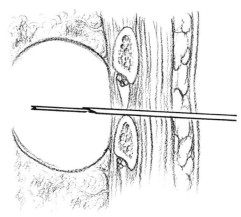

Advance the carrier needle over the forked needle, turn both 180 degrees and remove. The tissue will be in the groove of the forked needle (p. 158).

PLEURAL BIOPSY

The primary indication for pleural biopsy is unexplained pleural effusion. Needle biopsy of the pleura should not be attempted in the absence of demonstrable fluid by x-ray.

A full thoracentesis tray (page 242) plus a Cope pleural biopsy needle make up the necessary equipment. The Cope needle consists of an 11-gauge outer sleeve, a 13-gauge inner puncture needle with a fitted stylet and a hook-type curette. The puncture needle and the curette each fit into the sleeve and extend beyond the end of it.

The tap should be made into the area of the greatest fluid accumulation. Place the patient in a semirecumbent position or in an upright position as for a posterior thoracentesis (page 242). The position will depend upon the site selected for insertion of the needle.

Prepare the skin with alcohol and tincture of Zephiran. Make a skin wheal with procaine and infiltrate the deeper tissues. Make a small incision in the skin with a bayonet tip scalpel blade. Insert the 13-gauge inner puncture needle with its fitted stylet through the outer 11-gauge sleeve. This should fit snugly and protrude beyond the sleeve. Insert the two through the skin incision and into the pleural space, passing low in the interspace to avoid the intercostal blood vessels.

When you estimate that the pleural cavity has been entered, remove the stylet, attach a syringe and aspirate. If the needle is in proper position, fluid will be aspirated. Reinsert the stylet. Remove the inner needle and stylet from the sleeve and replace it with the hook-tipped curette, occluding the sleeve with your thumb while changing needles.

The pleura can now be biopsied along the lower half of the interspace. Turn the curette so that the hook points to either side or downward. The curette is slowly withdrawn until the pleura is snared. While maintaining traction on the biopsy snare, push the outer sleeve forward. The beveled edge of the outer sleeve transects the specimen. The outer sleeve is left in place and the curette with the biopsy is withdrawn. The biopsy is removed from the curette. The inner needle is reinserted, the stylet removed and a conventional thoracentesis performed.

COMPLICATIONS

The two most important complications of needle biopsy of the chest are hemorrhage and tension pneumothorax.

Hemorrhage

Hemorrhage may occur from any of the major vessels or from an intercostal vessel. The best means of avoiding bleeding from the major vessels is to stay away from them. It is too hazardous to attempt this procedure on a mass which is near a major vessel. Bleeding from an intercostal vessel can be avoided by inserting the needle low in the intercostal space. The vessels lie close to the rib above. If hemorrhage does occur, attempt to control it by inflating the lung by thoracentesis or by intercostal tube drainage (p. 245) and replacing blood when necessary. When falling blood pressure indicates that you are having difficulty keeping up with blood loss, immediate thoracotomy should be undertaken.

Tension Pneumothorax

If the tumor was adherent to the chest wall and the aspirating needle entered through that area, pneumothorax cannot occur. On the other hand, there could frequently be some leakage of air in a pneumothorax resulting from the needle's having crossed a free pleural space and entered normal lung before encountering the tumor. Immediately after the biopsy, examine the patient to determine the presence or absence of a pneumothorax. Regardless of whether this is immediately evident, the patient should be watched for the next four to six hours. A small air leak may culminate in a tension pneumothorax after one-half to several hours. When this occurs, the patient is markedly dyspneic, there is very little motion of the chest on the affected side, the interspaces are widened, the trachea is deviated to the other side and the breath sounds are distant. Treatment consists of immediate thoracentesis (p. 245) followed by intercostal tube drainage.

Chapter Seventeen

The Abdomen

TRAUMA

Trauma to the abdomen may be divided into two types: trauma to the abdominal wall and trauma to the abdominal contents.

ABDOMINAL WALL

Contusion

Contusions of the abdominal wall are caused by blunt force. When you see a patient with this type of trauma first ascertain that there has been no associated intra-abdominal injury. The signs are described later in this chapter. If there is no intra-abdominal injury, the problem is merely the treatment of a local contusion. There may be some ecchymosis or accumulation of blood in the soft tissues and the mass of blood may simulate a tumor. If the mass continues to increase in size, external pressure can be applied to control it. Cold applications may help at this time. If there is a large hematoma, it may be aspirated, although this is rarely necessary. Usually the area of ecchymosis spreads extensively before it is re-absorbed. Occasionally a collection may proceed to abscess formation and external drainage is then required.

Laceration

Any wound of the abdominal wall which penetrates, or is thought to have penetrated, the abdominal cavity should be explored. Under no circumstances should the wound be probed to decide whether or not the peritoneal cavity has been entered. Probing it may make a penetrating wound out of one which originally was not. If the abdominal cavity was not penetrated, merely cleanse the wound, suture it loosely, and drain it.

Trauma to Abdominal Contents

Perforation of Intraperitoneal Viscus

Evidence of damage to the abdominal wall may or may not accompany injury to the abdominal contents. Rupture of the spleen or liver with serious bleeding, or rupture of any hollow viscus within the peritoneal cavity may occur with little or no bruising of the abdominal wall. Penetrating wounds of the abdomen can also injure any one of these structures. When injuries are due to flying missiles and bullets the damage usually involves several organs. In the care of such patients it is of utmost importance to decide whether or not the intra-abdominal contents have been damaged; if so, the patient is prepared for immediate operation. If there is serious intra-abdominal hemorrhage, the patient will exhibit signs of peritoneal irritation with a falling red blood cell count and ultimately the classical clinical picture of hemorrhagic shock. If a viscus has been perforated, the signs of peritoneal irritation will be evident early. These include pain, tenderness, muscle guarding, rigidity, rebound tenderness, and a silent distended abdomen if generalized peritonitis has developed. When the shock is well advanced, the patient has a tachycardia and temperature elevation. There will also be leukocytosis and a relative increase in neutrophils. In most cases you will see the patient soon after the trauma and these advanced signs of peritonitis will not yet have appeared. In the early phases of small perforation, only less well defined signs will be present. Whenever there is any suspicion that a missile has entered the abdominal cavity, operation is mandatory.

Stab Wounds of the Abdomen

A stab wound of the abdomen can test the diagnostic ability of the surgeon. The external orifice of a stab wound usually appears relatively innocent. There is a great temptation to probe the wound to ascertain its depth. This is a deadly error because the probe may convert a wound of the abdominal wall into a wound perforating a viscus. The proper handling of such a wound is to carefully examine the wound and the abdomen. Reconstruct the direction of the blow and consider the weapon used. Carefully check the abdomen for signs of peritoneal irritation. If there is any suggestion that the instrument entered the peritoneal cavity the abdomen must be explored. The exploration should not be through the stab wound but through a separate incision.

Thoraco-abdominal Injuries

Any wound of the thorax which might have traversed the left leaf of the diaphragm, or the right leaf and liver, must be explored. This includes injuries where diaphragmatic injury may be postulated from the direction of access of the injuring agent or in chest injuries where there is clinical evidence of peritoneal irritation. You must appreciate that an abdominal viscus which ruptures into the chest will demonstrate its findings in the chest.

Postoperative Hemorrhage

It is routine in the postoperative care of all patients to be alert to the possibility of hemorrhage. The situation may not be evident on inspection if the bleeding is intra-abdominal, and particularly so after an operation in which no drain was inserted. But routine check of the vital signs—pulse, respiration, and blood pressure—will call the facts of bleeding to your attention. Whenever such a possibility arises the operating surgeon should be notified immediately. A single unit of blood may be enough to avoid reoperation. If one transfusion does not correct the problem or if it should recur, reoperation becomes necessary.

If there is a drain in the wound or if the bleeding is superficial it will be detected on inspection. The area of the operation should be routinely inspected; this need not include uncovering the incision but does necessitate careful examination of the dressing. If the condition of the dressing suggests considerable blood loss the wound should be uncovered and examined. If excessive blood is coming through the drain the surgeon should be notified. In all instances of bleeding from a wound it is a good idea to have the nurse set aside the bloody dressing for later examination by the surgeon so that the extent of blood loss may be gauged.

A surprising number of patients who bleed postoperatively are losing blood from a small vessel in the skin. Often the vessel is in the stab incision made for placement of the drain. If examination reveals that the point of bleeding or oozing is in the skin, the simplest method of control is to inject one-half per cent procaine solution into the area with a syringe and a hypodermic needle. The fluid distends the tissues and compresses the blood vessels, effecting hemostasis.

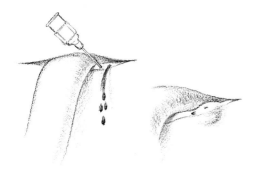

INFECTION

Superficial infections in the abdominal wall are handled in the same manner as in any other part of the body. Intra-abdominal infections require drainage after they have become localized. Intra-abdominal procedures are beyond the scope of the book.

DIAGNOSTIC PROCEDURES

Diagnostic procedures are now often performed through the abdominal wall. The main advantage is that the procedure often obviates the necessity of laparotomy.

Liver Biopsy

The liver is probably the organ for which needle biopsy has found widest application. In addition to simplifying the diagnosis of primary or secondary malignancy of the liver, needle biopsy makes it possible to learn the cause of hepatomegaly, differentiate the various causes of jaundice, and follow the progression of hepatic disease and its response to treatment.

The contraindications are an uncooperative patient, prothrombin activity below 50 per cent of normal, obstructive jaundice, suspected blood vessel tumors of the liver, and infection in the right hemithorax.

Technique

Place the patient in the prone position. Prepare the skin of the right hemithorax with alcohol and tincture of Zephiran. Infiltrate a point overlying the ninth intercostal space in the posterior axillary line with 1 per cent procaine solution. Make a small incision in the skin with a bayonet tip scalpel blade. Insert the forked needle in the carrier needle in such a way that the inner needle does not extend beyond the end of the outer. Insert these through the chest wall but not through the diaphragm.

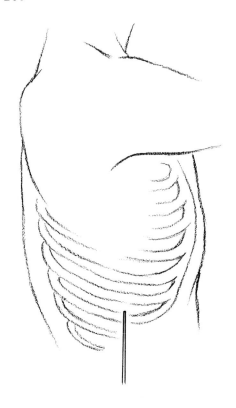

Ask the patient to take three deep breaths, exhale, and then hold his breath. While he is holding his breath, advance the needle about 5 cm. Push the forked needle beyond the carrier.

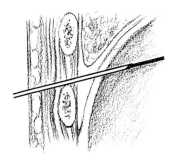

Advance the carrier over the forked needle, rotate both 180 degrees and withdraw them; the specimen will be in the groove of the forked needle. The patient may then resume breathing. The patient should be checked periodically for the next several hours to rule out the possibility of hemorrhage or bile peritonitis.

SPLENIC PUNCTURE

Percutaneous puncture of the spleen is of value in diagnosing various types of hematologic disorders and in delineating the cause of portal hypertension.

Technique

The patient is placed in a comfortable position on an x-ray table either prone or supine, depending upon the size of the spleen. He is positioned so that x-rays can be taken later as indicated. The skin over his lower left thoracic cage is prepared with alcohol and tincture of Zephiran. The point of puncture is infiltrated with 1 per cent procaine. A bayonet tip scalpel blade is used to penetrate the skin and subcutaneous tissues. The needle with stylet in place is pushed through the chest wall. Before pushing the needle into the diaphragm, ask the patient to hold his breath, then rapidly advance the needle to a point which you visualize as being within the spleen. Remove the stylet; if the needle is properly placed, there should be a slow drip of blood from the end of the needle. If there is no drip of blood, reposition the needle. Collect 2 ml. of blood and send it to the laboratory for examination. Insert the stylet, release the needle and ask the patient to breathe slowly and shallowly. Whenever you plan to touch the needle, have the patient stop breathing and not resume until you are no longer manipulating the needle.

The intrasplenic pressure is measured by attaching a venous pressure manometer to the needle. Have the patient stop breathing. Attach the manometer, filled with sterile saline solution, and take a reading after the level ceases to fall. Remove the manometer and replace the stylet. A still more accurate method is to attach a strain gauge to the needle and measure the pressure on a recording apparatus. It is important that the patient hold his breath while you are touching the needle.

The needle can also be used to do a splenoportogram. Ask the patient to hold his breath; attach a syringe containing 30 ml. of Renografin, and rapidly inject this, taking an x-ray at the same time.

After the study is completed have the patient again hold his breath, rapidly remove the needle and apply a small dressing.

Complications

The most serious complication is bleeding. This is most likely to occur when the needle is handled while the patient is breathing; it is imperative that the patient stop breathing before you touch the needle and not breathe again until you are no longer touching it. After this procedure, the patient must be checked periodically for several hours. If there is any evidence of bleeding, laparotomy and splenectomy are indicated.

PARACENTESIS

When there is a collection of fluid in the abdomen, paracentesis is indicated both in order to establish the diagnosis and to relieve the associated discomfort. The equipment necessary includes the usual material for preparation of the patient, i.e., antiseptic solution, sponges, and towels for draping. For local infiltration the following are required: a syringe, a short 26-gauge needle and a larger 23-gauge 1½-inch needle for the injection of the anesthetic solution as well as a container to hold it. Specific instruments include a scalpel with a bayonet tip blade, a trocar, test tubes for collecting fluid for culture, 2 hemostats, 1 tissue forceps, suture material and a container for the aspirated fluid.

Technique

Have the patient void immediately before the procedure in order to lower the bladder below the intended point of puncture. Seat the patient on the side of the bed or in a chair in as comfortable a position as possible.

Expose the abdomen and prepare the skin with alcohol and tincture of Zephiran; drape with a sterile towel. The trocar may be inserted in either iliac fossa or in the midline 2 or 3 inches below the umbilicus. Infiltrate the area of choice with 1 per cent procaine solution; make a 2 cm. vertical incision in the skin and carry this down through the fascia. Before inserting the trocar ascertain that the plunger moves freely and that the various ostia are patent. Insert the trocar into the incision and with continuous pressure and a boring motion, push it into the peritoneal cavity. As soon as you know that it is in the cavity by the fact that resistance decreases, remove the stylet to allow the fluid to flow.

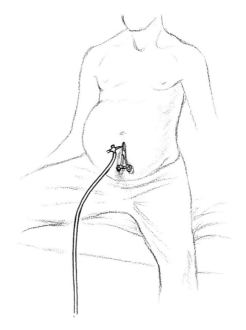

Fill both test tubes with fluid, tape one to the patient's bed and send the other to the laboratory for microscopic study, culture, smear, and protein measurement. Drain off as much fluid as possible. Drainage can be encouraged by repositioning the patient as the flow slows down so as to keep the needle in a dependent position. Drainage is also assisted by wrapping a sheet about the patient's abdomen and gradually tightening this to compress the intra-abdominal contents. After all fluid has been removed, withdraw the trocar, establish hemostasis and close the wound with a few interrupted sutures.

Complications

1. **Perforation of bladder.** Insertion of the trocar into the bladder may occur if the bladder is distended. The complication is prevented by having the patient empty his bladder prior to paracentesis. If the bladder is perforated, an immediate operation must be undertaken to close the opening.

2. **Perforation of intestine.** Insertion of the trocar into a loop of the intestine is more likely to occur if the paracentesis is done on a patient who has distended loops of intestine, or in a patient who has adhesions due to multiple previous paracenteses or previous abdominal operations. This procedure should not be attempted in the presence of marked distention of the bowel and special care must be taken when tapping an abdomen which may have adhesions. If the intestine is perforated, the patient must have an immediate laparotomy and repair of the perforation.

3. **Dizziness or shock.** The patient may become dizzy or actually go into shock during paracentesis. This is due to the fact that removal of a large amount of fluid takes some of the pressure off the circulatory system, allowing the vessels to distend rapidly. Insufficient blood volume within the circulation to compensate for the loss of fluid can result in shock. The patient should be treated as one would treat any patient in shock (p. 101). The complication is less likely if the fluid is withdrawn more slowly. But since it occurs only rarely and is easily treated, the fluid can be allowed to run out as fast as it will, provided you have the means available to treat shock.

4. **Leakage from the wound.** Occasionally there may be leakage of ascitic fluid from the wound for several weeks. This rarely results in any serious complication and requires no treatment other than changing the dressings as needed.

DRAINAGE THROUGH ABDOMINAL WALL

Simple Drainage

Either the subcutaneous space or the peritoneal cavity may be drained if there is a localized infection or if one anticipates that there will be an excessive accumulation of fluid in a wound. If one encounters purulent material deep in the belly, even though the peritoneal space may be closed, it is wise to drain the subcutaneous tissues or leave the wound open (p. 99)

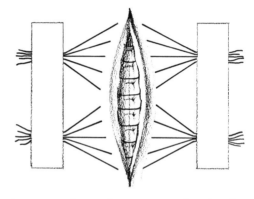

because the subcutaneous fat is the tissue most susceptible to injury. The drain most commonly used is a thin-walled rubber drain, obtainable in three different widths. All have gauze wicks which many surgeons remove. Some feel that the purpose of the wick is to increase drainage. This is not so. The wick is used to give added strength to the tube. If a long drain is used, the wick insures against tearing the drain and leaving part of it deep in the wound. The drain is best inserted through a separate stab wound rather than the laparotomy wound. The end of the drain should be sutured to the skin, leaving the end of this suture long to simplify its identification. The length of time the drain is left in place depends upon the individual problem and the practices of the surgeon in charge. It is best not to disturb the drain without first checking with the surgeon. If the drain is long it should not be removed all at one time, but should be shortened twice. Remove the skin suture holding the drain. Gently tug on the drain until you have removed one-third of its length. To be certain that the remaining portion of the drain does not slip into the wound, insert a large sterile safety pin into the end. Grasp the pin with a hemostat and the drain with a dressing forceps or another hemostat. Insert the pin into the drain distal to where you are holding it with forceps.

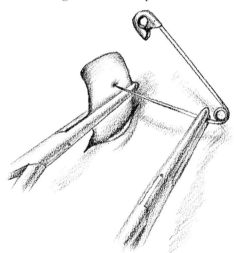

If you insert the pin in the drain between the forceps and the skin you may pull the drain out of the wound.

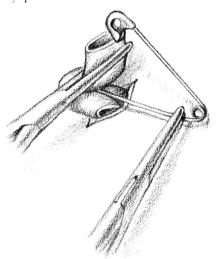

Always mention in the operative note that a drain has been inserted. When the drain is shortened or removed, this must be noted in the progress notes. Detailed notes relevant to removal of the drain may protect the patient and later prevent medicolegal problems.

CHOLECYSTOSTOMY

In elderly patients who are quite ill or in younger patients in whom marked inflammation obscures the structures, acute cholecystitis is sometimes treated by simple drainage of the gall bladder (cholecystostomy). A hollow rubber tube is sewn into the gall bladder and brought out through the abdominal wall. The tube is attached to a routine postoperative drainage bottle. After the inflammation subsides, the drainage should diminish, allowing one to clamp the tube. If the patient tolerates clamping of the tube, it can probably be removed with safety. In most cases, however, cholecystostomy should be followed by cholecystectomy at an elective time. It is best to keep the cholecystostomy tube in place until the time of removal of the gall bladder.

"T" TUBE DRAINAGE OF COMMON DUCT

Most surgeons drain the common duct after choledochostomy. While any hollow tube would be effective, the most commonly used tube is a "T" tube, a specially made, soft rubber, thin-walled, hollow tube in the shape of a "T." Each limb of the "T" is inserted into one end of the common duct and the long limb is brought to the exterior through the opening in the common duct, preferably through a stab wound in the skin separate from the abdominal wound and the drain. Since the drainage comes through it and not around it, the tube should be attached to a drainage bottle. The "T" tube should not be removed until there is evidence that the bile is flowing satisfactorily through the common duct and that the patient can get along without the "T" tube. Removal is accomplished as follows: The limb of the drainage tube is raised approximately 10 cm. above the level of the common duct. With the tube in this position, the bile is encouraged to go through the ampulla, where there should be less resistance, rather than through the tube. In this procedure a vent must be established in the drainage tube, otherwise the descending limb of the tube will create suction by siphonage. This is best provided by attaching a glass "Y" connector to an IV pole at the high point in the loop.

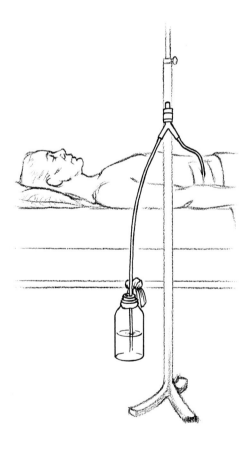

When bile is flowing through an open ampulla, less than 20 ml. of bile will collect in the drainage bottle. If there is this evidence of ampullar drainage, the patency of the duct and the absence of stones should be checked by a "T" tube cholangiogram. If this is negative the "T" tube should be clamped and the attending nurse instructed to unclamp it if the patient should have pain in the upper abdomen. If the patient tolerates the tube's being clamped for 24 hours without discomfort it can be removed. Remove the skin suture holding the tube in place and exert gentle traction on the tube. Make no effort to close the opening in the skin. Apply a dry dressing; the wound will seal itself.

If the ampulla remains blocked and prolonged "T" tube drainage (for more than a week) is required, correction must be made for the large amount of bile being lost through the "T" tube. The simplest solution is to return the drained bile to the patient's gastrointestinal tract. Since bile is not palatable, it is best returned through a nasogastric tube. Sometimes the taste can be sufficiently altered by the addition of orange or pineapple juice to allow oral ingestion. An occasional hardy soul will prefer to drink the plain bile.

PANCREATIC DRAINAGE

Occasionally drainage from an abdominal wound contains pancreatic secretions as a result of damage or operations involving the pancreas. This is quite irritating to the skin. The surface of the skin becomes macerated, markedly erythematous, and exquisitely tender unless it is protected from the secretions. This can be done by applying a protective covering to the skin and by removing the secretions before they reach the skin. The skin is coated with a protective coating of an ointment or a paste which is not affected by the pancreatic secretions. Aluminum paste or one of the commercial protective ointments, such as Protogel, is effective. The ointment should be applied liberally daily and the dressings changed frequently to prevent maceration of the skin from wet dressings. The drainage can be picked up before it reaches the skin by inserting a sump drain into the wound. If none is handy, the insertion of a catheter, so placed that its outermost hole is at the skin edge, will work very well. If this is kept at this level the tube cannot clog by sucking the wall against the opening, and it can remove any secretions which reach the surface.

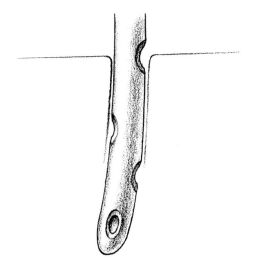

ILEOSTOMY

An ileostomy is a type of enterostomy difficult to care for because of the changes it produces in fluid and electrolyte balance and because of the effect of the drainage on the skin. Consequently, this procedure is limited to cases in which it is the only solution. To prevent the development of these complications, therapy must be instituted as soon as the operation is completed. The properly executed ileostomy should extend at least an inch beyond the skin. The skin should be protected immediately. A permanent bag is not fitted until the ileostomy stump has contracted to its permanent size. A temporary bag which has an adhesive plaster top which can be cut to fit the individual ileostomy is attached to the skin. Such a bag should be attached at the end of the operation.

These are replaced when they loosen, which is usually in three to five days. Some surgeons feel that the permanent bag can be fitted at the end of a week, while others feel a month should elapse for adequate shrinkage of the ileostomy. The permanent ileostomy bag consists of a rubber covered brass facing with an opening made to fit the individual ileostomy and a rubber bag to hold the drainage.

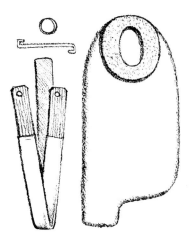

The facing is cemented to the skin and the bag is emptied through an opening in the lower end.

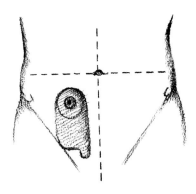

The patient re-cements the bag to the skin every three to seven days as necessary.

When the ileostomy first begins to function, there is an excessive loss of fluids and electrolytes. The function of the terminal portion of the ileum adjusts to correct this problem but the patient's fluid and electrolyte balance must be watched carefully until this readjustment has occurred. As soon as the ileostomy begins to function, one must increase the intake of fluid and electrolytes. The patient should receive a liter of normal saline containing 2 gm. potassium chloride for every liter of ileostomy drainage in addition to the normal daily fluid and electrolyte requirements. The electrolytes of the blood should be measured at least twice a week and treatment adjusted accordingly. After 48 hours the patient can be fed orally. Diet must be supplemented with oral potassium chloride. Supplementary intravenous therapy must be continued for approximately a week. The oral supplement can be gradually decreased, but the patient must not be discharged until blood electrolyte measurements have been normal for one week.

CECOSTOMY

This is usually performed as a temporary procedure either to relieve an obstruction farther along in the intestinal tract, or to protect a distal colon anastomosis. A tube is inserted into the cecum and brought to the exterior. This is attached to a drainage bottle and nothing further need be done. After a week to ten days some drainage will begin to appear around the tube. The surgeon must resist the great temptation to explore because of his concern that a peritonitis might be developing. Actually, drainage is coming out along the foreign body tract and will cause no peritonitis unless unwise exploration exposes the peritoneal cavity. Skillful neglect is the proper course here.

After the distal obstruction has been removed, there will be very little drainage from the cecostomy. The tube is left in place until the patient is having normal bowel movements. In most instances one merely has to withdraw the tube and cover the wound with a dry dressing. The wound will usually close without further treatment.

COLOSTOMY

Colostomy is commonly used as a temporary measure in the transverse colon for obstruction in the left colon and as a permanent procedure in the left colon after resection of the rectum.

When done for an obstruction in the left colon, the intact transverse colon may be brought out in a loop over a glass bar. If the patient's condition permits it is better to allow the skin wound to seal before opening the colon. This can be done anytime after six hours beyond the operation. If it is considered unwise to wait this long, a catheter may be inserted into the colon via a purse-string incision after the skin wound has been closed. The wound should be protected from the secretions by a covering of petrolatum gauze. The colon has few sensory fibers. If the colostomy is opened subsequent to the primary operation, it can be done in the patient's room without anesthesia. Cautery is most commonly used but a scalpel or scissors is satisfactory. For the first five days, care of the colostomy should consist of changing the dressing about the colostomy as it becomes soiled. One should then begin to train the patient to irrigate the colostomy. If they learn to care properly for their colostomy, the only dressing most patients need is a square of gauze over the opening. The time for them to learn is before they leave the hospital. Initially they can use an enema can attached to a 24 or 26 F. catheter and allow the drainage to run into a pan held against the abdomen. There are colostomy irrigation sets available which allow one to fasten a cup over the colostomy. This cup has a small orifice where the catheter is inserted and a drain which carries the fluid coming out of the colostomy between the patient's legs into the toilet.

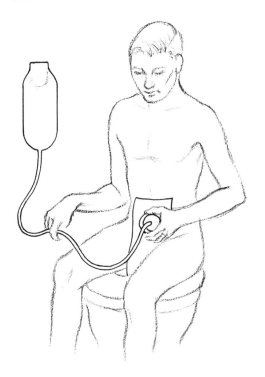

The enema can is filled with a quart of warm tap water which is then placed 18 to 24 inches above the level of the colostomy. A clamp on the tube prevents the water from running out. When the colostomy is irrigated the patient is on the toilet.

The tip of the catheter is lubricated with surgical jelly or petrolatum. The clamp is loosened and, after all air has been expelled from the catheter, with the fluid still running the catheter is inserted 2 or 3 inches into the colon and moved back and forth to clean the terminal portion. It is then advanced another few inches and the remainder of the fluid is run in. The catheter is removed and the fluid is allowed to drain. At least a half hour should be allowed for the drainage. Drainage can be helped by massaging the abdomen. Each patient will learn from experience ways of improving the results. The procedure should be done at approximately the same time daily at an hour when the patient will not be rushed. Some patients learn to do this so well that an irrigation is needed only every 2 or 3 days. In the interim they need only cover the colostomy opening with a gauze square.

The diet of the patient can affect the function of the colostomy. Either diarrhea or constipation may occur. The former is the more bothersome. Foods which bothered the patient prior to colostomy are most likely to continue to bother him and should be avoided. Again experience will tell the patients which foods cause trouble. The American Cancer Society publishes a very good pamphlet for the colostomy patient entitled *Care of Your Colostomy.*

Chapter Eighteen

The Anorectal Region

EXAMINATION

DIGITAL

A routine physical examination should include a digital examination of the rectum. If a patient has complaints which suggest disease of the rectum an endoscopic examination should be performed.

There are special tables available for proctoscopic examinations which are hinged in the middle and allow one to drop the head of the table.

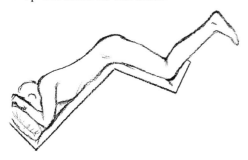

A satisfactory examination may be done with the patient on his side in the Sims position

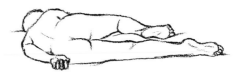

or in the knee-chest position.

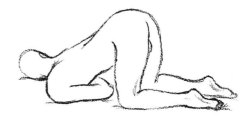

To inspect the exterior surface place a hand on each of the patient's buttocks near the anus and gently separate them. To examine the rectum digitally, use either a rubber glove or a finger cot. Lubricate the index finger. Place the finger tip against the anal orifice and after a slight hesitation apply gentle pressure: anal spasm may occur if the finger is forced abruptly into the canal. As you insert the finger, carefully palpate the anal canal, paying particular attention to the posterior wall. This may prove painful to the patient. Anal fissures which occur here are particularly painful. If the pain interferes with examination an anesthetic ointment may be helpful, but occasionally caudal or spinal anesthesia is needed.

When the finger is in the rectum apply counterpressure from the exterior with the thumb of the same hand in order to examine the sphincters. This maneuver is helpful in following the cord-like tract of a fistula. Finally, pass the finger to its full length into the rectum and palpate the entire interior of the wall. You can palpate any abnormal masses and note any change in the size and contour of the prostate. Put your finger as high as possible and ask the patient to strain. You can then palpate lesions which are otherwise beyond reach. When the digital examination is complete, withdraw the finger slowly.

Anoscopic Examination

The anoscope is a short hollow tube with an obturator. With the obturator in place, lubricate the instrument with lubricating gel and gently pass it into the anal canal with the tip aimed at the umbilicus. After its full length has been inserted remove the obturator. Have the patient bear down; this will cause any internal hemorrhoids to come into view. Next slowly withdraw the instrument, carefully examining the wall of the canal as you go. Pay particular attention to papillae, crypts, fissures, and hemorrhoids. Many different types of pathology may be seen in this limited area.

Sigmoidoscopic Examination

Longer instruments permit examination of the rectum (proctoscopy) and the sigmoid (sigmoidoscopy). These are passed through the anal canal with the obturator in place. Place lubricant on the tip of the instrument and spread it over the distal half. Gently and slowly

pass the scope into the rectum, aiming at the umbilicus. After the tip of the instrument is through the anal canal and into the rectum remove the obturator. Attach the glass shield with attached insufflator bulb and turn on the light. You can pass the scope from this point under direct vision. Fluid may collect at the end of the scope; it can be removed with a long aspirator or with cotton balls on long applicators. For the intermediate portion of its passage, the scope is usually pointed toward the hollow of the sacrum. If folds of bowel get in the way, insufflate some air to move these away from the advancing scope. The most difficult angle to pass is usually at the rectosigmoid junction, 16 cm. from the dentate line. The sigmoid can be recognized by its multiple tranverse mucosal folds as compared to the smooth surface of the rectum. When the scope is completely inserted its angle of direction is intermediate between the previous two. In the accompanying figure the successive positions of the scope are expressed by increasing shading.

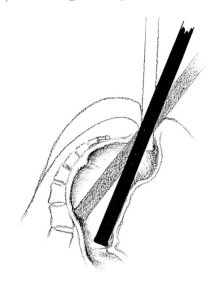

Examination is performed during withdrawal and not during insertion of the instrument. Examine the interior of the bowel carefully. Note the character of the mucosa, any abnormal bleeding, and any masses (polyps or carcinoma) as the instrument is withdrawn. Before removing the instrument from the rectum, be certain to examine the blind area just above the anorectal ring posteriorly. Finally, remove the glass shield to release some of the insufflated gas before withdrawing the scope.

INJURY

INSTRUMENTAL INJURY

The anal canal or rectum may be injured by a thermometer, by the tip of an enema nozzle, or by a proctoscope. The commonest injuries are simple abrasions or lacerations. If the entire thickness of the bowel wall is not transversed, these lesions rarely require much treatment. Occasionally a troublesome bleeding vessel may have to be clamped and ligated. If the rectum is perforated below the peritoneal reflection, the patient should be given streptomycin (0.5 gm. b.i.d.) and penicillin (600,000 u.b.i.d.). If an abscess develops it must be drained. If the perforation is above the peritoneal reflection, a proximal colostomy must be established.

PERFORATIONS

If the patient sustains an impalement type of injury, the rectum is usually perforated into the peritoneal cavity. This requires laparotomy and colostomy.

During World War II there was a rash of injuries caused by pranksters directing the flow of a high pressure air hose at the perineum of co-workers in industrial plants. These usually caused multiple bowel perforations. For this sort of injury laparotomy, repair of the perforations, and proximal colostomy must be performed.

FOREIGN BODIES

Foreign bodies as large as bottles and drinking glasses have been removed from the rectum. These are usually found after the patient has been on an alcoholic binge. The foreign body is readily palpable on digital examination.

Removal requires spinal or caudal anesthesia; sometimes obstetrical forceps are needed, and occasionally a laparotomy is required.

Small foreign bodies ingested orally may perforate the rectal mucosa, causing inflammation and abscess formation in the perirectal area. Such problems require hospitalization and drainage of the abscess, preferably under spinal or caudal anesthesia.

POSTOPERATIVE HEMORRHAGE

Patients may bleed immediately after anorectal operations or several days later. If the immediate bleeding is external it is obvious from staining of the first dressings. Pressure over the area is often adequate to control bleeding, but if this is not sufficient a catgut ligature will usually solve the problem.

Internal bleeding may not be detected until the patient has a copious, bloody bowel movement. If more than 500 ml., the blood loss must be replaced and the patient returned to the operating room where the bleeding vessel can be identified and ligated.

INFLAMMATORY LESIONS

ANAL CRYPTITIS AND PAPILLITIS

Anal crypts, because of their contour, are the site of lodgment of food particles which initiate an inflammatory process. Inflammation of the crypt rapidly spreads to the papilla. Chronic inflammation of the papilla causes it to hypertrophy. Anal papillae are symptomatic only during an acute phase of infection or after they have enlarged sufficiently to be grasped by the anal sphincter. They may become as large as several centimeters in diameter. Those with large bulbous ends are sometimes misdiagnosed as rectal polyps.

An infected crypt should be opened. To do this insert a hooked probe into the crypt, lift it to outline the crypt and excise the roof.

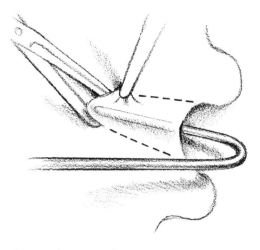

Leave the wound open.

The papilla can be excised under local anesthesia. Insert the anoscope and the polyp will fall into view when the obturator is removed. After cleansing the base with a swab and an antiseptic solution, infiltrate the area with 1 percent procaine solution. Grasp the base of the papilla with a forceps, lift it, and cut it off at its base with a scissors.

Compress the area for a few moments. Ligate any remaining bleeders with 3-0 catgut and leave the wound open.

ANAL FISSURE

An anal fissure, commonly thought of as a crack in the anal skin, is really an anal ulcer. The condition causes pain during and after defecation. The pain is out of proportion to the appearance of the lesion. There may be a small amount of bleeding on the surface of the stool. Examination reveals an irregularly oval shaped ulcer with its long diameter parallel with the direction of the anal canal. There is undermining of the ulcer and there is bulbous swelling distal to the ulcer called the sentinel pile. The tenderness varies from exquisite in acute lesions to very little in the chronic. If the lesion is palpable one can feel varying degrees of fibrosis.

Treatment is surgical excision. Expose the fissure. Excise an ellipse of mucosa.

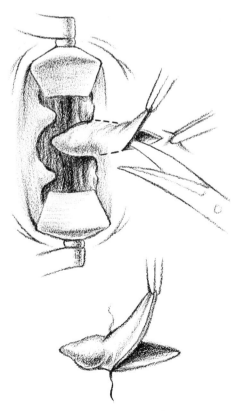

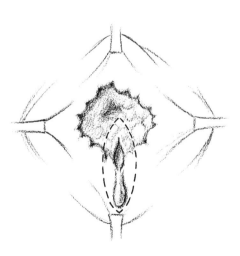

Carry the incision down to the muscle and leave the wound wide open to granulate.

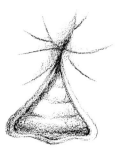

SPECIFIC LESIONS

HEMORRHOIDS

These are really varicosities of the hemorrhoidal veins. Anatomically they are divided into external (originating below the pectinate line) and internal (originating above the pectinate line).

External Hemorrhoids

Uncomplicated external hemorrhoids rarely cause symptoms other than itching. However, when they become thrombosed they are quite painful. A sharp constant pain of increasing severity develops in the anal area. Examination reveals a globular, bluish, firm, exquisitely tender mass projecting above the skin at the anus. Nonoperative treatment consists of codeine and aspirin for pain, rest in bed, hot or cold compresses to the anus, mineral oil orally, Sitz baths, and anesthetic ointment locally.

Much more dramatic benefits may be achieved by evacuating the clot. After properly preparing the area infiltrate the skin over the lesion with a small amount of procaine solution. Incise the mass or excise an ellipse of skin

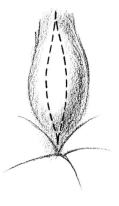

and evacuate the clot.

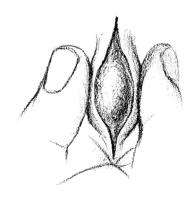

Bleeding is rarely a problem and, if present, will cease after light pressure for about 10 minutes. Sitz baths and local compresses plus codeine and aspirin provide relief until the lesion heals (a few days).

Internal Hemorrhoids

The treatment of internal hemorrhoids depends upon the particular problems presented. Asymptomatic internal hemorrhoids seen on a routine anoscopic examination require no treatment. Symptomatic internal hemorrhoids in patients who have other problems contraindicating operation can be treated by nonsurgical means.

If the hemorrhoidal mass is protruding it should be reduced by exerting mild pressure with gloved fingers, to prevent strangulation by pressure of the sphincters. If strangulation has occurred the area will be markedly tender and the protruding mass quite edematous. This patient must have a narcotic before the area can be manipulated. Hold the hemorrhoid between your fingers and compress it with gradually increasing pressure. Pressure should be continued until sphincters relax, allowing you to push the mass up into the rectum. The tendency to protrude should be controlled by doubling up several gauze dressings, packing them against the anus, and holding them in place by taping the buttocks together. If the reduction is too painful to the patient the sphincters can be first injected with procaine solution. The patient should be put to bed in a prone position with a pillow under his hips and the foot of the bed elevated. Continuous warm saline compresses will provide considerable comfort if this area is inflamed. The bowel function should be adjusted with mineral oil or a bulk laxative. The mineral oil should be given in the morning; mineral oil at bedtime predisposes to lipoid pneumonia. The patient should be placed on a low residue diet with no seasoned food or alcohol. Local applications of an astringent analgesic ointment are helpful. With this regimen the condition in the nonstrangulated case will subside in a few days, but the advanced strangulated case may require several weeks of treatment. In such cases, considerable time can be saved by excising the hemorrhoids early.

INJECTION TREATMENT. In some cases internal hemorrhoids respond to treatment by injection. A sclerosing solution is instilled into the submucosal layer of the rectum; this diffuses about the hemorrhoidal veins, producing an inflammatory reaction which shrinks the vessels.

This treatment is the treatment of choice for bleeding hemorrhoids which do not protrude down beyond the pectinate line. It can be used in bleeding hemorrhoids which prolapse in patients who have problems which make operations hazardous, as well as in the patient who wants to postpone surgical excision. It must be remembered that this treatment in such cases will give only temporary relief.

Injection treatment should not be used in (1) external hemorrhoids, (2) severe prolapsing internal hemorrhoids, and (3) cases with associated inflammatory disease of the anal canal.

The necessary equipment includes a small Luer-Lok syringe with finger rings, a long 25-gauge needle, and an anoscope. The sclerosing solution may be quinine and urea hydrochloride in 5 per cent aqueous solution or a 5 per cent solution of phenol in clear vegetable oil.

The patient is placed in position for endoscopic examination and the anoscope passed to its full length. Only one hemorrhoid should be injected at a time. Begin by injecting the largest. Gradually withdraw the anoscope until the most proximal portion of the hemorrhoid comes into view. Make the injection into the pedicle rather than into the bulbous portion of the hemorrhoid. Clean the site of injection with a swab and apply antiseptic solution. Insert the needle through the mucosa; advance it in the loose areolar tissue of the submucosal layer and inject the solution.

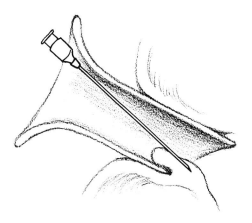

If the area at the end of the needle blanches immediately, you are injecting intramucosally and the needle should be repositioned. The injection will cause some ballooning of the tissues. Continue until the mucosa overlying the infiltrated area begins to blanch; the amount of fluid required varies from 1 to 3 ml., depending upon the local situation. After completing the injection, withdraw the needle and the anoscope. Any bleeding can be controlled by pressure over the area with cotton swabs. No special aftercare is necessary other than proper control of bowel movements with mineral oil. Injections are done every 1 to 2 weeks. A hemorrhoid should not be reinjected until all inflammation has subsided.

COMPLICATIONS. *Pain.* Injecting hemorrhoids should be a relatively painless procedure because of the nature of the nerve supply of the rectum. The patient should experience, at most, a feeling of fullness which disappears as the fluid diffuses. If real pain develops, the injection was made too close to the pectinate line, allowing the fluid to diffuse below the line where there is a sensory innervation. This is avoided by injecting sufficiently far above the pectinate line.

Slough. A slough at the site of injection may be due to (1) use of too much solution, (2) injection into the mucosa, or (3) injection into an inflamed area. If a slough occurs, the patient should be seen twice a week and the surface cleansed. Constipation must be prevented by bulk laxatives.

SURGICAL EXCISION. Surgical excision is the treatment of choice in (1) prolapsing internal hemorrhoids, (2) internal hemorrhoids with accompanying external hemorrhoids, or (3) strangulated internal hemorrhoids. Some recommend nonsurgical treatment as already detailed for strangulated internal hemorrhoids, but the period of disability can be considerably shortened by early surgical excision. This operation must be done in a hospital under anesthesia.

PROLAPSE OF RECTUM

Prolapse of the rectum may be incomplete (only mucosa protruding) or complete (all layers of the bowel protruding). In incomplete prolapse the protrusion is usually 2 to 3 cm. and rarely more than 5 cm. This is the more common of the two types and occurs most often in infancy and childhood

and in old age. With a finger inserted into the lumen, allowing counterpressure against the thumb, one can determine the number of layers by palpation.

The prolapse must be reduced to prevent strangulation. Place the patient in a knee-chest position. Place gauze over the mass and grasp it in your hand at the apex. Continue to exert pressure to reduce first the edema and then the prolapse. Prevent recurrence by placing cotton or gauze against the anus and taping the buttocks together. Later recurrences can be prevented by a long painstaking routine. The patient should defecate while in a recumbent position. Manual pressure on either side of the anus during defecation helps prevent recurrence. Proper control of the bowels and good general care to build up the nutrition of the patient is helpful. Any proctitis should be treated. If this routine is unsuccessful, injection of sclerosing solution, as was done for internal hemorrhoids, should be attempted to fix the rectum by fibrosis of the submucosal layer. One milliliter of solution is injected in each of four quadrants. This should be repeated in a week to 10 days if necessary. The nonsurgical routine outlined above should be continued until fixation occurs. If the measures are inadequate, the patient should be hospitalized for more radical treatment.

FECAL IMPACTION

Fecal impaction may occur as a result of reduced motility of the bowel or from any type of obstruction. It occurs in many seriously ill patients bedridden in the hospital. The initial symptom is constipation, frequently followed by diarrhea. The patient has a persistent desire to defecate and his efforts produce only small, diarrheal stools. The diagnosis is readily made on digital examination. Occasionally, the problem can be solved with a few good saline enemas. If the mass is hard and inspissated, insert 6 to 8 oz. of mineral oil and attempt to break up the mass digitally. Follow this in 2 hours with a vigorous saline enema. The efficacy of each treatment should be checked by a digital examination. The treatment should be repeated after a few hours if the impaction is not removed. Occasionally, the impaction may be so resistant that it must be broken up and removed digitally. This can be done in the patient's room, without anesthesia. Afterward the cause should be determined and the patient placed on a preventive routine.

Chapter Nineteen

The Lower Extremity

TRAUMA

THIGH

The commonest traumatic lesion of the upper leg is contusion of the thigh resulting from blunt trauma. It usually produces a hematoma which, if it continues to enlarge, should be controlled by applying pressure to the area. After a day or two, warm applications sometimes hasten its dissolution. If need be the hematoma can be aspirated; otherwise it will gradually spread and ultimately be absorbed. Occasionally, the hematoma will become infected and require external drainage.

Lacerations of the thigh are treated as one would treat lacerations of any other part of the body. Avulsions of the skin are treated as discussed on page 271.

KNEE

The knee is subjected to severe trauma more often than any other point. Fortunately it has a strong capsule and additional valuable support from the attached muscles. One should have a thorough knowledge of the anatomy of the joint and the motions possible in the joints. The main motions are flexion and extension, with some slight rotation in semiflexion.

When examining the joint, first ask the patient to walk. If the knee is injured the ability to walk is impaired. With the knee in extension any abnormal swelling or dislocation is evident. Determine whether there is any limitation of extension or flexion. Check for any lateral motion. Palpate the joint for areas of tenderness. Most injuries to the knee joint cause pain and swelling of the area and effusion or hemorrhage into the joint. Motion, particularly of a type which puts tension on the injured structures, is painful.

Treatment consists of placing the joint at rest and removing excessive effusions. Apply a posterior splint from the upper thigh to the ankle and wrap the entire extremity snugly. If there is any reason to suspect a fracture, an x-ray of the joint should be made. Occasionally the joint may lock in partial flexion. If this occurs put the patient at rest in bed; when the associated spasm disappears the joint will extend. Have the patient keep the leg elevated for 24 to 48 hours. The pain can usually be relieved by salicylates or codeine.

Effusions may occur in the knee joint or in the patellar bursa. The exact sites can be identified by the nature of the swelling. The main portion of the patellar bursa is between the lower portion of the patella and the skin. The distended bursa is evident as a fluctuant mass in front of the patella. Fluid in the joint is behind the patella and bulges out above and about the sides of the patella. When the knee is extended a large effusion will lift the patella away from the femoral condyles. Small effusions are treated by a pressure dressing. Large effusions must be evacuated to relieve the pain of the distended capsule and to remove a possible source of irritation to the joint.

ASPIRATION OF THE KNEE JOINT. Have the patient lie comfortably on a table with his knee elevated on a pillow. Prepare the skin with alcohol and tincture of Zephiran. The joint may be aspirated through either of two sites: 1 cm. medial to the lower half of the patella, or the distended suprapatellar portion of the joint capsule lateral to and above the patella. Make a skin wheal with 1 per cent procaine at the site chosen for aspiration. Insert a large bore (16 to 18 gauge) needle attached to a 20 ml. syringe through the wheal and direct it toward the center of the joint. Advance the needle until the tip is in the middle of the joint. Remove as much fluid as possible and withdraw the needle. After removing the needle apply a posterior splint and a pressure bandage about the knee. Foam rubber incorporated into the dressing on each side of the patella improves the pressure dressing. The joint may be reaspirated if the effusion recurs.

The patellar bursa may become distended acutely or as a result of chronic irritation. Acute effusions respond to aspiration of the fluid. This is accomplished by a needle inserted directly into the distended bursa. Chronic effusions will recur. These must be treated by obliteration of the bursa. Aspirate all fluid from the bursa and insert a sclerosing solution (1 ml. 5 per cent sodium morrhuate) and apply a pressure dressing. If there is any further accumulation of fluid the procedure should be repeated in 5 days. Eventually many bursae become markedly thickened and are a constant source of discomfort. When this occurs the bursa should be excised. The incision should be so placed that it will not be on the weight-bearing surface of the knee.

INJURY TO THE FOOT AND ANKLE

Lacerations

These should be treated as lacerations elsewhere. In other words, the wound should be debrided, thoroughly cleaned, and closed without drainage with interrupted sutures. A pressure bandage should be applied and the patient allowed to walk if he can.

Puncture Wounds

The foot is a very common site of puncture wounds, usually caused when the patient steps on a nail or some sharp object. The patient may consult you immediately or may not come in for several days afterwards.

Treatment. If the wound appears to be clean, and there is no evidence of infection, clean the local area and apply a dressing. Anti-tetanus treatment should be given as recommended on page 105. If there is any evidence of infection about the wound, it should be laid open in order to allow it to drain. If it is considered necessary to probe the depths of the wound for a suspected foreign body, this should be done after providing hemostasis with a blood pressure cuff as a tourniquet below the knee.

Foreign Bodies

If the patient has a sliver in his foot, it is usually easy to follow its path and locate the foreign body and remove it. If it is quite superficial, the wound should be left open to granulate.

Sharp pointed objects, such as needles, can move around for a considerable distance in the foot. Consequently, they are best localized by means of an x-ray. To prevent movement of the foreign body after the x-ray is made, do not allow the patient to walk. Remove the needle under local anesthesia, providing hemostasis with a blood pressure cuff at the level of the knee.

Sprains of the Ankle

Any of the ligaments about the ankle joints may be sprained but the most vulnerable are the lateral ligaments. Sudden inversion of the foot causes some tearing of these. The patient limps and has considerable pain. Swelling, ecchymosis, and tenderness of the ankle appear on the side where the ligament is torn. The sprain will show point tenderness and movements of the ankle joint which put strain upon the damaged ligament will cause pain at the site of injury. It is important to determine the extent of the injury. Infiltrate the area of tenderness with 1 per cent procaine solution and measure the extent of motion of ankle joint. If the range of motion of the ankle joint is increased there is a reasonable possibility that a ligament has been severed or ruptured. In such an injury an x-ray should be made to rule out the possibility of fracture.

In simple sprains, the ankle joint can be supported by taping. Sometimes, however, it is only necessary to inject the points of tenderness and allow the patient to use his foot. The injections can be repeated as often as daily to relieve the pain. Obviously, however, this procedure should only be used in those patients in whom there is no severe ligament injury.

There are two popular types of strapping; the most commonly used one is the Gibney boot. Have the patient seated comfortably opposite you and support the heel of his injured foot on your knee. Have him hold his foot in a normal position, using a 3-inch gauze bandage as a halter about the toes to pull the foot back to proper position.

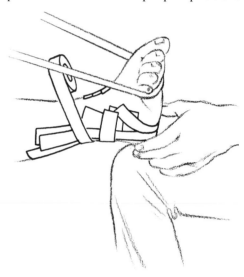

Apply 1-inch adhesive plaster, strapping in alternate longitudinal (vertical) and transverse (horizontal) strips. The longitudinal strips should extend from approximately halfway between the ankle and the knee, down one side of the ankle and foot, beneath the foot, and up the other side of the ankle. The alternate transverse strip should then extend from the lateral side of the foot back around the ankle to the medial side of the foot. These transverse strips should be applied in such a way that they never meet, allowing a clear area of skin in the midline and thus preventing any circular adhesive compression. The bandage should be completed with a single longitudinal strip on the anterior end of the horizontal strips on each side to cover the edges.

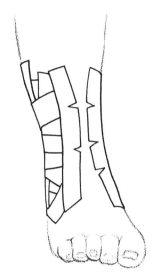

The bandage should not be disturbed until it becomes loose, at which time it should be renewed. Elevation of the foot and application of ice bags for 24 to 48 hours will relieve a good bit of the swelling.

Another method of application is to apply 1-inch strips of adhesive beginning beneath the medial malleolus and running under the foot up the lateral side of the foot and diagonally crossing the lower leg around the shins. Multiple strips of adhesive plaster are applied in this manner and they can be further reinforced with a covering of cotton elastic bandage.

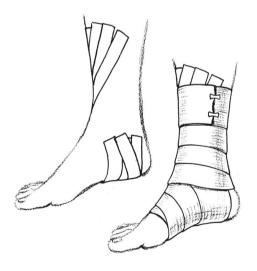

When there is evidence of abnormal mobility of the joint or evidence of a severe fracture, more prolonged immobilization is necessary. Either the patient should be put to bed with the foot elevated for several days until the edema disappears, or lateral splints should be applied until the edema subsides, at which time a walking cast should be applied. Take 3-inch plaster of Paris bandage and form a posterior plaster slab which extends from the level of the knee out to the end of the toes. It is wise to extend it beyond the end of the toes to preclude the danger of bumping the toe. After forming the slab, place a piece of cotton wadding or felt at the upper level of the cast to prevent irritation and wrap the foot and ankle with cotton wadding.

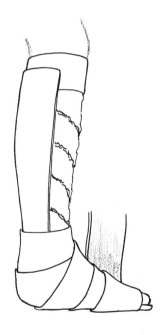

Dip the posterior splint in water, remove the excess water and apply it to the leg. Then hold this in place with multiple circular turns of 3-inch plaster of paris bandage until the cast has been properly applied. The patient should be

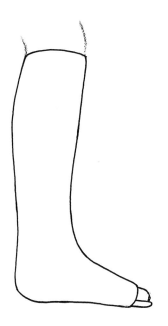

kept off his feet for 24 hours and then a walking iron or a heel is applied to the cast. The patient can then be allowed to

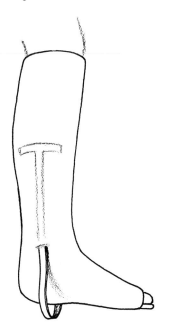

walk and, if the cast remains satisfactory, it can be left on for 6 weeks. If necessary, the cast can be changed, but a total immobilization period of 6 weeks is advisable.

INFECTION

Under normal circulatory conditions, acute bacterial infections of the lower extremity are treated in the same manner as infections elsewhere in the body.

ULCERS

The lower extremity may be the site of chronic ulceration. The two most common causes are anaerobic infections and varicose veins.

Anaerobic Ulcers

These are distinguished by their punched out or undermined margins. Proper treatment requires unroofing plus exposure of the tissues to oxygen, using zinc peroxide dressing as described on page 119.

Varicose Ulcers

The commonest ulcers of the leg are varicose ulcers which occur secondary to varicose veins. They are found most frequently on the medial aspect of the leg. Inadequate venous return produces increased pressure in the leg veins which ultimately produces edema. The edema impairs the oxygen transfer between the circulating blood and the tissues and eventually leads to an indolent ulcer. Unless the veins are properly treated, the ulcer will persist, get worse, or continually recur. Proper treatment is directed to the veins themselves; they should be either ligated or stripped. The initial treatment of the ulcer, particularly if it shows some evidence of infection, is external support. The simplest type of external support is a cotton elastic bandage. Clean the area of the ulcer. Apply a single layer of nonadherent dressing, merely large enough to cover the raw area. Cover this with a square of gauze bandage and apply a 3-

inch elastic bandage. The elastic bandage should extend from the toes to the level of the knee. Use a circular bandage on the foot, a figure-of-eight bandage over the ankle joint, and a circular bandage up to the knee. The bandage should not be stretched to the full extent of elasticity and should be slightly snugger below than above. This provides satisfactory external support.

A better method of providing support, which has been used for many years, is the Unna paste boot. The boot has the advantage of providing constant compression, whereas the elastic bandage may loosen and must be periodically removed for washing.

Unna's gelatin mixture is made as follows: gelatin 200 gm., powdered zinc oxide 100 gm., glycerine 400 ml., and hot water 375 ml. are mixed in a double boiler on an electric stove. Dissolve the gelatin in hot water; mix the glycerine and zinc oxide powder until smooth and add to the dissolved gelatin. Cook the mixture for one-half hour. This should make enough paste for four or five boots.

Seat the patient comfortably and support the foot of the extended leg with a heel rest. Clean the ulcerated area with soap and water, and with hydrogen peroxide if necessary, to remove dried serum. Cover the raw area with a single layer of petrolatum gauze, backed by a gauze square. Warm the paste but test it to make sure that it is not too hot. Using a 2-inch paint brush, paint the leg with gelatin paste from the toes to the knee, and cover this with 2-inch wide-mesh gauze around the foot and ankle and 3-inch wide-mesh gauze from the ankle up to the knee. Apply the gauze snugly over the paste. If there is edema the bandage can be applied fairly tightly because as the edema subsides the pressure will decrease. On the other hand, if you are treating an ulcer without significant edema and particularly in a patient with arteriosclerosis, the bandage should not be applied too tightly. Begin the bandage at the toes to prevent edema distal to the bandage. Paint the

entire bandage with a second layer of paste and cover with another layer of gauze bandage. It is sometimes worthwhile to add a third layer to give added support. If you anticipate a great deal of drainage from the ulcer, a piece of wax paper may be incorporated between the layers of the boot. After the final bandage has been applied, secure it with longitudinal strips of half-inch adhesive plaster covered by circular strips of half-inch adhesive plaster.

A boot is usually left on for two to three weeks. If there is considerable edema when the boot is first applied it should probably be changed at the end of one week. If the boot is not soiled and is fitting snugly it need not be changed. Occasionally, secretion from the ulcer will cause maceration of the surrounding tissues. In this case the boot should be changed more frequently and the skin around the ulcer protected with zinc oxide ointment before a new boot is applied. As the primary method of treatment, the boot should be used continuously for at least six weeks after the ulcer has completely healed, but it must be borne in mind that the effect of the boot is only to control the ulcer and not to cure the disease. Surgical treatment of the varicose veins is the only sure means of preventing recurrence.

There are several types of gelatin bandage available commercially which can be used in place of the Unna's paste boot. Instructions are supplied as to how to apply these and the effect accomplished is essentially the same as with the Unna boot. The only advantage of the commercial product is that it simplifies application.

ARTERIAL INSUFFICIENCY

The lower extremity is particularly subject to lesions resulting from inadequate blood supply. Some concept of the adequacy of the blood supply can be obtained by noting the presence or absence of pulsations and the character of the pulsations if present. In a patient with impaired blood supply even the most minor trauma or infection requires special care to prevent its ultimately resulting in a catastrophe—the loss of the limb.

The patient should take meticulous care of the extremity. Montgomery* gives the following instructions to all his patients with arterial insufficiency:

IMPORTANT PREVENTIVE
MEASURES AND INSTRUCTIONS
FOR FOOT CARE (Arterial)

To keep the circulation open and the skin in good condition.

General Advice
1. Never use tobacco in any form. Tobacco contracts blood vessels and so reduces circulation.
2. Keep warm. Cold contracts blood vessels and reduces circulation.
3. Do not bathe in ocean or cold water, or in water that is uncomfortably warm to the hand. Avoid sunburn of feet.
4. Do not wear circular garters or rubber bands.
5. Do not sit with knees crossed; this may shut off the circulation.
6. Never walk barefooted even in your bedroom.

Care and Hygiene
1. Use loose fitting socks at night if feet are cold. Never use a hot water bottle, electric pad, or hot water on feet.
2. If weight of bed clothes is uncomfortable place a pillow beyond the feet to hold the bed clothes above the feet.
3. Wear soft, wide, round-toed loose fitting shoes. Have all shoes checked by your chiropodist. Change hose daily.
4. Wash feet daily with warm water and soap. Dry gently but thoroughly, especially between toes, with a clean towel.
5. It is preferable to have nails cut by your chiropodist. Otherwise before cutting nails, soak feet in warm (not hot) water for ten minutes to soften nails. Cut straight across. Don't cut down into the corners. Do not cut them close to the flesh.

Any special directions dictated by the individual problem are added to these instructions. Warm compresses, when required, should be applied only for short periods and the solution must be at room temperature. The slightest trauma should be treated as an emergency. If a minor lesion does not

* Dr. Hugh Montgomery, Professor of Medicine, University of Pennsylvania.

heal rapidly, order complete bed rest. Vasodilators are of questionable value because the healthy arteries dilate to a far greater degree than do the diseased vessels. Most of the good results ascribed to vasodilators actually result from meticulous local care instituted at the same time. Paravertebral block (p. 85) and subsequent lumbar sympathectomy have been useful in many cases.

The patients with severe insufficiency should be evaluated to determine whether a direct attack on the arteries with endarterectomy or vascular shunt would be helpful. This is done by arteriogram of the extremity. Lack of a satisfactory run-off contraindicates operation on the arteries, whereas localized blockage encourages operation.

Excisional surgery in these patients is to be avoided whenever possible. Given the patient with an infection at the end of a digit, one is tempted to solve the problem by amputating that digit. Unfortunately, the amputation wound rarely heals and must be followed by subsequent procedures until a mid-thigh amputation has been performed. Many surgeons feel that when excisional surgery of any type is indicated the first procedure should be mid-thigh amputation. Certainly this saves many such patients hospital time because, in reality, you are condemning most patients to mid-thigh amputation when you excise the first toe. Thus, every effort should be made to avoid any amputation.

Recent work has demonstrated that early ambulation after operation makes it possible to limit the extent of many of these amputations to below the knee. A plaster of Paris dressing is applied at operation. The patient is ambulated early, bearing weight on the plaster dressing.

INGROWN TOENAIL

The soft tissue about the toenail becomes inflamed when the edge of the nail grows into the tissue. The nail acts as a foreign body in the soft tissues, creating and sustaining an inflammatory reaction.

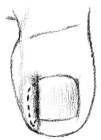

In mild cases this can be treated by packing the tissue away from the nail. In the more severe and recurrent cases, part of the nail must be removed.

To pack the tissue away from the nail, first have the patient soak his foot in warm saline. This will diminish the tenderness before you manipulate the affected area. Take a small pledget of cotton and, with a narrow instrument, insert it under the middle of the toenail and work it medially until the nail edge is raised from the tissue.

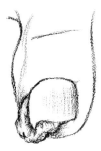

Leave the cotton in place. Have the patient soak his toe several times daily. Replace the cotton every other day until the nail has grown to a length which puts it beyond the edge of the covering skin. If the patient maintains the nail at this length, the condition should not recur.

An ingrown toenail is surgically removed as follows: Anesthetize the toe with a digital block as described on page 94. Place a sterile rubber band about the base of the toe as a tourniquet. The base of the nail must be removed as well as the nail itself. Make a linear incision parallel with and just medial to the inner edge of the toenail. Carry this

from the base of the nail (beneath the skin) up to the end of the toe. This should penetrate to the bone. Make another incision parallel to this in the nail approximately 0.5 to 1 cm. medial to the initial incision.

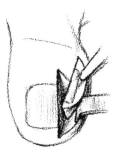

The exact position depends upon the amount of nail you wish to remove. Carry the incision down to the bone so as to remove a wedge of nail and adjacent tissue the length of the nail.

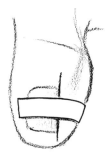

Curette the base. Now approximate the edges of the defect. It is possible to put sutures at either end, but the simplest way is to pull the skin edges together with narrow strips of adhesive.

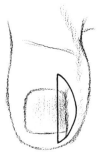

Remove the elastic tourniquet and wrap the toe with a recurrent type of bandage.

Chapter Twenty

The Urinary Tract

TRAUMA

Lacerations of the external genitalia are treated as one would treat lacerations of any other part of the body.

Contusions require no special treatment unless there is associated edema or hematoma which obstructs the urinary tract. A hematoma obstructing the urinary tract should be aspirated. If you are certain that the urethra is intact a small catheter can be threaded beyond the obstruction which is treated initially with cold compresses and later with warm applications.

DAMAGE TO THE URETHRA

If the urethra has been damaged it is probably not possible to pass a catheter into the bladder; the patient should have a suprapubic cystostomy.

TRAUMA TO THE KIDNEY

Whenever there is a possibility of trauma to the kidney the urine should be examined. If the kidney has been damaged the patient will have hematuria. Hematuria and localized pain over the kidney are not of themselves indications for operation. If no further signs develop and the hematuria gradually disappears, no treatment is needed. On the other hand, the presence of hematuria with progressive signs of hemorrhage or the appearance of a mass in the loin is an indication for operation.

OBSTRUCTION

The commonest cause of infection in the urinary tract is obstruction. This may occur at any level.

Phimosis

This occurs when the distal end of the foreskin is narrow, preventing retraction of the foreskin from the glans. If the orifice is so small that it is interfering with urinary flow it must be relieved. Definitive treatment is circumcision, but the condition can be relieved temporarily by a dorsal slit. Insert a groove director between the foreskin and the glans penis in the dorsal line of the penis. Infiltrate the skin overlying the groove director with 1 per cent procaine and divide the foreskin by cutting down on the groove director. Bleeding is controlled by suturing the inner and outer layers of the foreskin together, creating a V-shaped defect in the foreskin. At a later date circumcision must be performed.

Some patients with a tight foreskin develop paraphimosis. The skin is pulled back behind the glans and, because of the constricting bands of the foreskin and associated edema, cannot be reduced. The condition continues to get worse until reduction is accomplished. The simplest treatment is manual reduction and this should be attempted first. Take hold of the penis by grasping the edematous area on each side between the thumb and the index and middle fingers. While putting pressure on the glans with the thumb, attempt to slide the foreskin over the glans with the other four fingers. Another satisfactory method is to inject a small amount of hyaluronidase into the area of the constriction, as described by Wilbonis and Nichols.*

Obstruction of Meatus

The obstruction may be at the external meatus owing to congenital narrowing in the child or to previous infection in the adult. The condition readily responds to meatotomy, which consists of dividing the narrowed portion at the distal end of the urethra.

---

* Wilbonis, T. H., and Nichols, R. K.: A Method for Treating Paraphimosis. J. Med. Assoc. Alabama *21*:233–234, 1952.

Obstruction of Urethra

The obstruction may be physiologic as occurs after operation, or anatomic such as that due to prostatic hypertrophy or to stricture of the urethra. The problem is most often handled by urethral catheterization.

Urethral Catheterization

The most commonly employed urological procedure is catheterization of the bladder. This is indicated for patients who are unable to void, because either of urethral obstruction or of postoperative lack of return of tone to the bladder. Catheterization is also used to empty the bladder of patients before operations on the pelvic organs. The catheterization should be performed by a urologist when there is marked obstruction, a stricture of the urethra, or serious damage to the urethra.

CATHETERIZATION OF AN ADULT MALE. A routine male catheterization tray contains:

1 straight hemostatic clamp
1 large kidney basin
1 catheter clamp
2 beakers
1 5 ml. Luer-Lok syringe
1 20 gauge 1- to 1½-inch needle
1 Asepto syringe
1 urine specimen bottle with cap
1 Coudé catheter—15 Fr.
6 cotton balls—large
2 cotton tipped applicators
1 cystoscopic sheet
1 tube surgical lubricant
1 pair gloves

Place the patient in bed with his head and shoulders slightly elevated. Have him abduct his thighs and flex his knees. Stand on the left side of the patient. Cleanse the entire region of the genitalia with liquid soap and cotton balls. Pick up the penis with the left hand; retract the prepuce and scrub this area with liquid soap and cotton balls. The entire area should then be rinsed or swabbed with a disinfectant solution such as cyanide of mercury (1:1500). A cystoscopic sheet, which is nothing more than a small towel with a hole in it, is placed over the perineum, bringing the penis through the hole in the towel. Holding the penis in the left hand, irrigate the anterior urethra with 5 to 10 ml. of acroflavin solution (1:5000) or mercury oxycyanide solution (1:20,000), using a blunt tipped urethral syringe. Do not hold the syringe tightly against the external meatus because this will force material from the anterior urethra back into the bladder. Have your assistant deposit some sterile lubricant on the towel; pick up the catheter with the hemostat and dip the tip of the catheter into the lubricant. Holding the penis erect insert the catheter, without touching it, into the urethra, gradually advancing it until it enters the bladder as evidenced by the appearance of the urine from the end of the catheter. If this is to be an interval catheterization, the catheter is left in place until no more urine can be drained out.

Move the catheter about to be certain that the drainage has been completed; withdraw it, injecting 5 to 10 ml. of the antiseptic solution through the catheter into the bladder during the withdrawal.

Frequently, the catheterization does not go quite so smoothly. The size of the catheter to be used depends upon the size of the meatus. In the average adult, first try an 18 or 20 French soft rubber urethral catheter. If this does not pass into the bladder readily, one can then use a woven catheter which has a finer tip and, because of its woven construction, is much stiffer. Usually, it is possible to pass such a catheter. A woven catheter must be used with more care because of the greater likelihood of damage to the urethra. Such a catheter should not be left in place for a prolonged period. If you have difficulty passing this catheter use a filiform catheter. This is a small catheter which is passed into the bladder as a guide for the following drainage catheter. Since the filiform is quite small it may pass

readily into the bladder. If it becomes lodged in the urethra short of the bladder, leave it in place and attempt to pass another filiform catheter beyond it. If this becomes lodged repeat this until one passes into the bladder.

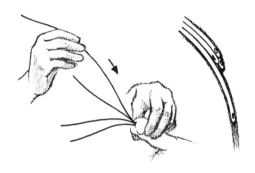

Leave this in place and remove the other filiform catheters. Now attach a following catheter to the filiform

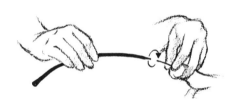

and pass it into the bladder. This can now drain the bladder.

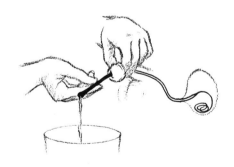

Handle the catheter drainage as you would with any other catheter.

Catheterization in the Female. Place the

patient in bed on her back with her head and shoulders slightly elevated; her knees should be flexed and the thighs abducted. Stand at her right side. Thoroughly cleanse the genitalia with liquid soap, using sterile cotton balls. Separate the labia and carefully cleanse the area, rinse off the soap with the disinfectant solution either by swabbing with cotton or by pouring the solution over the genitalia. Place a sterile towel on the bed between the patient's legs. Spread the labia apart and carefully sweep the pubic hairs away from the vulva. The urethra can then be seen; lift the catheter with the hemostatic clamp and after putting some sterile lubricating jelly on it, insert it into the urethra. Usually a 12 F. or 14 F. soft rubber catheter is used, although some use a glass catheter in females. The catheter should pass readily into the bladder as will be evidenced by the flow of urine from the end. Allow all of the urine to drain out. Manipulate the catheter to ascertain that all the urine has drained and withdraw the catheter. As you withdraw it insert 5 to 10 ml. of antiseptic solution through the catheter into the urethra.

Continuous Catheter Drainage

Continuous catheter drainage is indicated in the postoperative patient who is unable to void spontaneously and requires more than one catheterization after operation, in the patient who has obstruction in the urethra which interferes with the passage of urine, following injuries and surgical procedures on the urethra, and after certain operations on the bladder. The commonest type of instrument used for this procedure is a Foley bag type of self-retaining catheter. This catheter has two lumens: one at the end to drain the urine from the bladder, and the other a small lumen, which connects with a 5 or 10 ml. balloon near the end of the catheter. When the catheter is in place and the balloon is inflated against the vesical ori-

fice, the catheter cannot come out of the urethra.

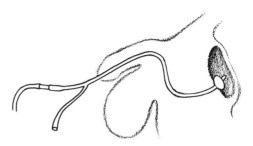

Before the catheter is inserted, fluid should be run into the balloon to be certain that it is expansible and that there are no leaks. If the balloon is not satisfactory another catheter can be obtained.

The passage of the Foley device is quite different from the passage of the soft rubber urethral catheter. You may, for instance, insert a stylet through this catheter to stiffen it. To pass the soft rubber urethral catheter one need merely hold the penis in a vertical position. The catheter with the stylet in place must be passed as if it were a sound. Since the stylet has a curve toward the end, the penis is held in a vertical position and the tip of the catheter is inserted with the major portion of the catheter horizontal to and parallel with the surface of the body. The penis is advanced over the catheter. As the tip of the catheter drops down below the pubic bone, the penis and the catheter are then brought back to the vertical position which puts the tip of the catheter facing directly cephalad at the beginning of the prostatic portion of the urethra. As the catheter is advanced further, the main portion is gradually depressed inferiorly. In this way, the tip easily follows the curve of the posterior urethra. Passage is helped somewhat by having the right hand make downward pressure over the root of the penis. Occasionally, it is helpful to insert the finger of the left hand into the rectum to guide the tip of the catheter through the membranous portion of the prostatic urethra.

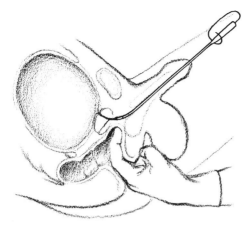

After the catheter has been inserted, 5 or 10 ml. of fluid is injected into the bag, and mild traction is applied to the catheter to make certain that it will remain in place.

Another method of fixing the urethral catheter is the pipe cleaner method. Sterile pipe cleaners are strapped around the circumference of the penis near its base. Each pipe cleaner is taped in place in a different quadrant, parallel with the penis, by 1-inch adhesive plaster placed 1 inch from the proximal end of the pipe cleaners. The distal ends of the pipe cleaners are then brought together around the catheter beyond the penis and held there with a small piece of adhesive plaster. A slight bow in each of the pipe cleaners keeps them away from the glans penis. The proximal ends of the pipe cleaners are then bent upon themselves so that they cannot pull out from under the adhesive plaster.

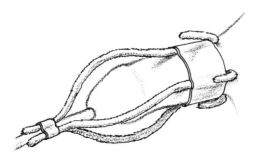

Retention catheters are uncomfortable for the first day but the discomfort disappears and the drainage can be continued for an indefinite period without discomfort provided the catheter is kept clean and is changed when it becomes sanded or blocked. You can tell whether the catheter is sanding by rolling it between the thumb and forefinger. Any gritty or calcareous deposits within can be felt. Usually the catheter is changed about every four to seven days but it can be left in place longer provided it is draining freely and has not become sandy. The catheter should be checked at least three times a day to be certain that it is in the proper position and that there is free flow of urine.

Do not insert the free end of the catheter into a urinal. This only tends to wet the external genitals and contaminate the end of the catheter. Infection then ascends along the catheter into the urinary tract. The catheter should be connected via a glass connector to a piece of rubber tubing and allowed to drain into a collection bottle which is hooked to the side of the bed. There are several different types of cages available to hold the bottle. When these are not available, gauze tied about the neck of the bottle can be tied to the frame of the bed. For the ambulatory patient, it is better to use some means of hooking the bottle to the bed which allows the bottle to be readily lifted free. When the bottle is emptied, it should be replaced by a clean empty one, the amount of urine measured and noted on the chart. The rubber tubing running between the catheter and the collection bottle should be pinned to the side of the patient's mattress. This is best accomplished by putting a piece of adhesive tape with a tab extension about the rubber tubing and fastening this tape with a safety pin to the mattress. This takes tension off the catheter, prevents its accidental removal, and avoids penile discomfort. The catheter should be irrigated periodically. The apparatus consists of a sterile Y tube inserted in the rubber tubing between the catheter and the drainage bottle. The other limb of the Y tube connects to a bottle containing irrigating solution which hangs on a pole at the patient's bed.

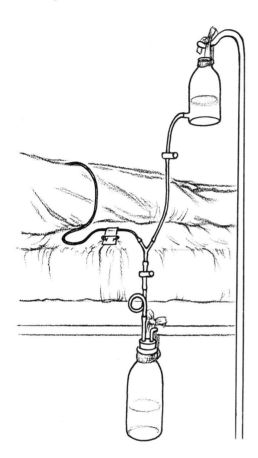

There is a clamp on the tubing running from the irrigating reservoir and another between the Y connector and the collection bottle. While the bladder is draining the clamp is closed on the tubing from the irrigating solution reservoir and the clamp is open on the tubing to the collecting bottle. Under these circumstances, any urine which is secreted runs directly into the collection bottle. To irrigate the bladder clamp the tubing leading to the collection bottle and release the clamp below the irrigating solution reservoir. Allow 50 to 100 ml. of the solution to run into the bladder. After clamping the tube from

the reservoir, the tubing to the collection bottle can be opened and the irrigating solution drained into the collection bottle. A record must be kept of the amount of irrigating solution used in order to know the exact amount of urine secreted. The bladder must be irrigated twice a day. The advantage of the special apparatus is that the entire system remains closed at all times and there is no chance of introducing infection during the course of the irrigation. It also takes less time for the irrigation.

Decompression of the Bladder

When a patient has a urethral obstruction due to a chronic prostatic enlargement, rapid removal of the accumulated urine can cause bleeding from the bladder wall. These chronic obstructions are best handled by gradual decompression of the bladder. When the catheter is inserted it should be attached to rubber tubing which runs through a regular intravenous drip chamber. A clamp on the tubing adjusts the flow to drip through the chamber at 40 to 60 drops a minute. At this rate it should take about two days to decompress the bladder. If you do not wish to use the drip arrangement drain off 100 ml. every hour.

Suprapubic Cystostomy

When urethral catheterization is unsuccessful, or when the urethra or the bladder has been damaged, it is advisable to drain the bladder through an incision in the lower abdomen.

A urethral catheter is far more likely to become occluded than a suprapubic drainage tube. A large catheter, usually with a mushroom tip or a Foley bag, is used. The suprapubic catheter is anchored to the skin so that an accidental pull on the catheter will not pull it out of the bladder. When this type of drainage is being used in a young child it is best to use hand restraints to keep the child from pulling it out.

When the wound is closed tightly about the catheter there will be no drainage around the tube. (There may be some little drainage shortly after the operation which will decrease as granulation tissue develops.) But, if the wound separates, more urine may come out through the wound than through the tube. If there is no drainage the wound will remain dry and require dressing infrequently, but if there is drainage about the tube the wet dressings must be changed before they become saturated. The frequency with which they should be changed will depend upon the amount of drainage, but it may be as often as every hour and certainly should be at least every four to five hours. The urine undergoes decomposition, producing a disagreeable odor particularly in warm weather. If the patient's dressings and bed clothes are not changed regularly, they will develop a very unpleasant and disturbing odor.

The suprapubic tube should be attached to a drainage bottle which is changed every day. The bladder should be irrigated with antiseptic solution twice a day. All glass tubing and connecting tubes should be changed and cleaned every two days or oftener if they become coated or blocked with mucus or pus. This coating can be removed by a weak solution of acid (¼ per cent acetic acid). If sand is felt the tubes should be changed.

Ureteral Drainage

The pelvis of the kidney and the ureters are drained by a ureteral catheter, a procedure which requires considerable care if infection is to be prevented. The catheter is held in the male by silk sutures tied to the catheter and held around the penis by a strip of ½-inch adhesive plaster immediately proximal to the glans.

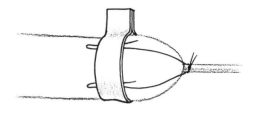

In the female the ureteral catheter can be held by tying it to a Foley bag urethral catheter which is in place. The free end of the catheter must be kept sterile. Davis* recommends placing the end of the catheter in a small sterile medicine bottle. This is held in place by a cork which has a notch cut out to allow the catheter to pass into the bottle.

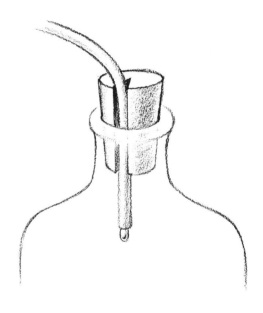

The bottle can be taped to the thigh and the patient allowed to walk. If the patient is kept in bed the catheter can be passed through the top of a sterile medi-

* Davis, D. M., and Warren, K. C.: Urological Nursing. Philadelphia, W. B. Saunders Co., 1959, p. 64.

cine dropper bulb which is attached to a drainage tube via a glass connector.

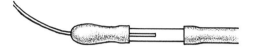

The catheter can be held in place by tying the bulb down on the tube. One can gain access to the catheter by removing the bulb from the glass connector. The catheter should be examined by a nurse every half hour to be certain that it is functioning. If the outflow of urine ceases, the nurse must attempt to clear the obstruction in the tube by aspiration with a syringe designed for that specific purpose.

Nephrostomy Tubes

Problems in the ureter may require the insertion of drainage tubes directly into the kidney. Such tubes are then brought out through the flank. It is quite important that these be kept in place because, obviously, if these become misplaced they are far more difficult to reinsert than other types of drainage tubes. They are attached to a drainage bottle and handled as any type of bladder drainage.

Chapter Twenty-one

The Circulatory System, Including Fluid and Electrolyte Therapy

ARTERIAL SYSTEM

ARTERIAL PUNCTURE

Arteries are punctured to sample arterial blood and to measure arterial blood pressure. The most commonly used artery is the brachial; the next are the radial and femoral arteries. Have the patient lie down with the arm extended and a towel beneath the elbow to allow slight hyperextension. Palpate the brachial artery.

A special needle is used for this purpose. This bears the name of Dr. André Cournand, who developed it. It is made up of three pieces. The outer needle is made so that either of the other two pieces project beyond the tip when they are in place. These latter two are of the same diameter, which allows either to fill the lumen of the outer needle. One of these is a sharp needle which, when in place in the outer shell, gives the pair a sharp point. The other is a blunt stylet which, when in place,

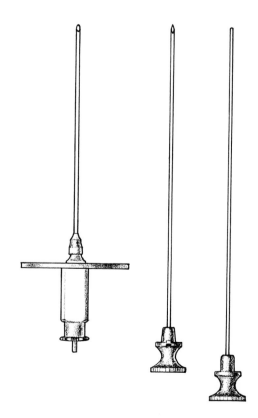

292

extends beyond the end of the outer needle, preventing the development of clot in the needle.

After you have located the artery by palpation prepare the skin with an antiseptic solution and insert the outer needle with the inner needle in place. Keeping the palpating finger of one hand on the artery, insert the needle into the artery. To do this you usually have to insert the needle deeper than originally seemed necessary. When the needle enters the artery there should be a slow drip of blood

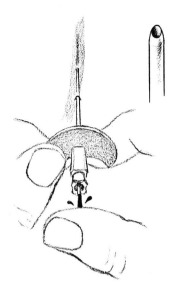

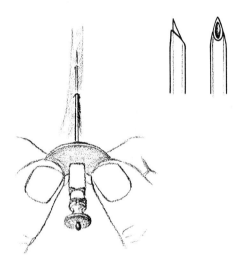

from the inner needle. Remove the inner needle. This should result in a pulsating spurt. If this does not occur push the needle in a bit further because the inner needle might have been in the lumen while the outer needle was only in the wall.

If no blood appears after the needle is inserted to its full length, remove the inner needle and slowly withdraw the outer needle. Keep your thumb approximately 1 cm. back of the orifice to prevent the blood from spurting on you. When a spurt has been achieved advance the needle, using the presence of the spurting blood as an indication that the needle remains in the lumen of the artery.

After the needle has been threaded well into the vessel (at least 2.5 cm.), insert the blunt stylet to its full depth. Tape the needle to the skin by attaching a 1-inch piece of adhesive plaster to the hub of the needle and running it along the skin over the needle. Apply a similar piece at right angles to this at the joint where the hub meets the skin.

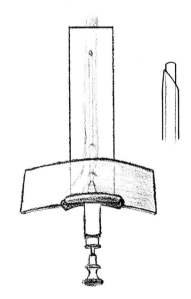

After you have completed the study withdraw the needle and maintain pressure over the site of puncture for 5 minutes *by the clock.*

INSERTION OF ARTERIAL CATHETER

Arterial catheters are inserted to monitor blood pressure, to insert dye for a contrast x-ray study of the arterial system, and for regional perfusion. A special needle is required for this. This needle also has three parts but it differs from the Cournand needle in that all three fit together at one time. The outer needle has no point. The inner needle has a sharp point which projects beyond the outer needle. A stylet fits within the inner needle extending to the point. The equipment is completed by a small spring 2 feet long which fits within the outer needle.

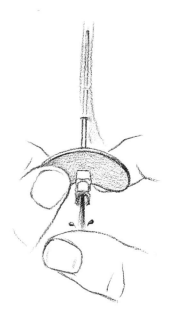

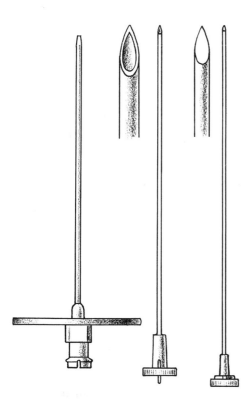

After proper preparation and palpation of the artery the needle is inserted through the skin. The stylet is removed and the needle is advanced into the vessel. This will be evident by blood dripping from the inner needle.

Remove the inner needle and advance the outer needle in the lumen while blood is spurting. Next pass the spring through the outer needle and up into the artery at least 6 inches. Put pressure over the spring

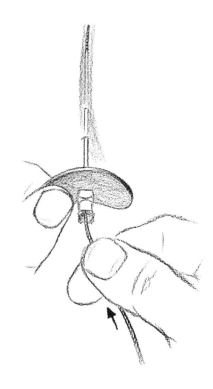

to hold it in place and remove the needle, sliding it back over the spring. Pass a piece of polyethylene tubing over the

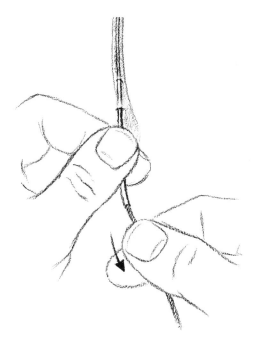

spring into the artery. After this is passed at least 6 inches hold the catheter in place and remove the spring. Attach the catheter to an adapter and connect this to whatever type of equipment is necessary to carry out the work planned.

VENOUS SYSTEM

VENIPUNCTURE

Venipuncture is used to obtain samples of blood for analysis or for crossmatching; to administer blood, fluids, or medications; and to perform specific tests which require the presence of a needle in a vein. The most common site of venipuncture is an antecubital vein. Support the arm in a comfortable position. Carefully cleanse the skin over the area with a piece of gauze soaked with alcohol. Apply a tourniquet on the

upper arm proximal to the site where you plan to do the venipuncture. This is most commonly a piece of rubber tubing. It should be applied sufficiently tight to interfere with the venous return, but not so tight as to shut off the arterial blood supply. Do not begin until the veins are distended. If the veins are slow in filling have the patient open and close his hand. Slapping the tissues over the vein may also be helpful. Use a 20-gauge needle for drawing blood or giving fluids and an 18-gauge needle if you plan to give blood. Examine the needle to see that it is sharp and has no burrs. Rub the needle against a piece of sterile gauze; if there is a burr it will pick up the gauze.

If there is a burr on the needle discard it and get another needle; otherwise the venipuncture will be needlessly painful. The median cubital vein or the cephalic vein may be used. Ascertain that there is satisfactory distention of the desired vein. If not choose another vein; you may find a better one at the wrist. If multiple venipunctures have preceded this one you may have to use a vein on the dorsum of the hand. After choosing the vein, insert the needle, with the bevel up, through the skin parallel to the vein.

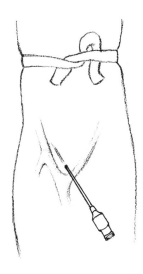

The needle is not inserted directly through the skin and into the vein.

Rather, after the needle is through the skin and beside the vein, change the direction and push the needle against the side of the vein and advance it until it slips through the wall and into the lumen.

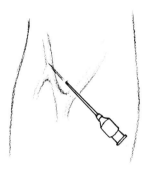

You can usually see the needle slip into the vein but penetration is always evident by the appearance of blood coming back into the syringe. Change the direction of the needle to that of the vein and thread it into the vein to prevent its slipping out. Remove the tourniquet to prevent extravasation of blood.

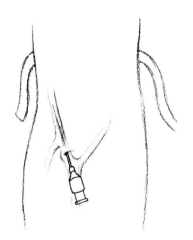

Sampling

If the purpose of the puncture is to sample blood, the desired amount of blood is drawn into the syringe. If the needle is properly placed, the blood should flow into the syringe readily. If considerable suction is required, un-desirable hemolysis may occur. This can be prevented by repositioning the needle. Occasionally it may be necessary to reapply the tourniquet. After the sample of blood has been withdrawn the needle can be removed. As the needle is withdrawn place a cotton sponge over the vein at the site of the venipuncture and have the patient hold this in place for approximately three minutes. By that time the puncture site should have stopped bleeding. If oozing from the skin persists the cotton sponge can be replaced and held in place with adhesive plaster.

Infusion

In many patients intravenous feedings must be continued for several days and it is wise to conserve the antecubital veins. Since intravenous feedings frequently cause a sterile phlebitis, with subsequent thrombosis, it is well to begin infusion in a distal segment of the vessel and to gradually move proximally. Any of the veins on the surface of the lower forearm are quite satisfactory. One of the branches of the cephalic vein over the head of the radius above the wrist is usually available and with the needle here the patient can move his arm. The veins over the back of the hands can be used. One should avoid the veins of the lower extremity for routine administration of fluid unless absolutely necessary because such use is associated with a very high incidence of thrombophlebitis.

Since the infusion must be kept in place for some time, it is best to immobilize the site of insertion. This is usually done with an arm board, an ordinary wooden board which extends from proximal to the elbow to beyond the hand. This may be unadorned or may be padded with cotton and covered with gauze. The board is placed beneath the arm which is loosely taped to it with adhesive plaster in such a way that the plaster does not impair the circulation.

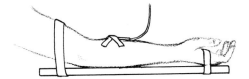

Before inserting the needle all air should be expelled from the tubing of the administration set. Air bubbles are clearly visible in the transparent tubing used today. Remove these by raising the needle at the end of the tubing above the level of the flask and gradually lowering it; the air will be forced out ahead of the fluid. Clamp the tubing which is then ready for use. After the needle has been inserted as described under venipuncture, it is positioned and immobilized. It is usually necessary to place a small piece of cotton under the hub of the needle in order to maintain it at the proper angle. Secure the needle in place with two strips of half-inch adhesive plaster crossing the needle at the hub.

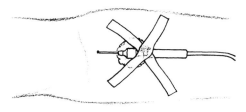

Anchor the tubing with an adhesive strip loosely to the skin so that any pull on the tubing will be absorbed without being transmitted to the needle itself. Open the clamp on the tubing widely to make sure that the fluid flows freely. If there is extravasation of the fluid into the tissues about the vein the needle is not properly positioned and should be reinserted. To ascertain whether the needle is still in the vein, lower the bottle of intravenous fluid below the level of the needle. If the needle is properly positioned in the vein blood will flow back into the tubing. The rate of flow of the solution is adjusted as indicated by the condition of the patient and the type of fluid being given. Most solutions are given at a rate of 250 to 350 ml. per hour. Blood is given more

slowly than electrolyte solutions. If the infusion is to run continuously the flow must be adjusted accordingly.

Regardless of how carefully you immobilize the arm the needle will in time either pull out from or penetrate the wall of the vein. When prolonged therapy is required a plastic catheter should be inserted. Several types are available commercially; they may be inserted percutaneously, thus eliminating the necessity of a cutdown and lessening the possibility of accidental removal.

Such units function well. The one to be described is a Bardic Deseret Intracath. The entire unit is available in a sterile condition. It consists of a needle protected by a plastic cap and a catheter (enclosed in a pliable plastic) which fits through the needle and whose proximal end locks in the needle. After proper preparation of the area apply a tourniquet, remove the plastic guard and insert the needle into the vein as you would any other needle (see A, p. 298). Remove the tourniquet and thread the catheter through the needle, using one hand to steady the needle and the other to advance the catheter. Pass the catheter several inches beyond the end of the needle. This can be done without opening the thin plastic envelope covering the proximal end of the catheter (see B, p. 298).

If the catheter seems to become impinged upon the vein as it passes through the needle this can sometimes be corrected by temporarily reapplying the tourniquet. This procedure distends the vein and may make it possible to thread the catheter into the vein.

Hold the catheter in place by pressing down on it in the vein beyond the needle while you withdraw the needle from the vein (see C, p. 298). Pull the needle back to where it engages the flared end of the catheter and attach it to an administration set (see D, p. 298). Apply a pressure bandage consisting of a dry sterile pledget held in place over the venipuncture by an encircling loop of one-inch adhesive plaster. Tape the needle to the skin.

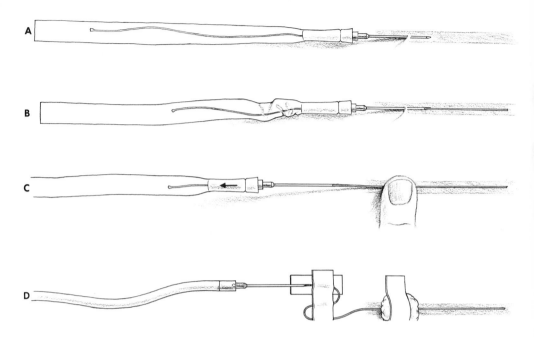

Cannulation of a Vein

Sometimes it is impossible to insert a needle percutaneously into a satisfactory vein. This occurs in the occasional patient who has no suitable vein and more commonly in the patient in whom prolonged intravenous therapy has resulted in thrombosis of available veins. (This situation can be postponed by using a percutaneous plastic catheter.) When no suitable vein is available you must expose a vein and insert a cannula. If the cannulation is planned for a short period of time the ideal vein is the long saphenous vein on the medial aspect of the ankle. This is one of the most constantly located veins in the body and in a patient in peripheral circulatory collapse you need not hesitate to cut down in this area even though you have not just been able to palpate the vein. It can always be found, except in the patient in whom the vein had been used for the same purpose previously.

Technique. Infiltrate the area directly over the vein with a small amount of local anesthetic solution. Make a transverse incision perpendicular to and directly over the vein, carrying it through the subcutaneous tissues.

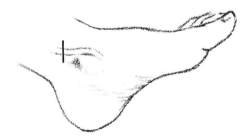

Using a hemostat separate the vein from the surrounding tissue. Since the bone underlies the vein it is a simple matter to slip the hemostat beneath the vein by putting the hemostat against the bone and pushing it through, lifting all tissue above it. Using a hemostat to pull them through, pass two ties about the vein, one at the proximal, the other at the distal edge of the incision.

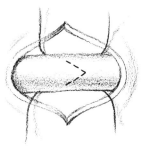

Make a V-shaped incision in the vein. If you have difficulty finding the lumen pick up the proximal edge of the incision in the vein with a fine point hemostat. Lift this flap to expose the lumen of the vein, facilitating insertion of the cannula.

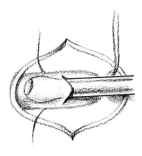

Use the proximal ligature to tie the vein down over the cannula.

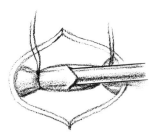

Attach the cannula to the adapter of an intravenous set and check the position by allowing the fluid to run rapidly for a moment. Close the subcutaneous tissues, using interrupted cotton sutures. A small dressing completes the cannulation, but the tubing should be strapped to the leg to prevent pull on the cannula if someone inadvertently drags on the tubing. The cannula allows the rapid administration of large amounts of fluids.

Cannulation of this vein carries the disadvantage that if it is used for more than 36 hours the patient will almost certainly develop chemical phlebitis. On the other hand, it is one of the most ideal veins for use in emergencies. One of the best veins to use for prolonged intravenous therapy is the external jugular vein. This is best done by inserting the catheter through a small nick in the vein, without tying off the vessel and threading it down into the superior vena cava. The intravenous fluids are thus passed into a large caliber vein through which a large amount of blood is continuously flowing. The dilution of the intravenous fluid with blood occurs so rapidly there is little or no opportunity for the fluid to cause a chemical irritation of the wall of the vein. It is possible to use such an arrangement for as long as a month without any complications.

PARENTERAL FEEDING

Materials Available

Solutions available for parenteral support are quite diversified. These are designed to supply the calories, electrolytes, and fluids needed by the patient.

Calories. The average patient requires 2,000 to 3,000 calories per day. The exact amount depends upon the general condition of the patient, his weight, body temperature, activity, and the specific disease. It is difficult to supply a patient with an adequate amount of calories by parenteral injection because of the limitation of the amount of fluid which the patient can tolerate. However, it is wise to try to give him as much as he can safely handle. Calories are most commonly supplied intravenously by glucose, usually in 5 or 10 per cent solution. The glucose may be in water or in physiologic salt solution. Ten per cent glucose in physiologic salt solution is irritating to the vein and when used for several days will cause a chemical phlebitis. (Glucose is occasionally given in 50 per cent solution, generally to elevate the osmotic pressure of the circulation so as to decrease cerebral edema.) Fructose is used in 5 or 10 per cent solution and it has the advantage that it can be added to a glucose solution, further increasing the caloric value. Each gram of glucose or fructose supplies 4 calories.

Ethyl alcohol is another means of supplying calories. One milliliter of 95 per cent alcohol supplies 1.4 calories. One can add as much as 60 ml. of 95 per cent alcohol to each liter of intravenous fluid. Such solutions should be given slowly to small individuals and should be avoided in patients with liver disease. It is probably safer to give only half this amount in each liter of fluid or put the full amount in alternate bottles. The addition of alcohol makes the intravenous fluid somewhat turgid, but does not impair its safety.

There are solutions of protein hydrolysates available which can be used to provide calories. Each gram of protein provides 4 calories. The hydrolysates may be used alone or in combination with 5 per cent glucose and saline. They provide the nitrogenous products necessary for protein anabolism. However, it does no good to give protein hydrolysates for building purposes unless one has covered the expected caloric requirements for the period of time by some other means—carbohydrate, fat, or alcohol.

Patients who are markedly undernourished or who required prolonged intravenous feeding as their main source of nutrition will benefit from parenteral hyperalimentation. This is described in detail on page 303.

ELECTROLYTES. The most commonly required electrolytes are sodium, potassium, and chloride. Sodium and chloride are available in a salt solution. The most commonly used is physiologic salt solution which is 0.9 per cent sodium chloride in water containing 154 mEq./L. of both sodium and chloride.

This may be given alone but it usually is given with glucose in 5 or 10 per cent concentrations and listed as 5 or 10 per cent glucose in physiologic saline. If large amounts of sodium and chloride are required but the amount of water is to be limited, sodium chloride can be given as 2.5 or 3 per cent sodium chloride in water. There are variations of physiologic salt solution containing small amounts of additional ions. Ringer's solution contains 147 mEq./L. of sodium, 4 mEq./L. of potassium, 4.5 mEq./L. of calcium, and 155 mEq./L. of chloride. Hartmann's lactated-Ringer's solution contains 130 mEq./L. of sodium, 5 mEq./L. of potassium, 3 mEq./L. of calcium, 2 mEq./L. of magnesium, 118 mEq./L. of chloride and 25 mEq./L. of lactate. Additional specific electrolytes can be added as needed. When one wishes to add only chloride ions without adding sodium, ammonium chloride can be used. Ammonium chloride in $\frac{1}{6}$ molar (0.9 per cent) solution contains 167 mEq./L. of ammonium and chloride. To add only sodium ions without adding chloride use sodium lactate. This is available in ampules in molar concentration. It should be diluted to one-sixth molar (1.9 per cent) before use. This contains 167 mEq./L. of sodium and lactate.

Potassium is added in the form of potassium chloride, which is available in concentrations of 1 gm. in 5 ml. of solution. One gram potassium is equivalent to 13.2 mEq.

Calcium may be provided as calcium chloride and as calcium gluconate. The calcium gluconate is the most commonly used solution, available as 10 per cent calcium gluconate in 10 ml. vials.

PROTEINS. If the albumin fraction of the plasma proteins is low (and this is a common situation when the patient has severe liver disease) the simplest and most rapid means of raising the albumin fraction is to give salt-free albumin, which is usually made up as 50 gm. in 100 ml. of solution. This is particularly valuable in these patients because the administration of large amounts of protein orally may induce hepatic coma by building up a high level of ammonium in the blood (the damaged liver is incapable of converting the nitrogen products to urea). Such a problem does not exist when one administers salt-free albumin.

PLASMA. Human plasma was widely used in shock to correct the large loss of plasma from the vascular system into the tissues, but plasma substitutes, such as dextran, are now preferred because they do not carry the risk of hepatitis. Plasma may be used where one is interested in building up the protein content of the plasma as a whole. However, since the most important fraction of the plasma proteins and the one which is usually deficient is albumin, the use of salt-free albumin is far more desirable.

WHOLE BLOOD. Whole blood is the best replacement for acute blood loss. A substitute such as plasma or a plasma volume expander should be used only until blood is available.

Whole blood is also used in patients who have lost a significant amount of weight; in such persons the blood count or hematocrit can be deceiving because the patient may have a diminished blood volume and the hematocrit merely gives one the concentration rather than an index of the total volume. A blood transfusion given to this type of patient may result in no improvement of the blood count, owing to the fact that the blood was needed to expand the diminished volume rather than to increase the concentration of cells, and this fact can be used as a rough index of the adequacy of the blood volume. When transfusions begin to increase the count, one knows that the volume has been restored to normal levels. A better means of assessing the situation is to measure the plasma volume.

Blood which has been lost through hemorrhage can be replaced rapidly until the blood pressure is back to normal and then given more slowly.

Blood given to the individual who has had no acute blood loss should not be given more rapidly than 90 to 120 minutes for a 500 ml. unit. Furthermore, this blood should be at room temperature; cold blood may cause a reaction if the patient should have cold agglutinins. Cold agglutinins would not be identified on a routine cross-matching of the blood and would be found only if one specifically examined for them. Allowing the blood to stand at room temperature for 30 minutes warms it sufficiently to avoid problems due to cold agglutinins.

Some patients represent risks for the administration of blood because of a poor cardiovascular status, yet need red cells to bring the total amount of hemoglobin up to a satisfactory level. The need can be safely met by giving small transfusions more frequently (250 ml. at a time), or by centrifuging the red cells from the plasma, and infusing the cells after resuspending them in a glucose solution. This should cause no increase in volume and no deleterious effects.

Daily Requirements

If the parenteral fluid is supplementing an oral intake the ability of the body to selectively absorb and discard electrolytes and fluid will correct for our inadequacy. On the other hand, if the patient is solely dependent upon the parenteral route for sustenance, the surgeon must calculate accurately. In this situation an indwelling urethral catheter must be inserted into the bladder to collect all urine, and a careful record of the intake and the output kept.

FLUID. The urinary output is the best means of determining the total amount of fluid to be administered to the patient. Man has an insensible loss (from the intestines, skin, and lungs) of 700 to 1000 ml. of fluid daily. This is increased by heat, sweating, hyperventilation, or elevation in body temperature, but still the urinary output is the best index of the adequacy of the hydration of the patient. The normal urinary output of the average patient is 800 to 1000 ml. per day and the patient should receive sufficient fluid to maintain his output at this level. To accomplish this the patient who has no abnormal losses should receive between 1500 and 3000 ml. of fluid daily.

The only exception is the occasional patient who is receiving excessive glucose rapidly. Under such circumstances the excess glucose in the urine may act as a diuretic. This happens only rarely and then is due to 10 per cent glucose being administered too rapidly. The situation is corrected by decreasing the rate of administration and/or using only 5 per cent glucose. More saline may be required.

Pure water depletion is treated by water either orally or parenterally. The volume required is calculated as follows:

The current total body water is 60 percent of the body weight ($0.6 \times$ body weight in Kg.)

The normal total body water (at serum sodium of 140 mEq. per liter is calculated by multiplying the current total body water by the measured concentration of serum sodium in mEq./L. and dividing this by 140.

The deficit is the difference between the normal and the current total body volume. This is the amount of water required to return the volume to normal. However, only one-third to one-half of this volume should be given in the first 24 hours.

ELECTROLYTES. Sodium and chloride are the electrolytes most commonly needed during parenteral alimentation. No sodium chloride is required in the immediate postoperative period because of the suppression of the excretion by the response to trauma. This lasts from two to five days. A good rule of thumb is to assume that sodium excretion begins with postoperative diuresis. This is not a precise index but does allow an estimate. Daily requirements of sodium are approximately 5 gm. per day. These are met with 500 ml. of normal saline daily.

If the patient develops a hyponatremia, the deficit may be calculated by multiplying the difference between the measured and normal sodium values by the total body water ($0.6 \times$ weight). One-third of the calculated deficit should be given in the next 24 hours. The following day the deficit should be recalculated and another one-third of the deficit given.

Potassium is not given in the immediate postoperative period, but should be started on the second postoperative day provided the patient has a satisfactory urinary output. The daily requirement of potassium is approximately 40 mEq. We meet this requirement by giving the patients 4 gm. of potassium chloride daily. It is preferable to put 2 gm. in each of two bottles of fluid.

Deficiencies in potassium cannot be measured as accurately. When evidence of potassium deficit is found either by analysis or the EKG, potassium must be given slowly either orally or parenterally. Parenteral administration should not exceed 20 mEq. per hour or more than 200 mEq. per 24 hours.

Treatment of hyperkalemia is more complicated and consists of (1) restriction of exogenous potassium, (2) sodium bicarbonate (if patient is acidotic), (3) fluids, (4) glucose and insulin, (5) ion exchange resins, (6) gastric suction and (7) renal dialysis.

If a patient has been sustained solely on intravenous therapy for more than a week he is probably deficient in calcium and magnesium. The calcium can be given as 10 ml. of 10 per cent calcium gluconate twice weekly. Incorporating Ringer's solution in place of saline into his fluid schedule supplies the necessary magnesium.

Replacement Therapy

If gastrointestinal secretions are being aspirated, compensation must be planned. Gastrointestinal drainage has an average of 10 mEq. potassium per liter. Substituting 1 L. of physiologic salt solution and 1 gm. of potassium chloride for each liter of gastric drainage is a satisfactory rule of thumb.

Patients on complete intravenous feeding should have their electrolytes evaluated twice weekly and any necessary adjustments made.

PARENTERAL HYPERALIMENTATION

A new technique of supplying adequate nutrition *via* the intravenous route has been worked out by Drs. Jonathan Rhoads and Stanley Dudrick.* Hyperalimentation is the intravenous administration of nitrogen, calories, and other nutrients in sufficient amounts to achieve tissue synthesis and anabolism in patients with normal or excessive nutritional needs. Rhoads and Dudrick accomplished this by infusing a high concentration of nutritives and electrolytes continuously at a constant rate that did not exceed the body's ability to tolerate infusion of these contents.

Since this technique involves the use of high concentrations, it must be given into a vessel large enough to allow immediate dilution, such as the vena cava. A long limb catheter is used. The patient is placed in a Trendelenburg position, and the cervical area is cleansed with acetone and an antibacterial agent. The catheter is placed percutaneously with sterile precautions into the subclavian vein and directed into the superior vena cava to a predetermined distance. The catheter is sutured to the skin. An antibiotic ointment is applied to the catheter at the point of entrance into the skin, and a sterile occlusive dressing is applied. The catheter is kept open with a slow drip of 5 per cent dextrose in water, while the patient is given a chest x-ray to check the position of the catheter and to determine any post-cannulation complications.

---

* Rhoads and Dudrick: Surgery 54:134, 1968.

The hyperalimentation infusion is then begun. The base solution can be prepared by adding 350 ml. of 50 per cent dextrose to a bottle containing 750 ml. of the commercially available 5 per cent fibrin in 5 per cent dextrose. The resultant 1100 ml. of fluid provides 1000 calories and 5.25 gm. of nitrogen, equivalent to approximately 30 to 35 gm. of protein.

To each bottle of solution is added approximately 40 to 50 mEq. of sodium, either as the chloride salt or as a mixture of the chloride and bicarbonate forms, 30 to 40 mEq. of potassium as the chloride salt and 4 to 8 mEq. of magnesium as the sulfate salt. To only one bottle of solution per day is added one ampule of MVI, the only vitamin mixture for parenteral use that contains vitamins A, D and E, three of the fat soluble vitamins, in addition to vitamin C and the B complex. Optional additives include vitamins K, B_{12} and folic acid, which can be added to the intravenous solution daily, in weekly supplements by vein or intramuscularly, depending upon the clinical situation. Iron is generally added as blood transfusion or by deep intramuscular injection of depot iron-dextran. Calcium and phosphorus are not routinely added to the adult hyperalimentation regimen because their increased urinary excretion can theoretically lead to nephrocalcinosis and nephrolithiasis. Therefore, calcium and phosphorus are added only when serum levels of either of these two elements fall below normal. Whenever one of these elements is added to the regimen, the other should also be added in order that a reciprocal reduction in the serum level of one of these elements is not precipitated as the serum level of the other rises.

On this routine the average adult is generally given 2 L. of solution, providing approximately 2000 calories over the first 24 hours, utilizing 12 hours for the infusion of each bottle and adding any extra required water either by piggyback technique into the central vein or by peripheral vein. If glycosuria is not excessive, that is, less than 3+ nitroprusside reaction, the daily ration is increased by 500 ml. over five to seven days until the usual adult ration of 3000 to 3500 calories is achieved. Starting at levels higher than this, or increasing the increments of glucose calories too rapidly or too high, may result in excessive glycosuria and secondary osmotic diuresis with resultant nonketotic hyperglycemic hyperosmolar dehydration. This is a very serious complication which may lead to coma, convulsions and deaths, but which can be easily avoided by careful attention to the rate of infusions, to urine sugar determinations every four to six hours and to the blood sugar. Generally insulin is not added routinely to the solutions except in patients who have diabetes mellitus. In nondiabetic patients insulin is added to the solutions in doses of 5 to 25 units per 1000 calories if it is felt that adequate calories to satisfy predicted requirements cannot be absorbed because of relative glucose intolerance or pancreatic insufficiency. This form of "forced feeding" must be practiced very cautiously with conscientious attention to glucose utilization in order to prevent hypoglycemic shock.

The parameters usually measured prior to starting intravenous hyperalimentation are body weight, water balance, routine vital signs, serum electrolytes, blood sugar, BUN, hemogram, prothrombin time, calcium, phosphorus, magnesium and serum proteins. After beginning intravenous hyperalimentation, body weight, strict intake and output measurements, and urine sugar determinations every four to six hours must be conscientiously monitored. Serum electrolytes are determined daily, while alterations are made in the total intravenous regimen and assessed two or three times a week thereafter throughout the course of hyperalimentation. BUN, blood sugar and hemogram are obtained weekly. The remainder of the initial studies are repeated every three weeks. Deviations from normal should be treated promptly as indicated. It must be remembered that total intravenous hyperalimentation is a form of intensive care that requires persistent vigilance on the part of the physician, and close attention must be paid to the patient and to the patient's responses to his disease process and feeding regimen.

The catheter requires meticulous care. A member of the house staff should be assigned to check the dressing daily and redress the catheter site every two to three days. If the same individual does the redressings, he will be better able to notice minor changes in the skin, the insertion site and the catheter. Strict surgical technique must be used. The IV administration set should be replaced at the time of each redressing.

Complications

INFECTION. This may begin at the site of insertion or at the tip of the catheter.

The strict sterile precautions listed earlier must be followed. One must realize that this constitutes an open surgical wound. Should fever occur without obvious cause, the infusate and intravenous tubing are replaced and cultures of the blood and fluid obtained. If the fever persists for more than a few hours, infusion is terminated, the catheter is removed and its tip cultured. Broad spectrum antibiotic therapy is seldom required, but may be instituted at this time as desired or indicated. Prophylactic antibiotics must never be added to the regimen of intravenous hyperalimentation as this may result in superinfection with resistant bacteria or fungi.

HYPERGLYCEMIA. The patient should be followed with fractional urinalyses. If he spills sugar in his urine, this can be controlled by slowing the infusion or adding insulin.

HYPOGLYCEMIA. Therapy must not be discontinued abruptly. Following hyperalimenation the patient must be maintained on intravenous infusions of 5 or 10 per cent glucose in water for at least 24 hours. Frequent measurements of serum glucose should be made.

HEART FAILURE. The cardiac status of the patient should be evaluated prior to treatment. The central venous pressure should be checked regularly. Watch must be maintained for gallop rhythm, basilar rales and pedal edema. A considerable diuresis is to be expected; should this not occur, congestive heart failure should be suspected.

HYPOKALEMIA. The usual 40 to 60 mEq. of potassium per 24 hours is generally insufficient to maintain normal serum potassium with the intracellular movement of this cation associated with anabolism. Adequate ions must be infused with precautions, which are listed on page 304.

PNEUMOTHORAX. This may be associated with percutaneous subclavian puncture. The patient may become dyspneic. Auscultation of the lungs on the routine chest x-ray should pick this up. Aspiration of the air should correct this.

HEMORRHAGE. This may occur at the time of percutaneous puncture. Local pressure should control it until it ceases. If not, the area can be opened and the bleeding controlled.

Contraindications

1. Renal failure
2. Hepatic failure
3. Severe diabetes mellitus

DIAGNOSTIC TESTS

Central Venous Pressure

With the marked increase in massive fluid therapy in seriously ill patients physicians have come to appreciate the safety afforded by the use of a central venous pressure catheter, which allows a continuous measurement to avoid overloading the circulation of the recipient.

Several different commercial plastic catheters are available. These are of sufficient length to reach from the antecubital or cervical area to the region of the right atrium. The distance from the site of the percutaneous sticks to the region of the atrium should be estimated and marked on the catheter before insertion. The skin is prepared surgically, and with sterile precautions the catheter is inserted *via* a large bore needle percutaneously into a vein in the antecubital area or the neck. The catheter is threaded into the vein for the predetermined distance. An x-ray of the chest is then taken to determine that the catheter, which is radio-opaque, is in the general area of the right atrium. The catheter is attached to a three-way stopcock which is communicating with a bottle of intravenous fluid and a calibrated tube which is positioned so that its 0 point is at the level of the atrium. Readings are taken by allowing the IV fluid to fill the calibrated tube which then is put in contact with the catheter. The level of fluid in the catheter will fall until it reflects the central venous pressure.

Circulation Time

The function of both sides of the heart can be evaluated by timing the transit of a drug from a peripheral vein through the heart to the lungs or the peripheral arterial circulation. To do this insert a needle into an antecubital vein and inject the testing solution. The time required for the patient to experience the bitter taste of Decholin is the arm to tongue time or time of transit through both sides of the heart and lungs. The time required for the patient to sense ether or paraldehyde in his lungs measures the arm to lungs time of transit through the right side of the heart.

Chapter Twenty-two

Resuscitation

Sudden respiratory or cardiac arrest in a patient is an acute emergency. The urgency of the situation is far more important than the need for special equipment. A clear airway must be established at once and ventilation and cardiac support supplied as needed. You must undertake emergency measures immediately; auxiliary equipment which will be needed later can be assembled by other persons.

RESPIRATORY ARREST

In any case of respiratory arrest, respiratory exchange must be restored quickly because the brain cells can tolerate anoxia for only 4 to 6 minutes. The first thing to do is to ascertain that the airway is open. If obstruction precipitated the respiratory arrest it must be removed. Any obstruction which cannot be removed must be bypassed by a tracheostomy (p. 202), but this is rarely necessary. The tongue is a common source of obstruction and every unconscious patient should be examined to make sure that he has not obstructed his airway by swallowing his tongue.

ARTIFICIAL RESPIRATION

Until oxygen and breathing apparatus is available you can ventilate the patient adequately with mouth-to-mouth breathing. Place one hand under the patient's chin and the other on top of his head. Lift up on the chin and push down on the top of the head to tilt the head backwards.

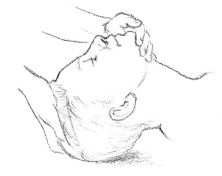

306

Put the thumb of the hand under the jaw into the patient's mouth; grasp the jaw and pull it forward.

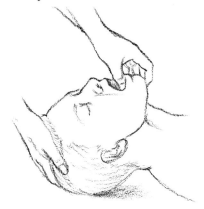

While holding the jaw forward pinch the nostrils closed with the other hand to prevent leakage of air through the nose.

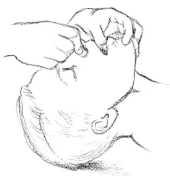

Take a deep breath; place your mouth tightly over the patient's and blow forcefully into his lungs.

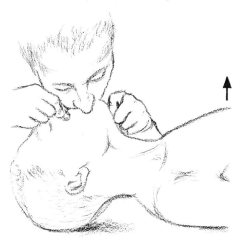

Blowing into the lungs causes the chest to expand. When the chest has expanded adequately remove your mouth from the patient's so that he can exhale.

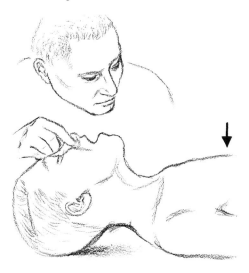

Repeat this sequence of maneuvers every 3 to 4 seconds until other means of ventilation are available.

If you cannot open his mouth blow through his nose. In infants cover both mouth and nose with your mouth. Blow gently into a child's mouth, and in infants use only small puffs from your cheeks.

Your first effort to blow up the lung will determine whether the trachea is blocked. If it is obstructed, attempt to grasp the obstructing object and remove it. If this effort is unsuccessful, turn the patient on his side and attempt to jar it loose with a sharp blow between the shoulder blades. If the victim is a child hold him by the heels or over your arm and give him a few pats between the shoulder blades.

Patients who are unconscious may have some vomitus in the pharynx; the patient may aspirate this or you may force it down into the lung by artificial respiration. Turn the patient's head to the side and wipe out all the vomitus with gauze sponges between periods of inflation.

When the proper equipment is ready you can replace the mouth-to-mouth respiration with a more conventional method. A face mask attached to an anesthesia machine with a breathing bag is available in every hospital. Apply the mask to the patient and provide ventilation by periodically compressing the breathing bag. When the patient begins to breathe the bag should be compressed at the same time that he inspires. When the chest expands remove your hand from the bag and allow the chest to contract.

Another means of providing ventilation is a bag attached to a face mask. Oxygen may be supplied through such a unit; as you compress the bag you force the oxygen into the lung. Special reinflatable bags can be used which do not require oxygen but depend on room air only. It is far more important to move air in and out of the lung than merely to direct a high oxygen mixture into the pharynx.

When the necessary equipment is available insert an endotracheal tube (p. 239) and attach it to an anesthesia machine or to an intermittent pressure breathing machine. The endotracheal tube prevents aspiration of vomitus and distention of the stomach by the inflating gas.

CARDIAC ARREST

Cardiac arrest may occur in a patient in any part of the hospital. The entire hospital staff should be trained to handle such an emergency. The limiting factor in such successful treatment of cardiac arrest is the short interval during which the cells of the brain can survive without oxygen. If circulation and oxygen transport to the brain is not re-established in 4 to 6 minutes, the patient will suffer irreversible brain damage and, in the majority of instances, death. Consequently, cardiac arrest requires immediate action by whoever is present at the time that it occurs. If a previously satisfactory pressure and pulse disappear, it is unnecessary to listen for faint sounds in the chest. Time

is better spent in re-establishing an airway and circulation. It is likewise senseless to worry about an electrocardiogram, and attempts to stimulate the heart by transthoracic injections of medication into the heart only waste treatment and time.

One should first establish an adequate airway. In most instances the arrest is brought on by anoxia which is usually due to some obstruction of the airway. An endotracheal tube should be inserted as soon as it is available.

There is an open, as well as a closed, method of treating cardiac arrest. The open method has been in use for some time and its efficiency is established by the number of people who are living a normal existence after having suffered this catastrophe. However, it should be performed only by individuals trained in the technique and who have had the experience of assisting.

CARDIAC MASSAGE

A relatively simple closed-chest method has been developed which allows anyone a reasonable opportunity to resuscitate a patient in cardiac arrest. The closed technique should be used by all who have not had experience doing a thoracotomy. It is worthwhile for even trained personnel to use this method for a brief initial period before resorting to the open method. The closed method should always be used until an endotracheal tube, an anesthesia machine, and proper help have arrived. If the patient is not in a hospital, or if you are alone and there is doubt that you will be able to get help rapidly, the closed method is the only method.

The closed method of cardiac massage through the intact chest wall was described in July, 1960, by Kouwenhoven, Jude, and Knickerbocker.* They presented convincing experimental

---

* Kouwenhoven, W. B., Jude, J. R., and Knickerbocker, G. G.: Closed Chest Cardiac Massage. J.A.M.A. *173:*1064, 1960.

work and reported experience with this method in five clinical cases. Since then, more clinical experience has accumulated. Two-thirds of all patients so treated were resuscitated. Results have been so gratifying that this method is now being widely publicized by the American Medical Association and the American Heart Association. The procedure takes advantage of the fact that pressure on the sternum compresses the heart between the sternum and the spinal column forcing blood from the ventricles into the lung and the peripheral circulation. Relaxation of the pressure allows the heart to fill. The thoracic cage in unconscious and anesthetized adults is surprisingly mobile. The patient is placed in a supine position on a rigid support so that there is no give under the patient as pressure is applied. The individual applying the pressure stands or kneels at right angles to the patient. He places the heel of one hand with the heel of the other on top of it on the sternum, just cephalad to the xiphoid process.

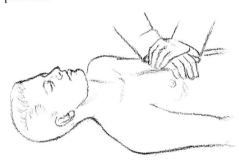

Firm pressure is applied vertically downward about 60 times a minute. At the end of each pressure stroke the hands are relaxed to permit full expansion of the chest. The position of the operator should be such that he can use his body weight while applying the pressure. Sufficient pressure should be exerted to move the sternum 3 or 4 cm. toward the vertebral column. Closed chest cardiac massage provides some ventilation of the lungs and when only one person is present in case of an arrest, attention should be concentrated on the massage, but stop massage every

2 minutes and give 3 to 4 breaths of respiration. If two or more persons are present, one should give massage to the heart while another gives mouth-to-mouth respiration coordinated with the massage.

Only moderate pressure by the finger tips on the middle third of the sternum should be used on infants.

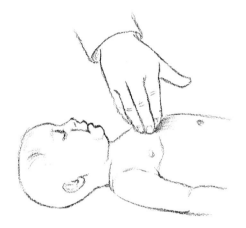

Children up to 10 years of age require the force of only one hand.

There is no question as to the adequacy of the circulation if a peripheral pulse is palpable. The absence of a palpable peripheral pulse is most likely due to improper massage. Either the technique must be corrected or the chest opened for direct massage within 1 minute of an imperceptible pulse if resuscitation is to be successful.

After an adequate airway has been established and the massage started, in many cases the heart either starts in normal rhythm or reverts to normal rhythm in which case nothing further need be done.

If cardiac action does not resume within a few minutes after institution of adequate ventilation and effective compression, one can assume that the heart is flabby and dilated. It is necessary to improve the tone of the cardiac muscle to increase perfusion pressure with further compression. Epinephrine is the drug of choice. Three to five ml. of a 1:10,000 solution of epinephrine are injected into the heart.

It is possible to produce ventricular fibrillation from the use of epinephrine in the presence of an anoxic myocardium; however, if ventilation and artificial circulation are adequate prior to the injection, the heart will be sufficiently oxygenated to prevent this complication. Even if ventricular fibrillation does develop it can be treated with electrical defibrillation.

Once cardiac action returns, 0.5 to 1 gm. of a 10 per cent solution of calcium chloride may be injected either intracardiac or intravenously if the heart beat is weak. These drugs may be repeated as needed during resuscitation.

The cardiac output produced by this technique is only about 30 to 50 per cent of the normal circulation. Reduced tissue perfusion rapidly produces a metabolic acidosis. Within five minutes, even with adequate closed chest cardiac resuscitation, the pH of the arterial blood has been measured between 7.0 and 7.05 in some patients. In this range catecholamines are relatively ineffective and the heart is more susceptible to ventricular fibrillation. The ventricular fibrillation threshold returns to normal when the pH is corrected with sodium bicarbonate or tromethamine (THAM).

If good cardiac action and blood pressure does not return with five minutes 50 ml. of sodium bicarbonate—3.75 gm. or 44.6 mEq.—should be injected and repeated every five to ten minutes throughout resuscitation in order to correct the metabolic acidosis. Fifty ml. of sodium bicarbonate solution will increase the pH of the blood approximately 0.1.

In patients with severe cardiac disease whose sodium intake should be restricted, THAM may be used instead of sodium bicarbonate. A rapid infusion of 500 ml. of a 0.3 per cent water solution of THAM, 18 gm. may be used.

Some hearts begin to fibrillate. This is an unsatisfactory contraction and must be corrected by stopping the heart and re-establishing a normal beat. This is most commonly accomplished by electrical defibrillation.

DEFIBRILLATION

The purpose of defibrillation is to stop the heart completely in order to start it again in a normal rhythm. This is usually accomplished by an electrical charge. In essence the patient is electrocuted and cardiac rhythm reestablished by cardiac massage. All hospitals should be equipped with a defibrillator. This consists of a supply unit, which allows adjustment of the intensity and the duration of the electrical shock, and two electrodes. The electrodes are flat circular surfaces, at least the size of a silver dollar, with well insulated handles. Newer defibrillators have electrodes specifically designed for external defibrillation. If such are not available, one can improvise with the old electrodes originally intended for open defibrillation. The various instruments differ to some extent, but all are provided with operating manuals. It would be wise to familiarize yourself with the manual available with the machine in your hospital before you are faced with the acute emergency of ventricular fibrillation.

Before doing anything you must be certain that the heart is fibrillating. When the chest wall is intact an electrocardiogram is the only means of ascertaining this. The brain cells are depending upon the cardiac massage and artificial ventilation for whatever oxygen they are receiving. Consequently it is very important to continue the massage until the moment you shock the patient. After the shock you must continue the massage (1) to provide some circulation if the heart is still fibrillating, and (2) to reinstitute cardiac contractions if the shock has been successful in stopping the heart.

The defibrillating instrument must first be adjusted. Many have separate adjustments for adults and infants. Set the machine to the appropriate adjustments for the size of the patient and for the duration and magnitude of the impulse. For the machine in use at our hospital an initial duration of impulse of 0.25 second with 440 volts is suggested.

Plug the electrodes into the jacks provided in the machine. Coat the contact surface of the electrodes with a generous amount of electrode paste. Connect the defibrillator to an electrical outlet. If possible connect the machine directly to the outlet because inserting a conventional electric extension cord may reduce the amount of current reaching the machine. Apply one electrode at the patient's sternal notch and the other over the apex of the heart. The electrodes must be held firmly with a pressure of at least 10 lb. Make certain that you are not in contact with the patient. Hold only the insulated handle of the electrode. Stop the massage. Make certain that no one has any physical contact with the patient. Turn off the electrocardiogram. Give the patient a single shock. If this does not stop the heart give three shocks close together. Resume massage. If the heart still does not stop increase the voltage on the machine and repeat the sequence of events listed above until the heart is stopped. Reinstitute regular rhythm by cardiac massage. If fibrillation recurs, the whole procedure must be repeated.

Failure to defibrillate the heart and reestablish normal rhythm may be due to:

1. Inadequate ventilation.
2. Inadequate massage. The most common error is failure to massage between episodes of defibrillation.
3. Inadequate electrical shock due to:
   a. Improperly placed electrodes.
   b. Improper contact caused by lack of electrode paste or insufficient pressure of the electrodes against the chest.
   c. Interposition of an ordinary electrical extension between the defibrillator and the source of current.

If the patient is not responding, investigate for these possibilities and make any necessary corrections. After a normal heart beat has been established observe the patient continuously for at least 30 minutes to be certain that normal rhythm persists. Once you are satisfied that a normal rhythm will persist, plans should be made to restore normal body temperature.

HYPOTHERMIA

Hypothermia has improved the salvage rate of patients who have sustained brain damage either from anoxia or from injury. The rationale for the use of this is twofold: (1) many of these patients die from the hyperthermia which follows brain damage, (2) the patient who sustains damage to his brain either from anoxia or injury develops edema of the brain. It has been shown experimentally that hypothermia reduces the volume of the brain thus preventing overdistention of the brain as well as lowering the temperature. Place the patient on an ice-water mattress; this mattress can be filled with ice water manually or cooled by a mechanical refrigerating unit. Wet the bedding between the patient and the mattress to improve conduction. Cooling can be accelerated by filling plastic bags with ice and applying these directly to the patient's skin. If the patient shivers as he is being cooled, this interferes with the cooling process. The shivering can be controlled by giving Phenergan intramuscularly—25 mg. at a time until as much as 100 mg. is given. The patient's temperature should be brought down to approximately 34° C. Once the temperature drops to 36° C. the ice bags can be removed and the patient covered with a sheet. The temperature will drift down to 35° or 34° C. It is possible to maintain this temperature with the ice water mattress.

The patient should be kept under hypothermia while he is unconscious. After he has recovered consciousness no effort should be made to warm him rapidly but the temperature can be allowed to gradually drift back to normal. These patients have difficulty with secretions from the lung which can be removed more easily with a tracheostomy.

INDEX